Synthetic Antidiarrheal Drugs

MODERN PHARMACOLOGY-TOXICOLOGY
A Series of Monographs and Textbooks

COORDINATING EDITOR

William F. Bousquet

Division of Biological Research
Searle Laboratories
G. D. Searle & Co.
Chicago, Illinois

ASSOCIATE EDITOR

Roger F. Palmer

University of Miami
School of Medicine
Miami, Florida

Volume 1 A Guide to Molecular Pharmacology-Toxicology, Parts I and II
Edited by R. M. Featherstone

Volume 2 Psychopharmacological Treatment: Theory and Practice
Edited by Herman C. B. Denber

Volume 3 Pre- and Postsynaptic Receptors
Edited by Earl Usdin and William E. Bunney, Jr.

Volume 4 Synaptic Receptors: Isolation and Molecular Biology
Eduardo De Robertis

Volume 5 Methods in Narcotics Research
Edited by Seymour Ehrenpreis and Amos Neidle

Volume 6 Horizons in Clinical Pharmacology
Edited by Roger F. Palmer

Volume 7 Synthetic Antidiarrheal Drugs: Synthesis—Preclinical and Clinical Pharmacology
Edited by Willem Van Bever and Harbans Lal

Additional Volumes in Preparation

Synthetic Antidiarrheal Drugs

Synthesis—Preclinical and Clinical Pharmacology

Edited by

Willem Van Bever

Department of Pharmacology
Janssen Pharmaceutica N.V.
Beerse, Belgium

Harbans Lal

Department of Pharmacology
and Toxicology
University of Rhode Island
Kingston, Rhode Island

MARCEL DEKKER, INC. New York and Basel

COPYRIGHT © 1976 by JANSSEN PHARMACEUTICA N. V.
2340 Beerse, Belgium

PUBLISHED by MARCEL DEKKER, INC.
270 Madison Avenue, New York, New York 10016

ALL RIGHTS RESERVED
Neither this book nor any part may be reproduced or transmitted in any
form or by any means, electronic or mechanical, including photocopying,
microfilming, and recording, or by any information storage and retrieval
system, without permission in writing from both the copyright holder and
the publisher.

LIBRARY OF CONGRESS CATALOG CARD NUMBER: 76-8605
ISBN: 0-8247-6370-X
Current printing (last digit):
10 9 8 7 6 5 4 3 2 1

PRINTED IN THE UNITED STATES OF AMERICA

FOREWORD

This monograph represents the individual research efforts by an unusually fine group of chemists, biologists, and clinicians with the goal of finding a better antidiarrheal agent. In 1956 this group discovered that the compound diphenoxylate possessed good antidiarrheal properties but, if taken orally, did not reveal its strong morphomimetic qualities. Since then, it has been used extensively and effectively over the world with no demonstrated cases of morphinelike dependence. Pursuing their research efforts further, these scientists determined the active principle of diphenoxylate to be difenoxin.

After extensive comparative clinical trials of diphenoxylate and difenoxin the latter has been shown to have five times the potency of the former. But difenoxin like diphenoxylate retains enough morphomimetic properties to be of some concern. Encouraged by their success with difenoxin, the group undertook the formidable task of finding a substance whose antidiarrheal properties were separated from its morphomimetic properties. This five-year search involved the synthesis of several thousand compounds.

The tenacity of purpose of the group is indicated by the fact that little success has attended previous efforts to separate analgesia from its dependence-producing properties with morphinelike drugs.

Lack of success in such efforts would serve to deter a less dedicated group from pursuing a long course of investigations of this type. It is all the more remarkable that success was achieved.

Best of all, it produced a most effective compound, loperamide. In loperamide they have produced a substance with such low morphomimetic properties that it has been shown to have no significance whatsoever either in laboratory or clinical studies. Loperamide has now had extensive clinical trial under controlled conditions and has been found to be a most highly effective agent during long-term, chronic use in otherwise intractable diarrhea. The project represents a fine example of what can be accomplished by concerted and unremitting effort.

The author is unaware of any other publication which deals so comprehensively with the problem of diarrhea. This contribution can be recommended highly not only for its scientific and clinical worthiness but as a classical example of what can be accomplished in solving a problem which has hitherto found little attention and been relatively of little interest to most investigators.

M. H. Seevers, M.D.

The University of Michigan
Medical School
Ann Arbor, Michigan

PREFACE

Diarrhea is a widespread condition that is often reported to the physicians for treatment, in addition to countless instances where diarrhea is treated by folklore medicine.

Nearly all practitioners of general medicine and often other medical specialities prescribe antidiarrheal drugs to their patients. Moreover, numerous inquiries on the treatment of diarrhea are daily referred by the patients directly to pharmacists, nurses, and other health professionals. The extent to which antidiarrheals are used is evident from the fact that of diphenoxylate, the only specific antidiarrheal available until recently, more than two billion doses have been prescribed in the last six years. Besides, there is widespread use of other nonspecific medications for diarrhea that are prescribed by physicians and can also be purchased directly from pharmacists.

In spite of such widespread use of antidiarrheals, readily available information for use to physicians and other health professionals is surprisingly scanty. Textbooks of pharmacology as well as those of medicine either do not mention them or refer to them only in passing. Because of this total lack of information on the various aspects of antidiarrheal action and their uses in medicine, we undertook to assemble a complete monograph on modern antidiarrheal drugs. We hope that our efforts will fulfill a long-standing need of the profession.

We limited the scope of this monograph to the extensive discussion of only those antidiarrheals which are specific for diarrhea and are used as such in modern human medicine. Many other pharmacological agents which reduce diarrhea only incidental to their other actions, or those drugs which are used in veterinary practice are not included here.

A glance over the contents of this book will easily reveal that the subject of antidiarrheal drugs has been discussed rather extensively by those who have been themselves involved in one or the other aspect of development, research, or clinical applications of those drugs. Only these contributors could impart a personal touch to the narration of many aspects of scientific endeavors which go into the making of an antidiarrheal drug.

The arrangement of presentation evolved to provide a scientific basis for rational therapy of diarrhea. Along with the data, critical description of methodology is given in order to bring about full appreciation of what goes into the making of a successful antidiarrheal drug. Although the research aspects are not fully elaborated, sufficient description of research methodology and current problems is included so that future research in various aspects of antidiarrheal drugs is facilitated.

We believe that this book will be useful to clinicians, pharmacologists in industry as well as in academia, advanced students in pharmaceutical and medical sciences, teachers in medical schools, and above all, to practicing physicians and drug-consultant pharmacists. We shall consider ourselves highly compensated for our efforts if the book can accomplish the above objectives.

Willem Van Bever

Harbans Lal

ACKNOWLEDGMENTS

The editors wish to express their gratitude and appreciation to all those who have given of their time, effort, and encouragement in the writing of this volume. Although it is impossible to acknowledge the contribution of all who helped us in compiling the present work, we would like to cite the valuable assistance given to us by the following people: Mr. H. Vanhove and Ms. V. van Kesteren for correcting the manuscript; Mr. J. Van Mierlo and Mr. R. Vermeer for drawing the figures; Mr. J. Dony and Mr. G. Claessen for the statistical analyses; Mrs. A. Nuyts and Mrs. R. Leys for typing part of the manuscript; Ms. C. Van Ghelder for finalization of the manuscript and secretarial assistance; and Mrs. M. J. Princen for proofreading.

The author A. Karim is indebted to many of his colleagues, especially to Mrs. Zagarella and Mr. J. Campion for the animal experimental data; to Doctors R. E. Ranney and T. Hutsell for assistance in the preparation of his chapter; and to Mrs. V. Bonnie for the secretarial assistance. The information on comparison of diphenoxylate and difenoxin absorption in man was kindly supplied by Doctors R. F. Palmer, M. J. Tidd, and M. Cohen (G. D. Searle & Co., High Wycombe, England).

The author A. Reyntjens is very grateful to Ms. M. Lestienne for her invaluable help in preparing the manuscript and tables of his chapter.

The editors wish to thank the contributors without whose support and excellent coverage of the material this book could not have been written. They also thank many investigators and publishers who generously provided their material with permission to publish in this book. Special thanks are due Dr. S. F. Phillips who provided extensive reviews of pathophysiology of diarrhea and granted permission to use his writings in preparing a chapter on that subject.

CONTENTS

FOREWORD iii

PREFACE v

ACKNOWLEDGMENTS vii

CONTRIBUTORS xiii

I. INTRODUCTION: Paul Janssen 1

II. PATHOPHYSIOLOGY OF DIARRHEA: Harbans Lal 7

    II.1. Introduction 7
    II.2. Gastrointestinal Functions 8
    II.3. Dysfunctions Causing Diarrhea 13
    II.4. Clinical Abnormalities Causing Diarrhea 19
    II.5. Conclusion 22

III. CHEMISTRY OF MODERN ANTIDIARRHEALS 23

III.1. Synthesis of Diphenoxylate, Difenoxin, Loperamide, and Related Compounds: Willem Van Bever, Raymond Stokbroeckx, Jan Vandenberk, and Maria Wouters . . 23

III.2. Physicochemical and Analytical Studies on Diphenoxylate, Difenoxin, and Loperamide: Willem Van Bever and Paul Demoen 37

III.3. Structure-Activity Relationships: Willem Van Bever, Karel Schellekens, and Carlos Niemegeers 49

IV. PRECLINICAL ANIMAL STUDIES OF MODERN ANTIDIARRHEALS 65

IV.1. In Vivo Pharmacology: Carlos Niemegeers, Fred Lenaerts, and Frans Awouters 65

IV.2. In Vitro Pharmacology: Study of the Peristaltic Reflex and Other Experiments on Isolated Tissues: Jan M. Van Nueten and Jeanine Fontaine 114

IV.3. Metabolism of Synthetic Antidiarrheal Drugs, Diphenoxylate, Difenoxin, and Loperamide: Aziz Karim and Jozef Heykants 132

IV.4. Safety Evaluation: Hermon Blaton, Carlos Niemegeers, and Robert Marsboom 155

V. MODERN ANTIDIARRHEALS IN MEDICAL PRACTICE: André Reyntjens and Harbans Lal 205

V.1. Introduction 205

V.2. Symptomatic Treatment of Acute Diarrhea in Clinical Practice 207

V.3. Symptomatic Treatment of Chronic Diarrhea 213

V.4. Pediatric Use of Modern Antidiarrheals 223

V.5. Indications for Decreasing the Intestinal Motility in Situations Other Than Diarrhea 224

V.6. The Use of Diphenoxylate in Detoxification of Heroin Addicts 224

Contents   xi

    V.7.   Abuse Potential of Antidiarrheals   225
    V.8.   Side Effects and Safety   227

VI. THE ABUSE POTENTIAL OF MODERN ANTIDIARRHEALS .   235

    VI.1. Facts and Falacies of Addiction Liability and Abuse
          Potential: Harbans Lal   235
    VI.2. Experimental Approach to the Evaluation of Drug-
          Abuse Liability: Francis Colpaert, Albert Wauquier,
          Harbans Lal, and Carlos Niemegeers   251

VII. CONCLUSION: Willem Van Bever   269

AUTHOR INDEX   273

SUBJECT INDEX   279

CONTRIBUTORS

FRANS AWOUTERS
Department of Pharmacology, Janssen Pharmaceutica, Beerse, Belgium

HERMAN BLATON
Department of Toxicology, Janssen Pharmaceutica, Beerse, Belgium

FRANCIS COLPAERT
Department of Pharmacology, Janssen Pharmaceutica, Beerse, Belgium

PAUL DEMOEN
Department of Chemical Analysis, Janssen Pharmaceutica,
Beerse, Belgium

JEANINE FONTAINE
Laboratory of Pharmacology, Institute of Pharmacy, Free University of
Brussels, Belgium

JOZEF HEYKANTS
Department of Metabolism, Janssen Pharmaceutica, Beerse, Belgium

PAUL JANSSEN
Director of Research, Janssen Pharmaceutica, Beerse, Belgium

AZIZ KARIM
Department of Drug Metabolism, G. D. Searle and Company,
Chicago, Illinois

HARBANS LAL
Professor of Pharmacology, Toxicology, and Psychology, University of Rhode Island, Kingston, Rhode Island

FRED LENAERTS
Department of Pharmacology, Janssen Pharmaceutica, Beerse, Belgium

ROBERT MARSBOOM
Department of Toxicology, Janssen Pharmaceutica, Beerse, Belgium

CARLOS NIEMEGEERS
Department of Pharmacology, Janssen Pharmaceutica, Beerse, Belgium

ANDRE REYNTJENS
Clinical Research Department, Janssen Pharmaceutica, Beerse, Belgium

KAREL SCHELLEKENS
Department of Research Coordination, Janssen Pharmaceutica, Beerse, Belgium

RAYMOND STOKBROECKX
Department of Chemical Synthesis, Janssen Pharmaceutica, Beerse, Belgium

WILLEM VAN BEVER
Department of Chemical Pharmacology, Janssen Pharmaceutica, Beerse, Belgium

JAN VANDENBERK
Department of Chemical Synthesis, Janssen Pharmaceutica, Beerse, Belgium

JAN VAN NUETEN
Department of In Vitro Pharmacology, Janssen Pharmaceutica, Beerse, Belgium

ALBERT WAUQUIER
Department of Pharmacology, Janssen Pharmaceutica, Beerse, Belgium

MARIA WOUTERS
Department of Chemical Synthesis, Janssen Pharmaceutica, Beerse, Belgium

Synthetic Antidiarrheal Drugs

CHAPTER I

INTRODUCTION

Paul Janssen

In 1956, the first synthetic antidiarrheal drug, diphenoxylate, R 1132 [4a], was discovered in our laboratory in the course of an experimental long-range program designed to explore systematically the relationship between the chemical structure of 3,3-diphenylpropylamines [1], related to methadone, and 4-phenylpiperidines [2], related to pethidine, and the pharmacological activity of these compounds.

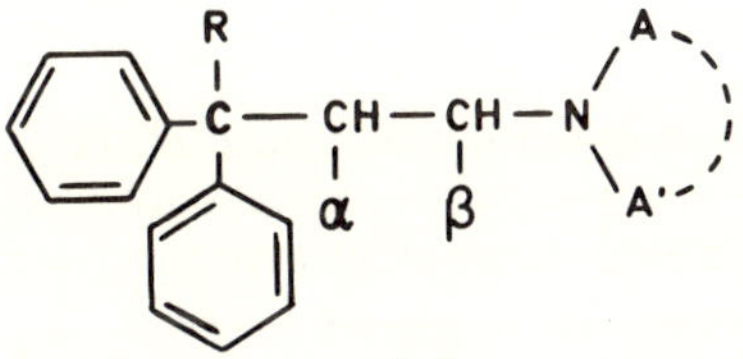

[1]

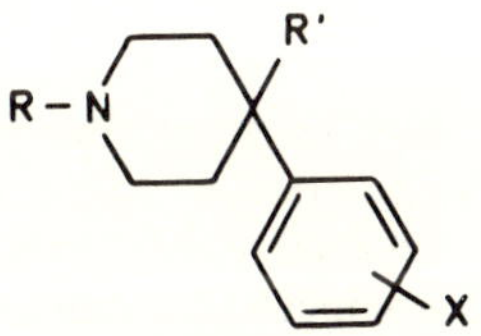

[2]

Diphenoxylate, the prototype of a series of hybrid molecules [3], chemically related to (1) and (2), was found to be an extremely potent constipating and antidiarrheal agent in laboratory animals as well as in man and to be relatively free of effects on the central nervous system (CNS) of the morphine-like type. The drug was brought on the market in 1960 and has been extensively used for the symptomatic treatment of diarrhea ever since, i.e., an estimated 3,200,000,000 tablets of 2.5 mg (Reasec, Lomotil, Diarsed, etc.) were sold in the 15-year period from 1960 to 1974.

The efficacy of the drug is undisputed and its safety margin excellent, particularly in adults. Tolerance is not a problem in chronically treated patients and the abuse liability of the drug is negligible; no serious cases of drug abuse have been reported up to the present day.

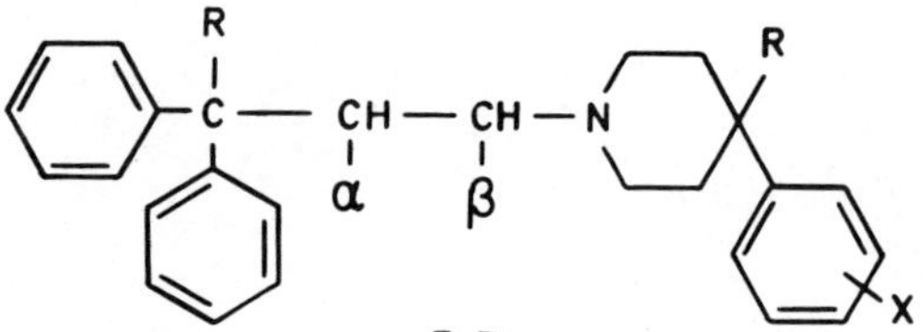

[3]

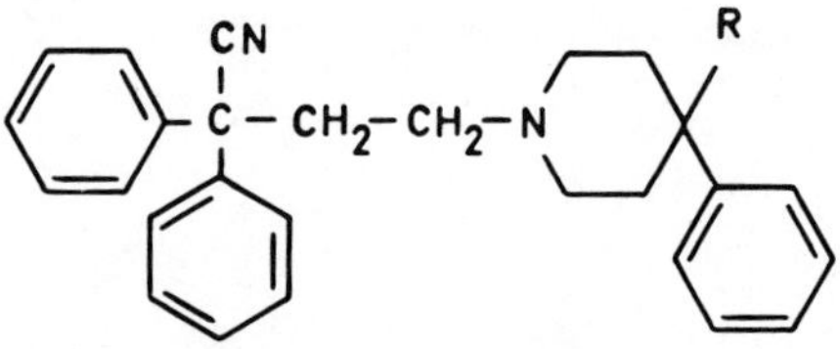

[4a] R = COOC$_2$H$_5$

diphenoxylate

[4b] R = COOH

difenoxin

It took us more than 10 years to realize fully that most of the antidiarrheal action of diphenoxylate is due to its major metabolite, difenoxin [4b], the aminoacid formed by hydrolysis of the ethyl ester part of the parent compound. Difenoxin was found to be about five times more potent than diphenoxylate (0.5 mg difenoxin tablets being at least as effective as 2.5 mg diphenoxylate tablets) and to have an even weaker effect on the CNS.

Between 1956 and 1968 several thousands of new derivatives of structures [1], [2], and [3] were prepared and pharmacologically investigated. Many of these compounds turned out to possess interesting morphinomimetic, anticholinergic, or neuroleptic properties, but all efforts to find specific antidiarrheals superior to diphenoxylate failed, the active molecules being either less potent, shorter-acting, or less specific, i.e., more active on the CNS. Superior compounds are indeed hard to discover in this field.

In 1969, when a new method for the synthesis of basic amides of type [5] was found, interest in the field of antidiarrheal drugs was revived. It was found that several members of the new series, but in particular loperamide [5a], chemically related to the classical neuroleptic haloperidol [6], and fluperamide [5b], chemically related to the long acting neuroleptic pentfluridol [7], were not only more potent and longer acting than diphenoxylate in animals and in man, but surprisingly free of morphine-like or

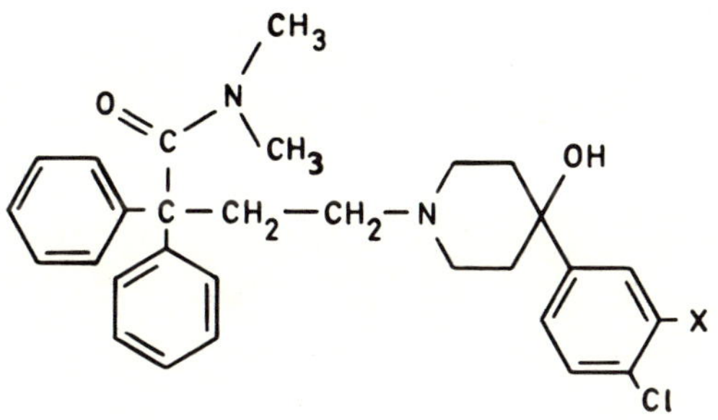

[5a] X = H

loperamide

[5b] X = CF$_3$

fluperamide

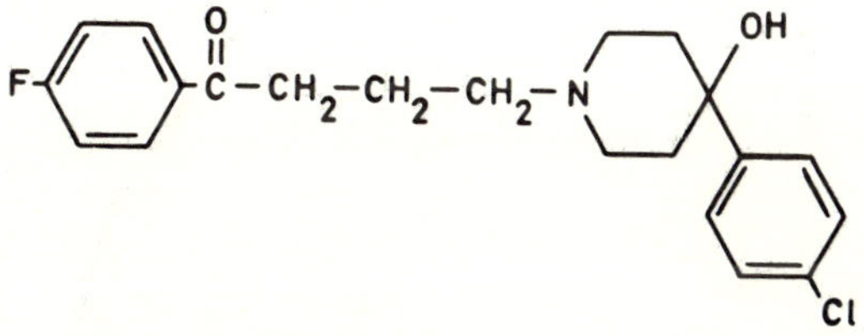

[6] haloperidol

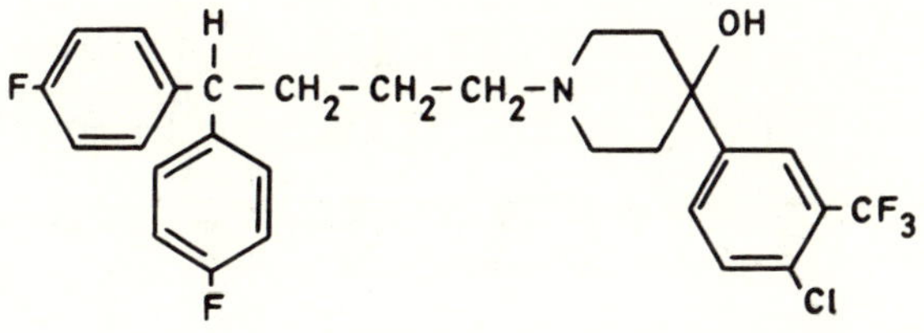

[7] penfluridol

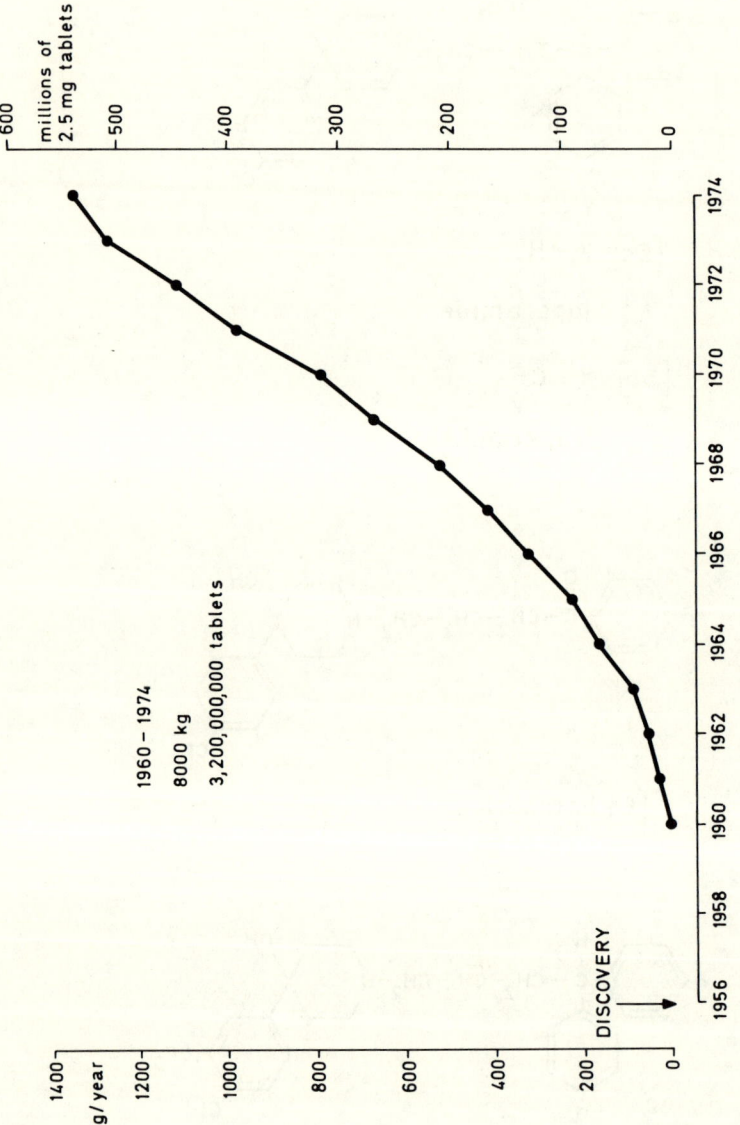

Fig. 1. Worldwide use of diphenoxylate in clinical practice.

Introduction

other CNS effects, even at very high subtoxic dose levels. A goal of completely separating antidiarrheal CNS activity had been realized. After 5 years of extensive pharmacological, toxicological, biochemical, and clinical investigations loperamide was brought on the market in 1974 in 2-mg capsules (Imodium) and is at present clearly the drug of choice for the symptomatic treatment of diarrhea.

The purpose of this book is to describe the genesis of these drugs in some detail by presenting the most important experimental evidence as it accumulated in the period of active investigation from 1956 to 1974 (Fig. 1).

The contributors of the chapters following are chemists, pharmacologists, toxicologists, and clinicians, many of whom collaborated together and made significant contributions to the discovery and development of these new exciting drugs. I wish to thank them most sincerely for an excellent job.

CHAPTER II

PATHOPHYSIOLOGY OF DIARRHEA

Harbans Lal

II.1. INTRODUCTION

1.1. GENERAL CONSIDERATIONS

The purpose of this chapter, devoted to a description of the pathophysiology of diarrhea, is to put the subject of diarrhea and the information on antidiarrheal drugs in their proper perspective and to provide a better understanding of the course of therapy. Since diarrhea is primarily a result of malfunctioning of one or more aspects of bowel physiology, the latter will also be briefly discussed, in order to give a better insight into diarrhea pathogenesis.

1.2. DIARRHEA

Diarrhea is a condition which results from failure of one or more functions of the alimentary canal. The alimentary canal receives, mixes, digests, and absorbs a wide variety and unpredictable amount of food with remarkable efficiency. What is left of the mixture of food at the end of the alimentary canal is finally excreted as a small and convenient volume of solid waste. Failure of one or more of the aforementioned processes results in the passage of inconveniently bulky and liquid stools at increased frequency and is termed "diarrhea."

The normal daily stools of a healthy adult weigh 100-200 g and contain 60% of water. Even small variations in weight (i.e., excretion of more than 200 g) and content (e.g., 60-90% of water) cause diarrhea and are due to any one of the following causes: abnormal motility, disturbances in intestinal permeability, or the presence of osmotically active, nonabsorbable substances in the human gut.

II.2. GASTROINTESTINAL FUNCTIONS

2.1. ANATOMY AND PHYSIOLOGY

Anatomically the gastrointestinal tract consists of the esophagus, stomach, small and large intestine, colon, and cecum. The esophagus is a muscular tube that rapidly transfers food from the pharynx to the stomach. Its walls include all the anatomical layers which are characteristic of the digestive tract in general.

The stomach, whose function is to store and digest food, reduces solid food to a fluid by virtue of the contraction of its muscular wall and the admixture of food with secretions from the glands of its mucous membrane. When the content of the stomach has been reduced to a pulplike fluid mass, known as chyme, it is soft enough to be transferred to the intestine in small portions.

The small intestine is the portion of the alimentary tract between the stomach and the large intestine. It is made up of the duodenum, the jejunum, and the ileum. The wall of the small intestine consists of five strata. These are, starting from the inside wall, the mucosa, the submucosa, the circular smooth muscle layer, the longitudinal smooth muscle, and the serosa. The mucosa consists of a single epithelial layer, the lamina propria, and a fine, smooth muscle coat known as the muscularis mucosae. The submucosa, a connective tissue, contains an autonomic nervous plexus, known as Meissner's plexus. Auerbach's plexus is located between the well-developed circular and longitudinal smooth muscle layers. The serosa, a layer of mesothelial cells and loose connective tissue, forms the outer surface of the intestinal wall.

Meissner's and Auerbach's plexi constitute the intrinsic neuronal control of gastrointestinal (GI) functions. The extrinsic nerve endings into the intestinal wall consist of preganglionic vagal fibers and postganglionic fibers of the sympathicus. The role of this extrinsic nervous system in normal GI functions is unknown.

The principal functions of the small intestine are: forward movement of chyme received from the stomach, continued digestion by means of special secretions from its intrinsic and accessory glands, and absorption of nutrients released by digestion into blood and lymph vessels of the mucosa.

The large intestine, the extension of the small intestine, is not folded except in the region of its terminal portion, the rectum. Here, villi cease and the mucosa consists of a smooth surface lined by simpler collumnar epithelium. In the anal, region, the wall of the intestine assumes the structure of the skin.

Pathophysiology

The movement of the gastrointestinal tract is due to the activity of smooth muscles. This tissue possesses extraordinary properties in that it can maintain constant tension over widely differing lengths. This property accounts for the fact that a large meal can be ingested in a short time without much alteration in intragastric or intraintestinal pressures, that is, the alimentary tract adapts itself to its contents whatever the bulk may be.

2.2. MOTILITY

Motility of the gastrointestinal tract (GIT) provides the mechanical impetus necessary for normal digestion, absorption, and transport of its intraluminal contents. Motor action of the intestine consists of rhythmic segmentation and peristaltic reflexes. Rhythmic segmentation enables the food to mix with digestive secretions and assists in absorption by bringing food into contact with the mucosa. It also promotes flow in blood and lymph vessels. Peristaltic reflex movements are involved in the transport of intestinal contents through the bowel in an aboral direction. This reflex is discussed in greater detail in Chapter IV.2.

Smooth muscle fibers in the GIT are spindle-shaped, approximately twenty times longer than their maximal diameter, and are unitary smooth muscle. This type of smooth muscle, sometimes known as visceral smooth muscle, exhibits spontaneous contractions, can be stimulated by stretch, and can conduct impulses independently of nerves. Among the factors influencing intestinal motility are the myogenic properties of the smooth muscle layers, intrinsic and extrinsic innervation, and local hormones.

2.3. ABSORPTION AND SECRETIONS

The normal small intestine contains practically no fluid in the fasting state. However, following ingestion of meals, large volumes of essentially isotonic fluids enter the lumen of the proximal bowel. The fluids contain liquids of the meal and, to a large extent, endogenous secretions of the upper digestive tract. The volume of fluids entering the proximal bowel exceeds the extracellular volume and its equivalent to a major proportion of the total body water. However, more than 90% of these fluids is reabsorbed, thereby completing an efficient enterosystemic cycle.

The gastrointestinal secretions predominate, commencing with saliva which provides a large volume of fluid which is hypotonic in relation to other body fluids, estimated to be at least 1,000 ml per day. The gastric secretory response to a normal meal approximates to that of maximal histamine stimulation. The contribution made by intestinal secretions, "succus entericus," is more debatable. The proximal small intestine contains specific secretory

(Brunner's) glands. These glands discharge alkaline fluid in the fasting state and are further stimulated by the ingestion of food or the administration of exogenous hormones. Total daily input into the gut amounts to 9 liters of essentially isotonic fluid. To this must be added variable quantities of fat, carbohydrate, and protein from the diet, protein in digestive secretions, and an unpredictable contribution by desquamated epithelial cells. Finally, electrolytes and water are secreted into the lumen of the bowel, presumably by transepithelial movement, even in areas devoid of specific secretory glands.

Although fecal water is the major determinant of fecal weight, the physicochemical means, by which gut contents are finally converted into solid and diarrheal stools, may not be solely responsible for fecal consistency. However, it is apparent that disturbances of water absorption and secretion provide the major clues to the pathophysiology of diarrhea. Adequate digestion and absorption of dietary macromolecules are essential to normal intestinal functions.

2.3.1. Osmolarity

The osmolarity of meals varies widely. Hypotonic saliva and isotonic gastric secretions modify the ionic strength of the gastric contents postprandially. Regardless of intragastric osmolarity, meals enter the duodenum where an isotonic chyme stimulates osmoreceptors, which are thought to reside in the distal duodenum. By this mechanism, and the intervention of humoral factors, gastric emptying is delayed. Isotonic gastric contents leave the stomach most rapidly; anisotonic meals are retained for longer periods. The process of osmotic equilibrium begins in the duodenum.

Hypotonic meals are rendered isotonic by the movement of water from the lumen and the concomitant movement of ions, mainly sodium and chloride, into the lumen. Dietary macromolecules are also hydrolyzed to smaller, osmotically active compounds. Water also moves rapidly into the small bowel to dilute the hypertonic contents. The duodenum reduces the osmolarity of its contents much faster than does the ileum. These rapid changes render the chyme essentially isotonic by the time it reaches the jejunum, where most absorption seems to occur. Subsequently, isotonicity is maintained during the distal progression of a meal; in addition, the contents of the fasting intestine are isotonic in the distal bowel. Throughout the intestine, chyme contains sodium as major cation, but potassium concentrations increase distally and can be greater than those of sodium in dialysates of feces.

Chloride is the major anion of jejunal contents, but its concentration decreases distally where it is partially replaced by bicarbonate in the ileum and organic anions in the colon.

Pathophysiology

2.3.2. Sodium and Water Absorption

Sodium can be absorbed across intestinal mucosal preparations by means of an energy-dependent phenomenon (active transport) that is able to transport sodium from the lumen against gradients of chemical concentration (activity) and against the negative electrical charge of intestinal mucosa, and, in certain circumstances, against the bylkflow of water.

In man, the electrochemical potentials against which sodium is absorbed increase aborally. Thus sodium is absorbed against greater gradients in the distal small bowel and particularly in the colon. Concomitantly, passive permeability of the bowel to sodium decreases distally. The size of the hypothetical water-filled mucosal pores, through which sodium and other polar solutes diffuse, is thought to decrease in the distal bowel. Thus, in the ileum and colon a less permeable membrane restricts the passive movements of sodium (and other water-soluble solutes), but active sodium absorption is more effective.

2.3.3. Absorption of Other Electrolytes

Fecal water contains high concentrations of potassium, and potassium excretion occurs commonly in diarrhea. Potassium movement across the jejunum and ileum can be explained by passive electrical (potential difference) and chemical concentration gradients. The negative mucosal electrical potential of 20 to 40 mv in the colon provides a passive force by which potassium can accumulate in the contents until concentrations two to three times those of plasma are achieved. Moreover, mineralocorticoid secretion may be stimulated by electrolyte losses in diarrhea, thereby increasing the negative colonic potential and augmenting passive losses of potassium. Stools may also contain mucus, desquamated cells, and bacteria, all of which could contribute to excretion of potassium. Finally, the water phase of feces may be distributed heterogeneously within solid stools. Compartmentalization of fecal water could explain the high local concentrations of potassium in fecal dialysates.

Intestinal absorption of anions is complex. Movements of chloride and bicarbonate are closely coupled, particularly in the distal bowel; chloride-bicarbonate exchange in the ileum is related to sodium and hydrogen ion transport. Chloride and bicarbonate can be absorbed together in the jejunum. However, in the ileum and colon, chloride is usually absorbed while bicarbonate is secreted. As chyme passes distally, chloride concentrations decrease, and bicarbonate concentrations and the pH rise. Organic anions (acetate, propionate, butyrate, and others) are prominent constituents of stool and comprise 70% of fecal anions.

2.3.4. Intestinal Secretion

The significance of transepithelial intestinal secretions (succus entericus) under normal circumstances is uncertain; but under certain pathological conditions, secretion of electrolytes and water is highly relevant to the production of diarrhea. Mucosal crypts of Lieberkuhn have been postulated as the site of secretion and this has been demonstrated under a variety of conditions:

a. Abnormal physical conditions, such as mechanical bowel obstruction, lowered pH, and postirradiation conditions.

b. In the presence of chemical stimulants, such as dihydroxy bile acids in the small intestine and colon, hydroxylated fatty acids, e.g., ricinoleic acid from castor oil, hydroxystearic acid, and cathartics of the anthraquinone group.

c. In the presence of bacterial toxins, such as those of Vibrio cholera, Staphylococcus aureus, Clostridium perfringens, certain shigellae, and Escherichia coli.

d. Stimulation by humoral factors. Mineralocorticoids, which augment sodium absorption and stimulate potassium secretion in the human colon, prostaglandins, gastrin, secretin, cholecystokinin, and newer polypeptide substances recently isolated from gut mucosa induce secretion in a variety of experimental models.

2.3.5. Mucosal Disease

Patients with nontropical sprue, intestinal scleroderma, and regional enteritis secrete sodium and water into the jejunum. Some bacteria which do not elaborate a recognizable enterotoxin invade the mucosa, produce changes in villus architecture and cause secretion of water.

The nature of the fluid secreted in response to these various stimuli remains constant for a particular region of the bowel; but fluids accumulating in the proximal and distal bowel have different compositions. It is not known for certain whether secretion arises from a new transport process that is initiated by this wide variety of insults, or whether an existing secretory mechanism, normally nonapparent in the healthy bowel, is stimulated.

In some secretory states, such as that induced experimentally by cholera toxin, mucosal structure and glucose absorption are normal. In clinical cholera, oral administration of glucose and glycine reduces the rate of water secretion. The probable explanation is that glucose absorption creates osmotic gradients for water absorption although a stimulatory effect of glucose on sodium transport has also been proposed. However, in sprue and experimental salmonellosis, the mucosal structure is abnormal and glucose does not modify the secretory state.

Pathophysiology

II.3. DYSFUNCTIONS CAUSING DIARRHEA

Three major categories of dysfunction can be distinguished:

Osmotic retardation of water absorption

Abnormal electrolyte and water transport

Disorders of transit

3.1. OSMOTIC FACTORS

3.1.1. Overload

Many patients relate diarrhea to dietary indiscretions, and physicians frequently ascribe these symptoms to "irritable bowel," yet dietary excess is poorly documented as a cause for diarrhea. However, individual and racial variations for digestion and absorption of carbohydrate are known and intakes in excess of intestinal capacity cause diarrhea. Ingestion of an artificial sweetening agent, sorbitol, a nonabsorbable sugar alcohol, has caused diarrhea. Therapeutically, delayed absorption of polyvalent ions (Mg^{2+}, PO_4^{3-}) and a nonhydrolyzable, nonabsorbable disaccharide (lactulose) is used to evoke catharsis. Some types of diarrhea, for which no other causes can be found, may occur when the normal compensatory capacity to digest and absorb is exceeded under certain dietary circumstances.

3.1.2. Malabsorption

Malabsorption of carbohydrate, fat, and protein may result from a wide variety of gastrointestinal diseases and diarrhea is a frequent symptom. The presence of certain unabsorbed dietary components in the bowel constitutes an abnormal osmotic load and the relationship between the malabsorption of food components and malabsorption of water warrants further examination.

Carbohydrate malabsorption occurs in primary disorders of digestion (e.g., lactase deficiency), secondary to mucosal disease of the small bowel (e.g., sprue). Hereditary disorders of monosaccharide transport (e.g., glucose-galactose malabsorption) are far less frequent.

Dietary lactose is incompletely hydrolyzed and poorly absorbed; barium and test meals are diluted in the small bowel, presumably by osmotic effects generated by nonabsorbable disaccharide. Fluid moving into the lumen consequently distends the small bowel and intestinal transit time is reduced.

Since long-chain fatty acids are virtually insoluble in water, even when fully ionized, these compounds, which comprise the bulk of fecal fats, cannot exert an osmotic effect on water movements. Intestinal bacteria are able to hydroxylate unsaturated fatty acids in the diet in vitro. This action is assumed to occur in vivo since fecal hydroxy fatty acid excretion can be reduced by antibiotic therapy or by removal of long-chain fats from the diet; moreover, considerable metabolism, presumably bacterial, of fats is known to occur in the colon. The relationship between fecal fat excretion and water malabsorption is most readily explicable by altered electrolyte and water transport (see below).

Malabsorption of protein is a frequent cause of diarrhea. A rare congenital deficiency of the mucosal enzyme, enterokinase, results in incomplete activation of trypsinogen and leads to protein maldigestion, malabsorption, and diarrhea.

3.2. ABNORMAL ELECTROLYTE AND WATER TRANSPORT

Although stimulation of intestinal secretion exemplifies altered electrolyte and water transport most dramatically, the consideration of normal physiological events suggests that even modest impairment of reabsorption in one area, if not compensated for by increased absorption in another area, can lead to diarrhea. Numerous toxic, chemical, humoral, and mucosal factors known to cause diarrhea have been shown to modify water reabsorption, but a complete evaluation of diarrheal disease is not yet available.

3.2.1. Bacterial Diarrhea

Dysenteric diseases continue to be a major worldwide problem. Those most vulnerable are the least prepared with respect to age, associated illness, and standards of social and medical care. The basis for the current comprehension of this subject was established by the study of cholera and the enterotoxin of V. cholera which causes diarrhea by the stimulation of small-bowel secretion.

Bacterial enteritis involves two separate pathogeneses for a wide variety of bacterial diarrheas:

Elaboration of filterable enterotoxins without mucosal damage
Mucosal injury by direct penetration

Some organisms appear to combine these properties. In both circumstances, abnormal intestinal secretion of electrolytes is demonstrable. The site of secretion is usually the small bowel.

Pathophysiology

Some bacteria also attack the colon, often with ulceration, but a detailed study of colonic water and electrolyte transport has not been made. Toxicogenic, enteropathic strains of <u>Eschericia coli</u> have no apparent effect on the colons of human volunteers. In the small bowel affected by cholera and nonspecific dysentery, net sodium and water absorption is decreased or net secretion occurs.

Unidirectional flux measurements have been interpreted as showing increased passive sodium permeability. Secretion of chloride and bicarbonate also occurs.

3.2.2. Bile Acids

Dihydroxy bile acids inhibit water absorption reversibly in the canine colon and provoke secretion in the human colon without producing morphological damage. This effect is independent of conjugation, is concentration-related, and is specific for dihydroxy compounds (cholic acid has no effect). The concentrations of bile acids required to impair absorption are similar to those occuring in the stools after ileal resection. Dihydroxy bile acids and their conjugates also provoke secretion in the jejunum.

Relationships between bile acids and bacteria may be important. Bacterial hydrolysis of their glycine and taurine conjugates is considered a prerequisite for bacterial dehydroxylation of the steroid moiety. Dehydroxylation of cholic acid (trihydroxy, inactive), yields deoxycholic acid (dihydroxy, active). Conversely, bacterial metabolism of chenodeoxycholic acid (active) yields lithocholic acid, which is insoluble under the usual in vivo conditions and presumably inactive. Although bile acid effects on the colon have been strongly incriminated in the diarrhea associated with ileal disease, the role of bile acids in the small bowel is more speculative. However, in states of jejunal bile acid deconjugation, such as bacterial overgrowth, an effect of the unconjugated forms on water transport could contribute to diarrhea.

3.2.3. Fatty Acids

The association between dietary fats, steatorrhea, and diarrhea, mentioned earlier, should be considered here, since fatty acids appear to induce diarrhea by impairment of sodium and water absorption. Ricinoleic acid (the active principle of castor oil) can be considered as a representative compound. This hydroxy fatty acid alters intestinal motility, increases mucus secretion, produces "chemical gastroenteritis," and also decreases sodium transport in vitro. Owing to chemical similarities between fecal hydroxy fatty acids and ricinoleic acid (see above), the diarrhea seen in fat malabsorption has been postulated as being caused by hydroxy fats.

Bile acid malabsorption can produce steatorrhea (and diarrhea). After resection of the major site of bile acid reabsorption, the colonic mucosa is exposed to greater amounts of dihydroxy bile acids (deoxycholic, chenodeoxycholic) which are present in concentrations that inhibit colonic water resorption. This mechanism has been held responsible for the diarrhea of ileal resection. In certain instances, treatment with cholestyramine or lignin, agents which render bile acids insoluble, lowers the effective concentration of bile acids in the colon, relieves diarrhea, but increases steatorrhea. Other patients, usually those with more severe steatorrhea, have smaller concentrations of bile acids in the aqueous phase of their stools but greater amounts of hydroxy and other fatty acids. In these patients, sequestration of bile acids does not reduce stool weight or frequency, but removal of long-chain fats from the diet is efficacious.

3.2.4. Humoral and Chemical Factors

Prostaglandins, when administered by arterial infusion, provoke secretion of isotonic fluid into the lumen of isolated intestinal loops; these agents also stimulate secretion of mucosal adenyl cyclase. High levels of prostaglandin $F_2\alpha$ have been demonstrated in tumors of patients with diarrhea associated with ganglioneuromas, pancreatic islet cell tumors, ileal carcinoids, and medullary thyroid tumors. Other gastrointestinal hormones, such as gastrin, secretin, cholecystokinin, and glucagon are also capable of modifying water absorption in man and experimental animals.

Hypersecretion of gastric juice is associated with diarrhea in many instances of the Zollinger-Ellison syndrome. Maldigestion of fat, leading to steatorrhea, is often demonstrable; under these circumstances, steatorrhea may contribute to diarrhea. In addition, electrolyte and water absorption in the jejunum may be abnormal in some patients and this abnormality may be related to jejunitis or an abnormal pH in the jejunum. Diarrhea is sometimes dramatically relieved by gastric aspiration. Changes in ileal function may aggravate diarrhea where an acid pH has been shown to impair vitamin-B_{12} and water absorption. But the pathophysiology of gastrin overproduction is even more complex, since gastrin may impair mucosal transport of electrolytes and water directly and may also influence intestinal motility.

In other cases of pancreatic islet cell tumor, diarrhea occurs without gastric hypersecretion and gastric aspiration does not ameliorate the symptoms. Marked choleresis, hypokalemia, and achlorhydria are observed in this syndrome. Bile flow is increased, probably by concomitant action on the hepatobiliary system of a humoral agent such as secretin. Further study of these metabolically active tumors should be revealing. Thus, overproduction of normal hormones or synthesis of abnormal active peptides by tumor cells has profound effects on many aspects of digestive function, including the stimulation of intestinal secretion. Moreover, it is possible that these

Pathophysiology   17

humoral agents and exogenous chemical stimuli (e.g., bacterial enterotoxins) may act on the enterocyte via a single intracellular mediator involving cyclic adenosine monophosphate and adenyl cyclase.

Among other chemical agents that modify water transport are certain absorbable cathartics, some diuretics, and antidiuretic hormones.

3.2.5. Miscellaneous Diseases

In the rare congenital abnormality chloridorrhea, excess chloride is secreted in the stool, leading to severe metabolic disturbances. Irregularity in the ileal exchange between chloride and bicarbonate has been proposed to account for the abnormality.

Villous and other tumors of the colon may secrete or exude mucus which is a complex mixture of mucopolysaccharides in an isotonic electrolyte solution, rich in potassium. Segments of colon containing villous tumours secrete sodium, potassium, and water.

Ulcerative, inflammatory, neoplastic, and allergic conditions may exude protein, blood, or mucus into the bowel. Electrolyte and water transport may be altered in inflammatory bowel disease. This abnormality can be corrected by steroid treatment.

Although exudation is an uncommon single cause of diarrhea, in some instances of colitis, frequent bowel movements may be due to a "pseudo-diarrhea," i.e., evacuations consist largely of exudate and blood whereas stasis of solid fecal matter is demonstrable in the proximal colon.

Diffuse mucosal disease, such as nontropical sprue, leads to gross abnormalities of electrolyte, water, and glucose absorption. Indeed secretion of sodium and water into the jejunum is prominent and abnormalities of mucosal permeability have been reported.

3.3. TRANSPORT DISORDERS

In order to allow normal absorption, the chyme must be mixed, properly digested, and adequately exposed to the mucosal surface for a critical minimum time.

3.3.1. Mucosal Factors

Evidence is accumulating that the bowel remaining after resection is capable of considerable compensatory hypertrophy of function and even of structure, particularly if normal nutrition can be maintained. Survival and normal development, despite lifelong diarrhea, have been reported after preservation of only a few centimeters of proximal small bowel. Fecal water losses after resections can be complicated by additional factors such as bile acid effects on the colon, steatorrhea, gastric hypersecretion, and changes in bacterial flora. In certain circumstances, delay of intestinal transit by mechanical or pharmacological means can facilitate absorption in the remaining bowel. Attempts to slow transit by antiperistaltic agents have been relatively successful.

3.3.2. Motor Factors

3.3.2.1. Hypomotility

Normal intestinal motor activity is an important determinant of the relative sterility of the small bowel. The consequences of hypomotility and stasis, whether due to strictures, blind loops, or neuromuscular disease, relate to bacterial overgrowth in the small bowel.

Steatorrhea is often present and is thought to result from bacterial deconjugation of bile acids, rapid absorption of free bile acids by nonionic diffusion, and jejunal bile acid deficiency.

Diarrhea has been related to excess of fat in the lumen of the small bowel and colon, possibly mediated by hydroxy fatty acids. An inhibitory action of free bile acids on jejunal water absorption and changes in jejunal morphology produced by unconjugated bile acids could also be partly responsible.

3.3.2.2. Hypermotility

When rapid transit and malabsorption coexist, the cause-effect relationships are poorly defined. Thus, increased volume in the lumen, due to incomplete absorption, may accelerate transit as in perfusion studies. Moreover, several factors cited earlier as modifying intestinal water transport (fatty acids, bile acids, and humoral agents), also affect the function of the intestinal smooth muscle. The relationships between volume flow rates and water malabsorption have been tested experimentally and termed "volumogenic diarrhea." With greater rates of infusion into the duodenum, total fluid absorption increases; however, the proportion of the infusion solution that is absorbed decreases and the absolute volume required to produce diarrhea decreases. Fluid loss from the rectum can be modified by the hydrodynamic restrictions on flow imposed by the ileocecal valve and the anal sphincter.

Pathophysiology

Hormonal and pharmacological stimuli of the intestinal smooth muscle have been named as possible causes of certain types of diarrhea. Prostaglandins stimulate the intestinal smooth muscle in vitro, decrease transit time, provoke diarrhea in volunteers, and have been implicated, clinically, in diarrhea. Other pharmacologically active agents (secretin, pancreozymin, gastrin, and 5-hydroxytryptamine) stimulate the intestinal smooth muscle and are secreted by certain tumors that may produce diarrhea. However, relationships between the activity of the intestinal smooth muscle, propulsion of contents, and absorption are extremely complex.

II.4. CLINICAL ABNORMALITIES CAUSING DIARRHEA

4.1. INFECTIONS AND INFESTATIONS

Acute viral infections are not well documented; in fact, the frequency of a viral etiology for nonspecific diarrhea has not been established. In a model of transmissible viral gastroenteritis in pigs, the onset of watery diarrhea coincides with atrophic changes in villous structure, similar to those in sprue. Acute infectious diarrhea occasionally produces transient steatorrhea and disaccharide deficiency which could represent additional pathophysiological mechanisms. Diarrhea caused by parasitic infestations is poorly defined. Mucosal changes may occur, and these can be associated with steatorrhea. Exudation of plasma proteins has been reported in capillariasis and changes in bacterial flora of the gut have been implicated in diarrhea caused by a number of infections.

4.2. IATROGENIC FACTORS

Use and abuse of drugs constitute a frequent cause of diarrhea. Laxative agents include nonabsorbable ionic cathartics and hydroxy fatty acids (ricinoleic acids, castor oil). The important anthraquinone laxatives cause secretion in the small bowel and colon of experimental animals. These drugs also undergo enterohepatic circulation. Unconjugated forms are absorbed in the small bowel and are conjugated with gluceronic acid in the liver. Other anions and conjugates may be secreted in the bile. Conjugation impairs absorption from the small bowel allowing the drug to reach the colon. Impaired sodium and water reabsorption in the colon has been suggested as the cause of catharsis. Chronic abuse of such laxatives can result in protein-losing gastroenteropathy, steatorrhea, electrolyte depletion, and secondary hyperaldosteronism.

4.3. GASTROINTESTINAL RESECTIONS

Gastroduodenal surgery results in maldigestion and malabsorption of fat in up to 50% of patients; relevant mechanisms of steatorrhea have been reviewed under Sect. 3.2.3. When steatorrhea is present, water malabsorption may result from mechanisms already discussed.

After gastroenterostomy, the small bowel can be the site of bacterial overgrowth, thereby functioning as a blind loop. Other factors which may contribute to diarrhea are, for example, rapid intestinal transit, attributed to postoperative "dumping" and emergence of latent lactose malabsorption. Resection of the small bowel has been discussed above.

Factors of varying degrees of importance include the length and functional status of the remaining bowel, intestinal stasis with bacterial overgrowth, and the site of resection. In this context, loss of the ileum is of particular importance since ileal resection depletes the bile acid pool, thereby aggravating any existing steatorrhea due to decreased absorptive surface. In addition, passage of excess of bile acids through the colon may induce water malabsorption there.

Ileostomy represents a special case of intestinal resection, but one in which the continued loss of excess water and sodium from the gut can be examined for long-term complications.

The pathophysiological sequelae of ileostomy include increased susceptibility to sodium depletion, dehydration, oliguria, and renal calculi. Such events are predictable from present concepts of intestinal and renal function and have been discussed previously in this context. Recently, interruption of the enterohepatic circulation of bile acids has been proposed as a causative factor in the increased incidence of cholelithiasis after ileal resection. Partial resection of the colon is commonly performed but has received little attention. The length of the residual large bowel is probably important, since stools from proximal colostomies are more liquid than those from distal stomas. However, when resection and anastomosis are performed, the anatomical consequences may be different; proximal colectomy is often accompanied by resection of the terminal ileum. Judging by what is known at present, removal of the proximal colon should impair water absorption to a greater degree than more distal resections.

4.4. VAGAL SECTION

Postvagotomy diarrhea is occasionally a troublesome complication of vagal section. Some researchers estimate the incidence as 20%, of which the vast majority of cases are transient or episodic. They feel that the

Pathophysiology

associated "gastric drainage procedure" is unimportant, that a close relationship between steatorrhea and diarrhea has not been established, and that the pathogenesis of diarrhea is still open to discussion. Selective vagotomy is associated with a lower incidence of diarrhea; thus, the extragastric effects of vagal denervation may be important. Changes in intestinal motility, bacterial overgrowth, impairment of pancreatic function and lactase deficiency have also been cited as possible causes.

4.5. STRUCTURAL DISEASE OF THE SMALL AND LARGE INTESTINE

Nontropical sprue is an example of the multiple ramifications resulting from the failure of the function of the small intestine. Brush-border digestive failure, impaired cholecystokinin-pancreozymin release with secondary pancreatic insufficiency and micelle formation, intestinal secretion, and exudation may all contribute to water malabsorption in the jejunum.

Granulomatous and ulcerative colitis reduce electrolyte and water absorption in the colon, but secretion remains normal. The efficiency of normal colonic water absorption (90% or more) and the relatively small increase in stool water required to produce diarrhea (100 to 200 ml per day) imply that subtle changes in colonic function could cause significant symptoms. In ulcerative colitis, changes in the histology and disaccharidase activity of the small bowel have been reported although their clinical significance is not clear.

4.6. METABOLIC DISEASES

Specific syndromes of diarrhea in primary endocrine dysfunction are poorly defined. Untreated Addison's disease may cause impaired fat absorption while mineralocorticoids promote potassium loss from the colon. Hypothyroidism reduces and hyperthyroidism increases the frequency of bowel movements. Hyperthyroidism increases the frequency of the "pacemaker potentials" which govern muscular activity in the small bowel. Juvenile diabetics with neuropathy may suffer intermittent bouts of diarrhea without apparent cause.

4.7. FUNCTIONAL ABNORMALITIES; IRRITABLE BOWEL SYNDROME

The symptoms are chronic, sometimes intermittent, aggravated by stress, and unrelated to any known structural disease of the gut.

II.5. SUMMARY

Diarrhea is a familiar and ubiquitous expression of digestive failure accompanied by abnormal stools. It has numerous causes and therefore the precise pathophysiology is hard to define in many cases. Because of the wide variety of causes, an equally wide variety of chemotherapeutic and other means would normally be required to treat each cause individually and to correct every single disturbed factor. However, advances in chemotherapeutic research have made it possible to provide effective symptomatic relief of diarrhea, no matter what its origin. Once the diarrhea is under control many pathophysiological processes correct themselves. In the remaining cases, more specific therapy can be applied with greater ease and effectiveness.

CHAPTER III

CHEMISTRY OF MODERN ANTIDIARRHEALS

III.1. SYNTHESIS OF DIPHENOXYLATE, DIFENOXIN, LOPERAMIDE, AND RELATED COMPOUNDS

Willem Van Bever, Raymond Stokbroeckx, Jan Vandenberk, and Maria Wouters

1.1. INTRODUCTION

The chemistry of synthetic antidiarrheal agents is essentially limited to a series of ester derivatives of 1-(3-cyano-3,3-diphenylpropyl)-4-phenyl-4-piperidinecarboxylic acid (Janssen, 1959a, 1970; Janssen et al., 1959b; Briggs,* 1972; Soudijn and van Wijngaarden, 1972) and a series of 4-aryl-4-hydroxy-α, α-diphenyl-1-piperidinebutanamides (Janssen et al., 1973; Stokbroekx et al., 1973). In the patent literature other series of compounds have been reported to possess antidiarrheal activity (Carabateas, 1972; Claude et al., 1972; Mervyn and Fothergill, 1972). Recently, the synthesis and preliminary evaluation of a series of 1-(disubstituted amino)-3-(3-dialkylaminoalkyl)-3-phenyloxindoles were reported (Butler et al., 1973). Oral antidiarrheal activity, evaluated according to the method of Kennedy et al. (1972), was from 5 to 50 times less than that of diphenoxylate. The related 3-phenylindoline derivative CI-750, presumably obtained by Wolff-Kishner reduction of the corresponding phenyloxindole, was reported to be

———
*4-[(2,5-dioxo-1-pyrrolidinyl)oxy]carbonyl-α, α,4-triphenyl-1-piperidinebutanenitrile monohydrochloride has been adopted by the United States Adopted Name Council as difenoximide hydrochloride (J. Am. Med. Assoc. 229, 1223, 1974).

approximately equipotent to diphenoxylate in the rat (Bass et al., 1973). However, since no clinical reports on CI-750 have appeared, its chemical synthesis is not discussed here. The synthesis of compounds that are described only in patent literature is also considered beyond the scope of this chapter.

1.2. DIPHENOXYLATE, DIFENOXIN, AND RELATED COMPOUNDS

The ester derivatives of 1-(3-cyano-3,3-diphenylpropyl)-4-phenyl-4-piperidinecarboxylic acid [1] are chemically related to pethidine [2] (Eisleb and Schaumann, 1939) and to nitriles of the isopropamide type [3] (Lands, 1951; de Jongh et al., 1955).

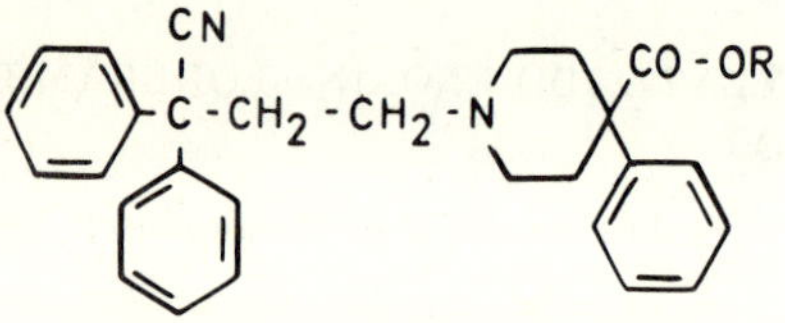

[1]

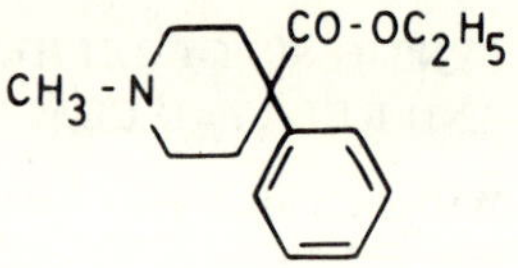

[2]

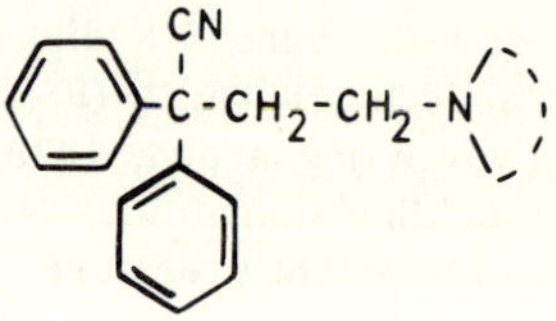

[3]

The synthesis of [1] is outlined in Scheme 1. Substitution of 4-bromo-2,2-diphenylbutanenitrile [5] with an appropriate 4-phenyl-4-piperidine-carboxylate affords [1]. Other 4-substituted piperidine derivatives such as 1-(4-phenyl-4-piperidyl)alkanones can be used as well. Since [5] is sterically severely crowded, substitution requires 72 hours reflux in methyl isobutyl ketone in the presence of sodium carbonate. Alternatively [1] can be obtained by alkylation of α-phenylbenzenacetonitrile [4] with an appropriate 1-(2-haloethyl)-4-phenyl-4-piperidinecarboxylate under reflux in an inert solvent in the presence of sodium amide. Since difenoxin [1] (R = H) cannot be synthesized by substitution of [5] with 4-phenyl-4-piperidinecarboxylic acid [8], it is prepared by selective hydrolysis of the ethyl or methyl ester of [1] (R = Et, Me) under basic conditions such as potassium hydroxide in isopropanol (Van Wijngaarden and Soudijn, 1972). The active compounds are listed in Table 1.

TABLE 1

1-(3-Cyano-3,3-diphenylpropyl)-4-phenyl-4-piperidinecarboxylates and 4-(1-oxoalkyl)-4-phenyl-α,α-diphenyl-1-piperidinebutanenitriles

Serial number	R	Solvent of crystallization	Yield %	Mp, °C	Formula
R 1132[a]	OCH_2CH_3	i-PrOH	55	222–223	$C_{30}H_{32}N_2O_2 \cdot HCl$
R 1326	OCH_3	i-PrOH	63	180–181	$C_{29}H_{30}N_2O_2 \cdot HCl$
R 1260	$OCH_2CH_2CH_3$	i-PrOH	60	204–205	$C_{31}H_{34}N_2O_2 \cdot HCl$
R 1261	$OCH(CH_3)_2$	i-PrOH	47	231–232	$C_{31}H_{34}N_2O_2 \cdot HCl$
R 1416	OCH_2CHCH_2	i-Pr$_2$O–i-PrOH	54	205–206	$C_{31}H_{32}N_2O_2 \cdot HCl$
R 1319[b]	$O(CH_2)_3CH_3$	Et$_2$O	65	200–201	$C_{32}H_{36}N_2O_2 \cdot HCl$
R 1355	$O(CH_2)_4CH_3$	i-PrOH	54	198–199	$C_{33}H_{38}N_2O_2 \cdot HCl$
R 1493	$O(CH_2)_5CH_3$	i-PrOH	49	189–190	$C_{34}H_{40}N_2O_2 \cdot HCl$
R 1357	$O-C_6H_{11}$[c]	i-Pr$_2$O–i-PrOH	51	218–220	$C_{34}H_{38}N_2O_2 \cdot HCl$
R 1500	$O(CH_2)_6CH_3$	i-PrOH	56	190–191	$C_{35}H_{42}N_2O_2 \cdot HCl$
R 1397	$OCH_2-C_6H_5$	i-PrOH	48	219–220	$C_{35}H_{34}N_2O_2 \cdot HCl$

TABLE 1 (Continued)

Serial number	R	Solvent of crystallization	Yield, %	Mp, °C	Formula
R 1375	$OCH_2CH_2-C_6H_5$	Me_2CO-i-PrOH	67	184–187	$C_{36}H_{36}N_2O_2 \cdot HCl$
R 1301	CH_2CH_3	Me_2CO-i-PrOH	62	229–231	$C_{30}H_{32}N_2O \cdot HCl$
R 1302	$CH_2CH_2CH_3$	Me_2CO-i-PrOH	64	227–228	$C_{31}H_{34}N_2O \cdot HCl$
R 12405	$OCH_2CH_2-C_4H_3S$[d]	Me_2CO-i-PrOH	59	188–189	$C_{34}H_{34}N_2O_2S \cdot HCl$
R 13558[e]	$OCH_2CH_2OC_6H_5$	i-PrOH	63	207–208	$C_{36}H_{36}N_2O_3 \cdot HCl$
R 15403[f]	OH	i-PrOH	75	289–290	$C_{28}H_{28}N_2O_2 \cdot HCl$

[a] Diphenoxylate.
[b] Butoxylate.
[c] C_6H_{11}: cyclohexyl.
[d] C_4H_3S: 2-thienyl.
[e] Fetoxylate.
[f] Difenoxin.

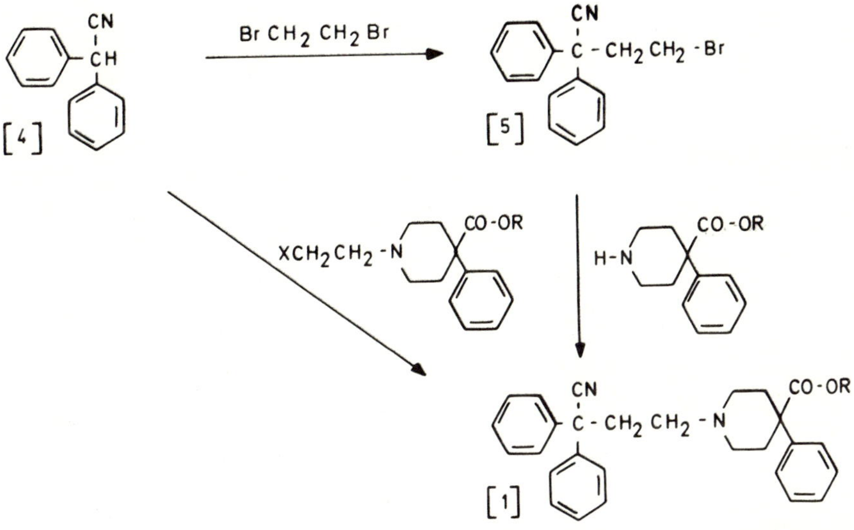

Chemistry: Synthesis

Scheme 1

4-Bromo-2,2-diphenylbutanenitrile [5] can be prepared by alkylation of [4] with 1,2-dibromoethane under Eisleb conditions (Bockmühl and Ehrhart, 1948; Dupre et al., 1949). However, better yields of [5] can be obtained by alkylation of [4] in 50% aqueous sodium hydroxide in the presence of benzyltriethylammonium chloride (Makosza and Serafin, 1965).

The synthesis of 4-phenyl-4-piperidinecarboxylates [11] and 1-(4-phenyl-4-piperidinyl)alkanones [13] is outlined in Scheme 2. Preparation of carboxylates [11] is analogous to the original synthesis of pethidine and related compounds, reported by Eisleb (Eisleb and Schaumann, 1939; Eisleb, 1941). Again, bisalkylation of N,N-bis(2-chloroethyl)benzenemethanamine [6] with benzenacetonitrile is improved by use of Makosza's conditions (Makosza and Serafin, 1965). Base hydrolysis of 4-phenyl-1-(phenylmethyl)-4-piperidinecarbonitrile [7], followed by standard esterification procedures with a suitable alcohol, affords the corresponding esters [9], which upon catalytic hydrogenation yield the desired ester derivatives [11]. Alternatively, hydrolysis and consequent dephenylmethylation of [7] yields 4-phenyl-4-piperidinecarboxylic acid [8]. Conversion of [8] to the corresponding acid chloride [10] by treatment with thionyl chloride and condensation of [10] with a suitable alcohol offers a somewhat more versatile pathway to compounds [11]. Alkanones [13] are synthesized by treatment of [7] with a suitable alkylmagnesium halide in tetrahydrofuran or hexamethylphosphortriamide, followed by removal of the protecting group by catalytic hydrogenation.

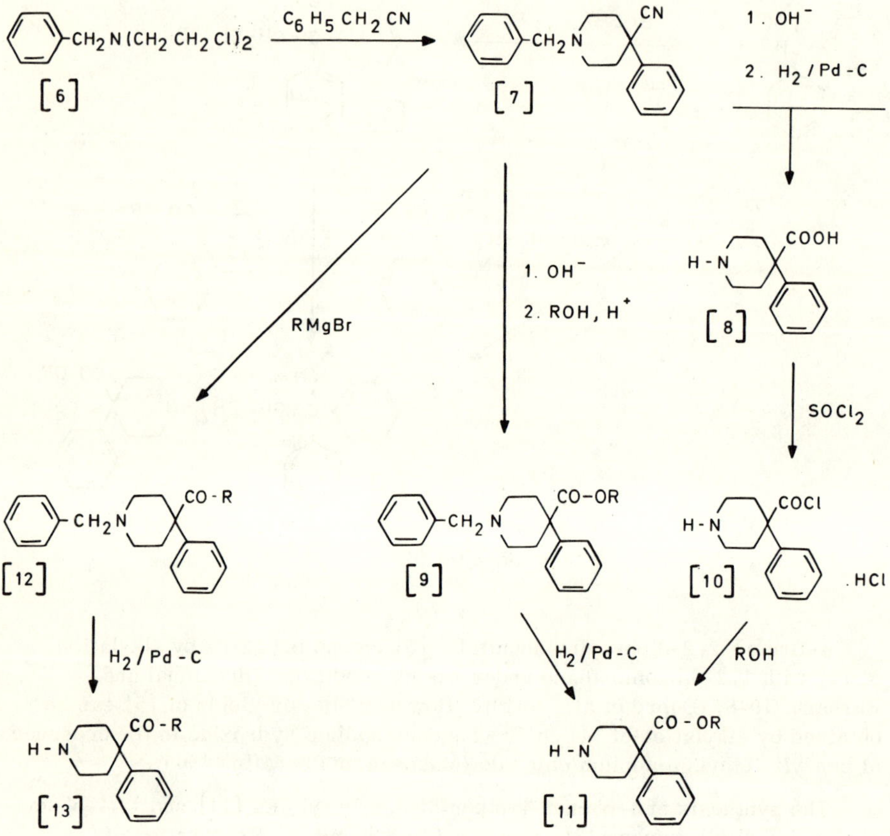

Scheme 2

1.3. LOPERAMIDE AND RELATED COMPOUNDS

The synthesis of 4-aryl-4-hydroxy-α, α-diphenyl-1-piperidinebutanamides [20], [23], and [25] is outlined in Scheme 3. Attempts to hydrolyze 4-bromo-2,2-diphenylbutanenitrile [5] under a variety of acidic and basic conditions to the corresponding butanoic acid [16] were unsuccessful. Therefore 4-bromo-2,2-diphenylbutanoic acid [16] was prepared from 3,3-diphenyl-2-iminotetrahydrofuran [14] (Attenburrow et al., 1949; Craig, 1952). Hydrolysis of [11] with aqueous hydrochloric acid affords

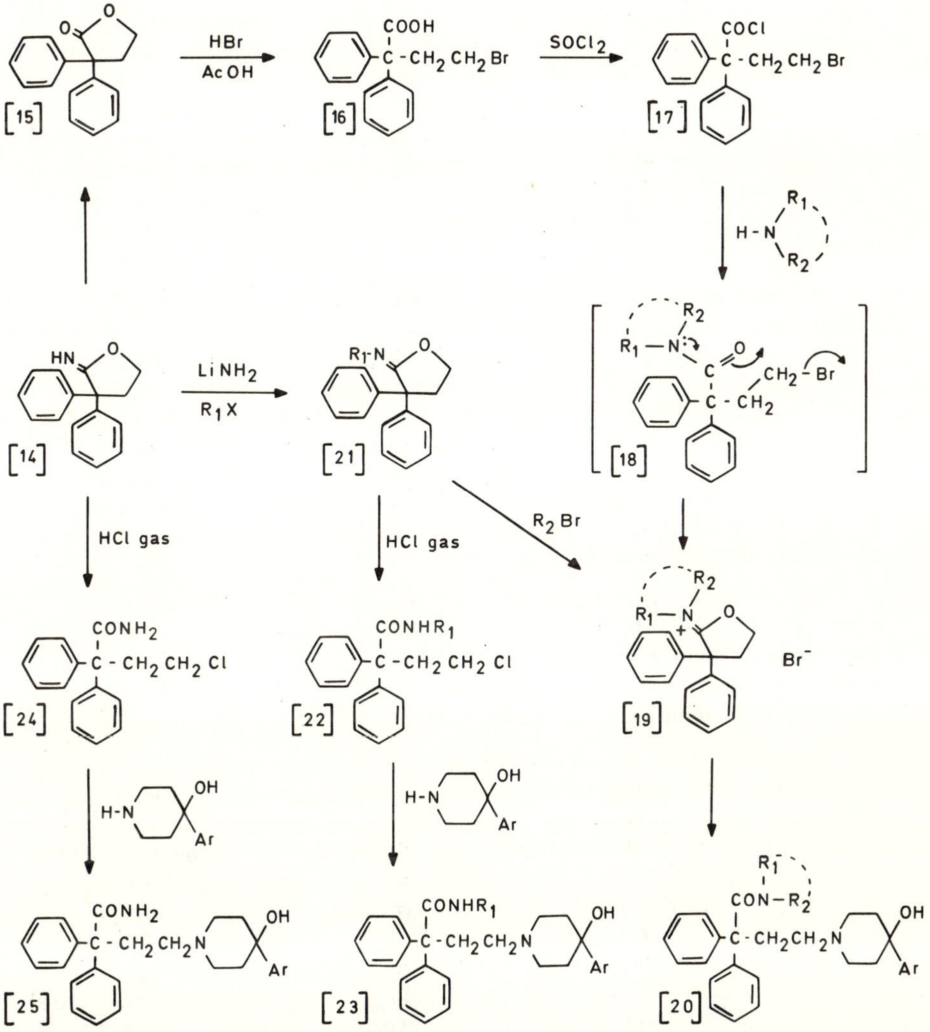

Chemistry: Synthesis

Scheme 3

the corresponding lactone [15] and subsequent ring opening with hydrobromic acid gas in acetic acid yields the acid [16]. Treatment of [16] with thionyl chloride followed by condensation of the resulting acid chloride [17] with an appropriate secondary amine affords intermediate butanamides [18], which rearrange spontaneously under the reaction conditions to form (tetrahydro-3,3-diphenyl-2-furylidene)ammonium bromides [19]. Ammonium salts [19] are highly reactive towards base and react practically instantaneously with 4-aryl-4-piperidinols to give tertiary butanamides [20]. The piperidinols are synthesized by addition of an appropriately substituted phenylmagnesium halide to ethyl 4-oxopiperidinecarboxylate and subsequent removal of the N-carbethoxygroup by treatment with potassium hydroxide in isopropanol (Hermans et al., 1970).

For the synthesis of secondary butanamides [23], 3,3-diphenyl-2-iminotetrahydrofuran [14] can be alkylated in the presence of a strong base (lithium or sodium amide) and a suitable alkyl halide to give N-alkylated compounds [21], which upon ring opening with gaseous hydrochloric acid yield N-alkyl-4-chloro-2,2-diphenylbutanamides [22]. Substitution of [22] with an appropriate 4-aryl-4-piperidinol affords desired end products [23]. Alternatively N-alkylated 2-iminotetrahydrofurans [21] can be quaternized with alkyl bromides to give ammonium salts [19]. This latter pathway is especially useful for the synthesis of tertiary butanamides [20] in which R_1 and R_2 are different.

The primary butanamides [25] are prepared by acid-catalyzed ring opening of [14] (Pagliarini et al., 1966), followed by substitution with an appropriate 4-aryl-4-piperidinol. The active compounds [20], [23], and [25] are summarized in Table 2. The 4-aryl-4-hydroxy-3-methyl-N,N-dimethyl-α,α-diphenyl-1-piperidinebutanamides are summarized in Table 3.

The synthesis of 4-aryl-4-hydroxy-β-methyl-α,α-diphenyl-1-piperidinebutanamides [29] is outlined in Scheme 4. Conversion of 4-cyano-3,3-diphenyl-2-methylbutanoic acid [26] (Salmon-Legagneur and Neveu, 1959) to the acid chloride with thionyl chloride, followed by reduction with sodium borohydride in dimethylformamide, affords the intermediate 2,2-diphenyl-4-hydroxy-3-methylbutanenitrile, which cyclizes in strong acid to 3,3-diphenyl-2-imino-4-methyltetrahydrofuran [27]. Its alkylation, followed by quaternization yields dimethyl(tetrahydro-3,3-diphenyl-4-methyl-2-furylidene)ammonium iodide [28]. Addition of 4-aryl-4-piperidinols to [28] affords [29]. The synthesis of 4-aryl-4-hydroxy-γ-methyl-α,α-diphenyl-1-piperidinebutanamides [3] is outlined in Scheme 5. Alkylation of an appropriately N,N-disubstituted-2,2-diphenylacetamide [30] with sodium amide in dimethylbenzene affords 2,2-diphenyl-4-pentenamide [31]. Cyclization of [31] with 30% hydrobromic acid in acetic acid yields dimethyl-(tetrahydro-3,3-diphenyl-5-methyl-2-furylidene)ammonium bromide [32], which upon addition of 4-aryl-4-piperidinols affords [33]. Compounds [29] and [33] are summarized in Table 4.

TABLE 2

4-Aryl-4-hydroxy-α,α-diphenyl-1-piperidinebutanamides

Serial number	$-N\begin{smallmatrix}R_1\\R_2\end{smallmatrix}$	R	Solvent of crystallization	Yield purified, %	Mp, °C	Formula
21 345	NH_2	4-Cl	i-BuCOMe	10	236-237	$C_{27}H_{29}ClN_2O_2 \cdot HCl$
21 531	$NHCH_3$	H	i-PrOH	40	218-219	$C_{28}H_{32}N_2O_2 \cdot HCl$
20 905	$NHCH_3$	4-Cl	i-BuCOMe	80	237-238	$C_{28}H_{31}ClN_2O_2 \cdot HCl$
18 936	$N(CH_3)_2$	H	PhMe	60	130-131	$C_{29}H_{34}N_2O_2$
18 976	$N(CH_3)_2$	4-F	i-PrOH	82	233-234	$C_{29}H_{33}FN_2O_2 \cdot HCl \cdot 0.5\,i\text{-PrOH}$
18 553[a]	$N(CH_3)_2$	4-Cl	i-PrOH	58	222-223	$C_{29}H_{33}ClN_2O_2 \cdot HCl$
18 937	$N(CH_3)_2$	4-Br	i-BuCOMe	64	123-124	$C_{29}H_{33}BrN_2O_2 \cdot HCl$
18 907	$N(CH_3)_2$	3,4-Cl_2	i-BuCOMe	80	239-240	$C_{29}H_{32}Cl_2N_2O_2 \cdot HCl$
18 910[b]	$N(CH_3)_2$	3-CF_3,4-Cl	i-PrOH	64	215-216	$C_{30}H_{32}ClF_3N_2O_2 \cdot HCl$
18 946	$N(CH_3)_2$	3-CF_3	i-BuCOMe	34	185-186	$C_{30}H_{33}F_3N_2O_2 \cdot HCl$
18 818	$N(CH_3)_2$	4-CH_3	Me_2CO	41	206-207	$C_{30}H_{36}N_2O_2 \cdot HCl$
19 391	$N(CH_3)_2$	2,4-$(CH_3)_2$	i-BuCOMe	43	126-127	$C_{31}H_{38}N_2O_2 \cdot HCl \cdot H_2O$
19 428	$N(CH_3)_2$	3,4,5-$(CH_3)_3$	i-PrOH	49	182-183	$C_{32}H_{40}N_2O_2 \cdot HCl \cdot 0.5\,i\text{-PrOH}$
19 685	$N(CH_3)_2$	2,5-$(OCH_3)_2$	THF[c]	40	180-181	$C_{31}H_{38}N_2O_4 \cdot HNO_3$

TABLE 2 (Continued)

Serial number	$-N\begin{matrix}R_1\\R_2\end{matrix}$	R	Solvent of crystallization	Yield purified, %	Mp, °C	Formula
18 898	$N(CH_2CH_3)_2$	H	i-PrOH	71	248-249	$C_{31}H_{38}N_2O_2 \cdot HCl \cdot 0.5i\text{-PrOH}$
18 885	$N(CH_2CH_3)_2$	4-F	i-BuCOMe	45	135-136	$C_{31}H_{37}FN_2O_2$
18 892	$N(CH_2CH_3)_2$	4-Cl	i-PrOH	44	236-237	$C_{31}H_{37}ClN_2O_2 \cdot HCl \cdot 0.5i\text{-PrOH}$
18 938	$N(CH_2CH_3)_2$	4-Br	i-BuCOMe	36	145-146	$C_{31}H_{37}BrN_2O_2 \cdot 0.5H_2O$
18 887	$N(CH_2CH_3)_2$	3,4-Cl_2	i-PrOH	60	245-246	$C_{31}H_{36}Cl_2N_2O_2 \cdot HCl$
18 860	$N(CH_2CH_3)_2$	3-CF_3, 4-Cl	i-BuCOMe	69	220-221	$C_{32}H_{36}ClF_3N_2O_2 \cdot HCl$
18 900	$N(CH_2CH_3)_2$	3-CF_3	i-BuCOMe	75	222-223	$C_{32}H_{37}F_3N_2O_2 \cdot HCl$
18 894	NC_4H_8 d	H	i-BuCOMe	56	187-188	$C_{31}H_{36}N_2O_2$
18 895	NC_4H_8 d	4-F	i-BuCOMe	62	192-193	$C_{31}H_{35}FN_2O_2$
18 356	NC_4H_8 d	4-Cl	i-BuCOMe	53	168-169	$C_{31}H_{35}ClN_2O_2$
18 939	NC_4H_8 d	3,4-Cl_2	EtOH	49	200-201	$C_{31}H_{34}Cl_2N_2O_2 \cdot HCl$
18 906	NC_4H_8 d	3-CF_3, 4-Cl	i-BuCOMe	30	188-189	$C_{32}H_{34}ClF_3N_2O_2 \cdot HCl$
18 947	NC_4H_8 d	3-CF_3	i-BuCOMe	40	117-118	$C_{32}H_{35}F_3N_2O_2 \cdot HCl \cdot 2H_2O$
18 899	NC_4H_8 d	4-CH_3	i-BuCOMe	38	165-170	$C_{32}H_{38}N_2O_2$
18 861	NC_5H_{10} e	H	i-BuCOMe	51	240-241	$C_{32}H_{38}N_2O_2 \cdot HCl$
18 580	NC_5H_{10} e	4-Cl	EtOH	66	251-253	$C_{32}H_{37}ClN_2O_2 \cdot HCl$
18 819	NC_5H_{10} e	3,4-Cl_2	Me_2CO	37	202-203	$C_{32}H_{36}Cl_2N_2O_2 \cdot HCl$
18 812	NC_5H_{10} e	3-CF_3, 4-Cl	i-BuCOMe	64	204-205	$C_{33}H_{36}ClF_3N_2O_2 \cdot HCl$
18 848	NC_5H_{10} e	3-CF_3	i-BuCOMe	62	200-201	$C_{33}H_{37}F_3N_2O_2 \cdot HCl$
18 798	NC_5H_{10} e	4-CH_3	Me_2CO	80	240-241	$C_{33}H_{40}N_2O_2 \cdot HCl$
18 897	NC_4H_8O f	H	i-PrOH	49	182-183	$C_{31}H_{36}N_2O_3 \cdot HCl \cdot 0.5i\text{-PrOH}$
18 491	NC_4H_8O f	4-Cl	Me_2CO	72	257-258	$C_{31}H_{35}ClN_2O_3 \cdot HCl$

#	NR₂	X	Solvent	Yield	mp	Formula
18 875	NC$_4$H$_8$O[f]	3,4-Cl$_2$	i-BuCOMe	78	242-243	C$_{31}$H$_{34}$Cl$_2$N$_2$O$_3$·HCl
18 869	NC$_4$H$_8$O[f]	3-CF$_3$, 4-Cl	i-BuCOMe	65	243-244	C$_{32}$H$_{34}$ClF$_3$N$_2$O$_3$·HCl
18 837	NC$_4$H$_8$O[f]	3-CF$_3$	i-BuCOMe	62	213-214	C$_{32}$H$_{35}$F$_3$N$_2$O$_3$·HCl
19 380	NC$_6$H$_{12}$O[g]	4-Cl	i-BuCOMe	36	241-242	C$_{33}$H$_{39}$ClN$_2$O$_3$·HCl
19 395	NC$_6$H$_{12}$[h]	4-Cl	i-BuCOMe	71	215-216	C$_{33}$H$_{39}$ClN$_2$O$_3$·HCl
19 424	NC$_6$H$_{12}$[i]	4-Cl	i-BuCOMe	85	235-236	C$_{33}$H$_{39}$ClN$_2$O$_2$·HCl
19 398	N(CH$_3$)CH$_2$CH$_3$	4-Cl	PhMe	30	215-216	C$_{30}$H$_{35}$ClN$_2$O$_2$·HCl
19 426	N(CH$_3$)CH$_2$C$_6$H$_5$	4-Cl	i-BuCOMe	60	225-226	C$_{35}$H$_{37}$ClN$_2$O$_2$·HCl
19 442	N(CH$_2$CHCH$_2$)$_2$	4-Cl	EtOH	60	258-259	C$_{33}$H$_{37}$ClN$_2$O$_2$·HCl
19 450	N(CH$_3$)CH$_2$CH$_2$CH$_3$	4-Cl	i-BuCOMe	78	190-191	C$_{31}$H$_{37}$ClN$_2$O$_2$·HCl
19 469	N(CH$_3$)CH(CH$_3$)$_2$	4-Cl	i-BuCOMe	73	225-226	C$_{31}$H$_{37}$ClN$_2$O$_2$·HCl
19 207	N(CH$_2$CH$_2$CH$_3$)$_2$	4-Cl	i-BuCOMe	76	258-261	C$_{33}$H$_{41}$ClN$_2$O$_2$·HCl

[a] Loperamide.
[b] Fluperamide.
[c] Tetrahydrofuran.
[d] -NC$_4$H$_8$: 1-pyrrolidinyl.
[e] -NC$_5$H$_{10}$: 1-piperidinyl.
[f] -NC$_4$H$_8$O: 1-morpholinyl.
[g] -NC$_6$H$_{12}$O: 4-(2,6-dimethylmorpholinyl).
[h] -NC$_6$H$_{12}$: 1-(4 methylpiperidinyl).
[i] -NC$_6$H$_{12}$: 1-(3-methylpiperidinyl).

TABLE 3

4-Aryl-4-hydroxy-3-methyl-N,N-dimethyl-α,α-diphenyl-1-piperidinebutanamides

Serial number	R	Solvent of crystallization	Yield purified, %	Mp, °C	Formula
19 470	H	i-BuCOMe	95	241–243	$C_{30}H_{36}N_2O_2 \cdot HCl$
19 510	4-Cl	(i-Pr)$_2$O	94.8	226–227	$C_{30}H_{35}ClN_2O_2 \cdot HCl$
19 427	3-CF$_3$, 4-Cl	i-BuCOMe	84	170–172	$C_{31}H_{34}ClF_3N_2O_2 \cdot HCl$
19 451	3-CF$_3$	i-BuCOMe	71	224–225	$C_{31}H_{35}F_3N_2O_2 \cdot HCl$

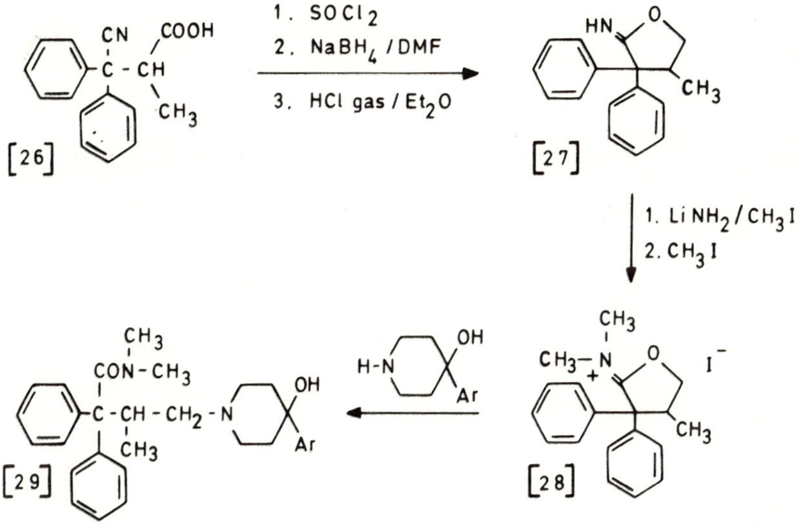

Chemistry: Synthesis

Scheme 4

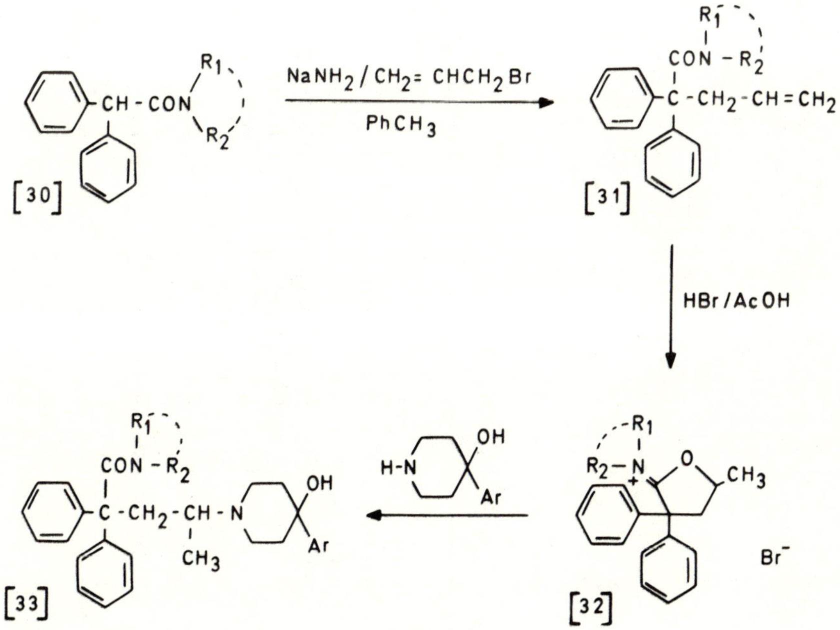

Scheme 5

TABLE 4

4-Aryl-4-hydroxy-β or γ-methyl-α,α-diphenyl-1-piperidinebutanamides

Serial number	-N⟨ ⟩	R_1	R_2	R_3	Solvent of crystallization	Yield purified, %	Mp, °C	Formula
18 921	$N(CH_3)_2$	H	CH_3	H	i-BuCOMe	43	193–194	$C_{30}H_{36}N_2O_2$
18 920	$N(CH_3)_2$	H	CH_3	4-F	i-BuCOMe	20	165–166	$C_{30}H_{35}FN_2O_2$
18 874	$N(CH_3)_2$	H	CH_3	4-Cl	EtOH	40	200–201	$C_{30}H_{35}ClN_2O_2$
19 029	$N(CH_3)_2$	H	CH_3	3-CF_3, 4-Cl	i-BuCOMe	45	207–208	$C_{31}H_{34}ClF_3N_2O_2 \cdot HCl$
18 855	$N(CH_3)_2$	H	CH_3	3-CF_3	i-BuCOMe	48	169–170	$C_{31}H_{35}F_3N_2O_2$
18 940	NC_4H_8[a]	H	CH_3	H	i-BuCOMe	57	168–169	$C_{32}H_{38}N_2O_2$
19 001	NC_4H_8[a]	H	CH_3	4-F	i-BuCOMe	27	186–187	$C_{32}H_{37}FN_2O_2$
18 948	NC_4H_8[a]	H	CH_3	4-Cl	i-BuCOMe	71	206–207	$C_{32}H_{37}ClN_2O_2$
19 014	NC_4H_8[a]	H	CH_3	3-CF_3	i-BuCOMe	30	133–134	$C_{33}H_{37}F_3N_2O_2 \cdot HCl \cdot 2H_2O$
21 108	$N(CH_3)_2$	CH_3	H	4-Cl	i-PrOH	54	196–197	$C_{30}H_{35}ClN_2O_2 \cdot HCl \cdot 0.5i\text{-PrOH}$
21 605	$N(CH_3)_2$	CH_3	H	3-CF_3, 4-Cl	i-PrOH	45	200–201	$C_{31}H_{34}ClF_3N_2O_2$
21 624	$N(CH_3)_2$	CH_3	H	3-CF_3	i-PrOH	40	252–253	$C_{31}H_{35}F_3N_2O_2 \cdot HCl$

[a] NC_4H_8: 1-pyrrolidinyl.

III.2. PHYSICOCHEMICAL AND ANALYTICAL STUDIES ON DIPHENOXYLATE, DIFENOXIN, AND LOPERAMIDE

Willem Van Bever and Paul Demoen

2.1. DIPHENOXYLATE

2.1.1. Description

Ethyl 1-(3-cyano-3,3-diphenylpropyl)-4-phenyl-4-piperidinecarboxylate hydrochloride (R 1132, Reasec, Lomotil, Diarsed, Retardin) is a white to nearly white, amorphous flocculent powder. It is odorless, tasteless, and stable to air and light. Molecular formula: $C_{30}H_{32}N_2 \cdot HCl$. Molecular weight: 489.04. Percentage composition: base, 92.54%; carbon, 73.67%; hydrogen, 6.80%; chloride, 7.25%; nitrogen, 5.73; oxygen, 6.54%. Structural formula:

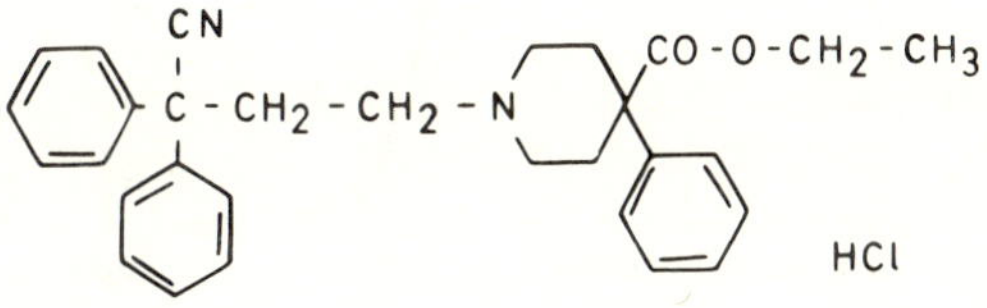

Crystallized from isopropanol it melts at 222-223° C (Tottoli apparatus). R 1132 is very soluble in chloroform; soluble in methanol, ethanol, propylene glycol, acetone, and tetrahydrofuran; slightly soluble in isopropanol, methyl isobutyl ketone, ethyl acetate, carbon tetrachloride, and benzene; practically insoluble in water, 0.1 N hydrochloric acid, 0.1 N sodium hydrochloride, hexane, ether, and diisopropyl ether. The corresponding base ($C_{30}H_{32}N_2O_2$; mol wt: 452.57) is a viscous semisolid, n_D^{20} between 1.560 and 1.561.

2.1.2. UV Absorption

Figure 1 shows the UV spectrum of R 1132 recorded with a Beckman DK-2A spectrophotometer. R 1132 (32 mg) was dissolved in 100 ml of a mixture of 10 ml 0.1 N hydrochloric acid and 90 ml isopropanol and the spectrum determined in a 1 cm cell, against a mixture of 0.1 N hydrochloric acid (1 vol) and isopropanol (9 vol). The absorption maxima and minima are given in Table 5.

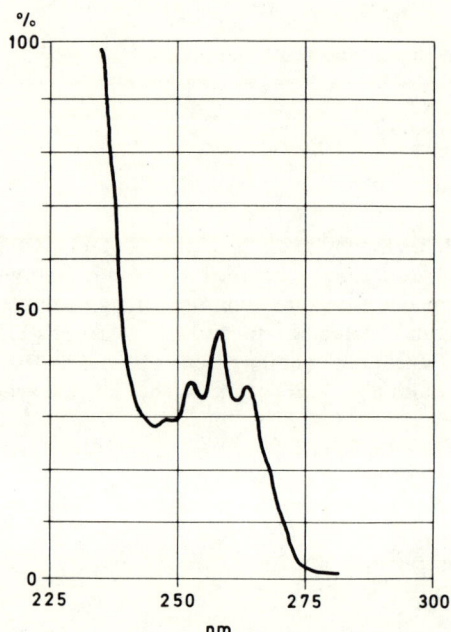

Fig. 1. UV spectrum of diphenoxylate hydrochloride in a mixture of 0.1 N HCl and isopropanol (1 : 9).

TABLE 5

UV Absorption maxima and
Minima of ϵ of R 1132 in a Mixture of
0.1 N HCl and Isopropanol (1 : 9)

Maxima		Minima	
λ, nm	ϵ	λ, nm	ϵ
251.5 ± 1	528	244.5 ± 1	403
257.5	648	254	469
263.5	508	262.5	468

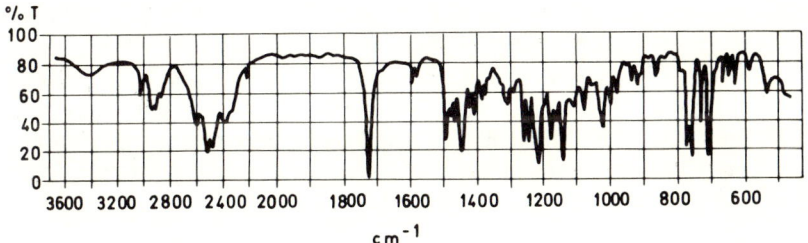

Fig. 2. IR spectrum of diphenoxylate hydrochloride (KBr pellet).

2.1.3. IR Absorption

Figure 2 shows the IR absorption spectrum of a potassium bromide dispersion of R 1132 recorded on a Perkin-Elmer 421 grating spectrometer. Strong absorption bands occur at 2550 ($^+$NH stretching), 1745 (carbonyl stretching), 1230 (C-O stretching vibrations), 720 and 695 cm^{-1} (monosubstituted benzene rings). A weak absorption band at 2225 cm^{-1} is attributed to nitrile stretching.

2.1.4. Quantitative analysis

Weigh accurately about 75 mg diphenoxylate hydrochloride and dissolve in 25 ml glacial acetic acid. Add 2 ml of a 3% solution of mercuric acetate and titrate with 0.02 N aqueous perchloric acid, either potentiometrically (glass-calomel electrodes) or visually (α-naphtolbenzeine). Each ml of 0.02 N HClO corresponds to 9.7808 mg R 1132.

2.1.5. Purity tests

a. Color and clarity of the solution: Dissolve 1 g R 1132 in 10 ml chloroform. The solution is clear and no more than slightly yellow. Filter (G4) and measure the transmittance in a 1 cm cell against chloroform at 400 nm, limit 80%.

b. Thin-layer chromatography: Dissolve 0.3 g R 1132 in 3 ml chloroform and spot 1 μl on an alkaline silica-gel plate. Develop with a mixture of equal volumes of chloroform and hexane in a chamber fitted with paper wicks. After drying the plate, visualize in a chamber containing iodine vapor. R 1132 shows a brown spot with an Rf-value of approximately 0.14.

c. Loss on drying: After 4 hr at 105°C the product loses no more than 0.5% of its weight.

d. Residue on ignition: Use about 1 g R 1132 in a porcelain crucible. R 1132 yields no more than 0.2% of residue on ignition.

e. Chloride: 7.25%. Weigh accurately about 25 mg R 1132, dissolve in 50 ml isopropanol, and add 0.5 ml 0.1 N nitric acid. Titrate with 0.01 N mercuric nitrate, in the presence of diphenylcarbazone as indicator. Each ml of 0.01 N $Hg(NO_3)_2$ corresponds to 0.35457 mg chloride.

2.2. DIFENOXIN

2.2.1. Description

1-(3-Cyano-3,3-diphenylpropyl)-4-phenyl-4-piperidinecarboxylic acid monohydrochloride (R 15 403) is a white, amorphous powder. Molecular formula: $C_{28}H_{28}N_2O_2 \cdot HCl$. Molecular weight: 460.98. Percentage composition: base, 92.09%; carbon, 72.95%; hydrogen, 6.34%; chlorine, 7.69%; nitrogen; 6.08%; oxygen, 6.94%. Structural formula:

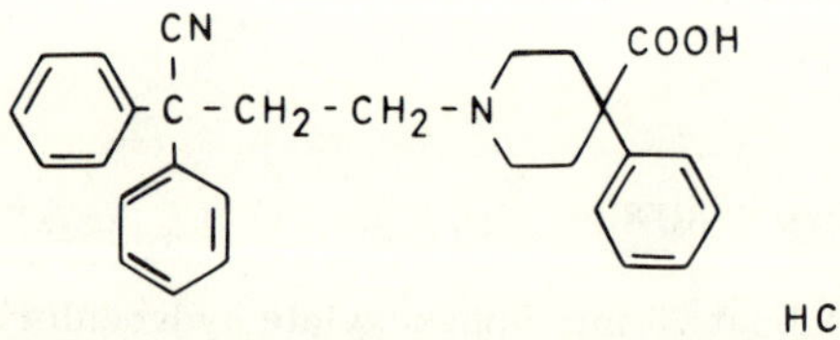

Crystallized from isopropanol it melts at 289-290°C (Tottoli apparatus). R 15 403 is very soluble in dimethylformamide, dimethylacetamide, and dimethylsulfoxide; soluble in chloroform, polyethylene glycol, and tetrahydrofuran; slightly soluble in hexane, 0.1 N sodium hydroxide, methanol, ethanol, propanol, butanol, isopropanol, hexanol, propylene glycol, and acetone; practically insoluble in water, 0.1 N hydrochloric acid, ether, ethyl acetate, and benzene. The corresponding base ($C_{28}H_{28}N_2O$; mol wt: 424-52) is a white, amorphous powder, melting between 235 and 240°C, and is less soluble in all solvents tested.

2.2.2. UV Absorption

Figure 3 shows the UV spectrum of R 15 403 recorded with a Beckman DK-2A spectrophotometer. R 15 403 (40 mg) was dissolved in a mixture of 10 ml 0.1 N hydrochloric acid and 90 ml isopropanol, and the spectrum determined in a 1 cm cell against a mixture of 0.1 N hydrochloric acid (1 vol) and isopropanol (9 vol). The absorption maxima and minima are given in Table 6.

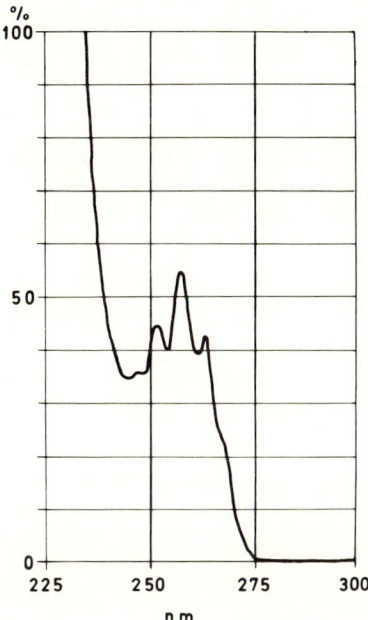

Fig. 3. UV spectrum of difenoxin hydrochloride in a mixture of 0.1 N HCl and isopropanol (1 : 9).

TABLE 6

UV Absorption Maxima and Minima and ϵ of R 15 403 in a Mixture of 0.1 N HCl and Isopropanol (1 : 9)

Maxima		Minima	
λ, nm	ϵ	λ, nm	ϵ
246	420	244	410
251	540	248	420
257	650	254	470
263	520	261	470

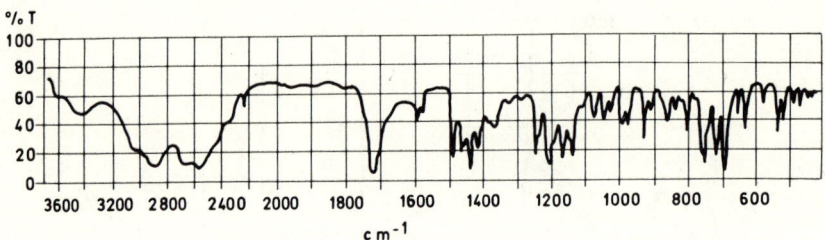

Fig. 4. IR spectrum of difenoxin hydrochloride (KBr pellet).

2.2.3. IR Absorption

Figure 4 shows the IR absorption spectrum of a potassium bromide dispersion of R 15403 recorded on a Perkin-Elmer 421 grating spectrometer. Strong absorption bands occur at 3000-2800 (CH_2 stretching and OH stretching of associated OH groups), 2560 ($^+$NH stretching), 1725 (acid carbonyl stretching), 1210 (C-O stretching vibration), and 723 and 695 cm^{-1} (monosubstituted benzene rings). A weak absorption band at 2230 is attributed to nitrile stretching.

2.2.4. Mass Spectrum

Figure 5 shows the mass spectrum recorded with a Varian MAT mass spectrometer (70 eV, source pressure 5.10^{-6} Torr, filament current 300 μA, sample rod temperature 120°C), m/e (%): 424(4), 219(17), 218(100), 193(5), 174(10), 172(7), 165(6), 91(8), 44(5), and 42(14).

2.2.5. Quantitative analysis

a. Base equivalent: Weigh accurately about 70 mg R 15403, dissolve in 25 ml glacial acetic acid, add 2 ml of a 3% mercuric acetate solution in the same solvent, and titrate with 0.02 N acetous perchloric acid, either potentiometrically (glass-calomel electrodes) or visually (α-naphtolbenzeine). Each ml 0.02 N $HClO_4$ corresponds to 9.2196 mg R 15403.

b. Acid equivalent: Weigh accurately about 35 mg R 15403, dissolve in 25 ml neutralized dimethylformamide, and titrate with 0.02 N sodium methoxide in the presence of thymol blue as indicator. Each ml 0.02 N NaOMe corresponds to 4.6098 mg R 15403.

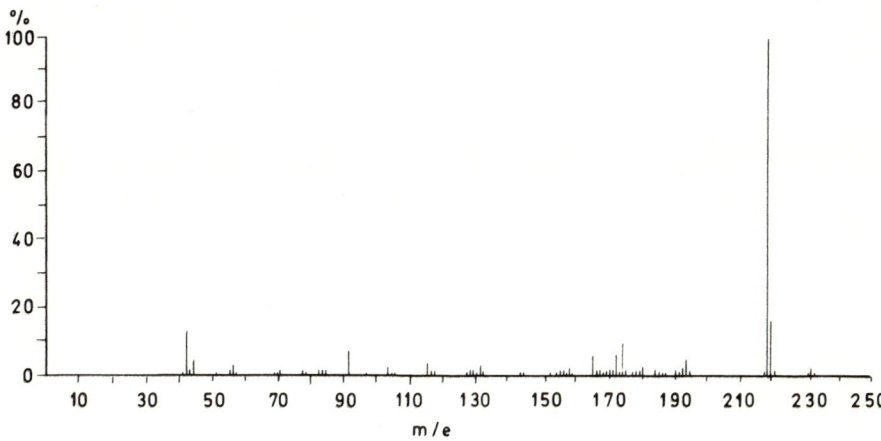
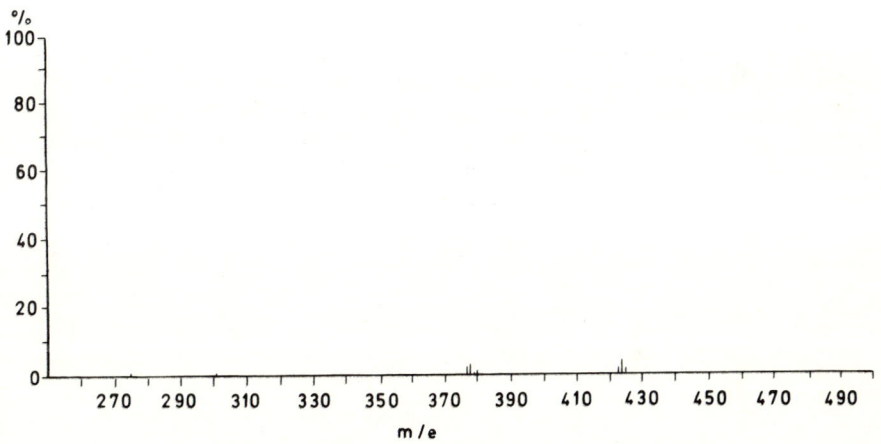

Fig. 5. Mass spectrum of difenoxin hydrochloride.

2.2.6. Purity tests

a. Color and clarity of the solution: Dissolve 500 mg R 15 403 in a mixture of 35 ml chloroform and 75 ml methanol. Filter and measure the transmittance in a 10 cm cell at 400 nm; limit 80%.

b. Thin-layer chromatography: Dissolve 30 mg R 15 403 in a mixture of 2 ml chloroform and 1 ml methanol and spot 10 μl on an alkaline silica-gel plate. Develop with a mixture of chloroform (17 vol) and methanol (3 vol). After drying the plate, visualize with Dragendorff's reagent or iodine vapor. R 15 403 has an Rf- value of approximately 0.70.

c. Loss on drying: After 4 hr at 105°C, the product loses no more than 0.5% of its weight.

d. Residue on ignition: R 15 403 yields no more than 0.2% of residue on ignition.

e. Chloride: 7.69%. Weigh accurately about 25 mg R 15 403, dissolve in 40 ml isopropanol, add 0.5 ml 0.1 N nitric acid, and titrate with 0.01 N mercuric nitrate in the presence of diphenylcarbazone as indicator. Each ml 0.01 N $Hg(NO_3)_2$ corresponds to 0.35457 mg chloride.

2.3. LOPERAMIDE

2.3.1. Description

4-(4-Chlorophenyl)-4-hydroxy-N,N-dimethyl-α,α-diphenyl-1-piperidine-butanamide hydrochloride (R 18 553, Imodium, Imosec) is a white to faintly yellow microcrystalline powder with a very bitter taste. It is stable in air and sunlight. Molecular formula: $C_{29}H_{33}ClN_2O_2 \cdot HCl$. Molecular weight: 513.49. Percentage composition: base, 92.90%; carbon, 67.83%; hydrogen, 6.67%; chloride, 6.91%; chlorine, 13.81%; nitrogen, 5.46%; oxygen, 6.23%. Structural formula:

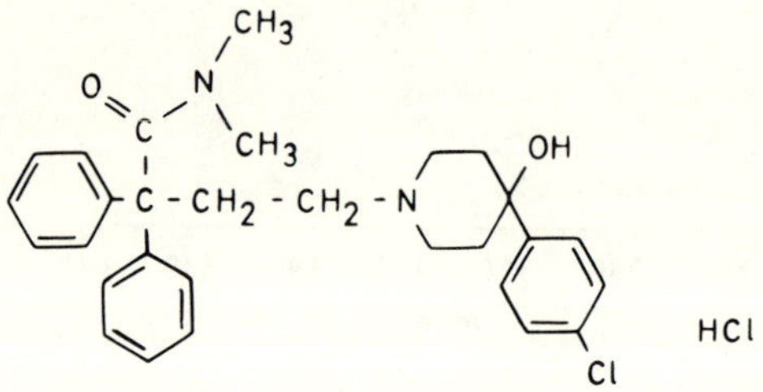

Crystallized from isopropanol it melts at 222-223°C (Tottoli apparatus). R 18 553 is very soluble in chloroform, methanol, dimethylformamide, and dimethyl sulfoxide; soluble in ethanol, isopropanol, propylene glycol, polyethylene glycol 200, benzene, and dimethylacetamide; slightly soluble in water, hexane, polyethylene glycol 600, acetone, and ethyl acetate; practically insoluble in 0.1 N hydrochloric acid, 0.1 N sodium hydrochloride, and ether.

2.3.2. UV Absorption

Figure 6 shows the UV spectrum of R 18 553 recorded with a Beckman DK-2A spectrometer. R 18 553 (40 mg) was dissolved in a mixture of 10 ml

Chemistry: Physicochemical and Analytical Data

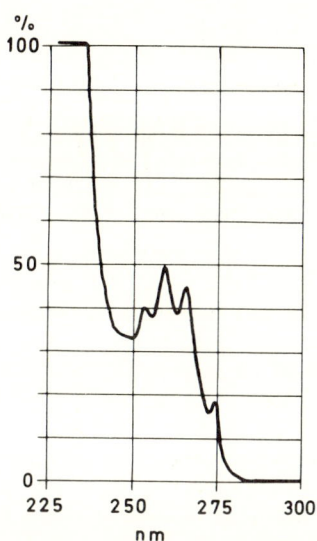

Fig. 6. UV spectrum of loperamide hydrochloride in a mixture of 0.1 N HCl and isopropanol (1 : 9).

0.1 N hydrochloric acid and 90 ml isopropanol, and the spectrum determined in a 1 cm cell against a mixture of 0.1 N hydrochloric acid (1 vol) and isopropanol (9 vol). The absorption maxima and minima are given in Table 7.

TABLE 7

UV Absorption Maxima and Minima and ϵ of R 18 553 in a Mixture of 0.1 N HCl and Isopropanol (1 : 9)

Maxima		Minima	
λ, nm	ϵ	λ, nm	ϵ
254	520	250	426
260	640	256	483
266	576	263	494
274	236		

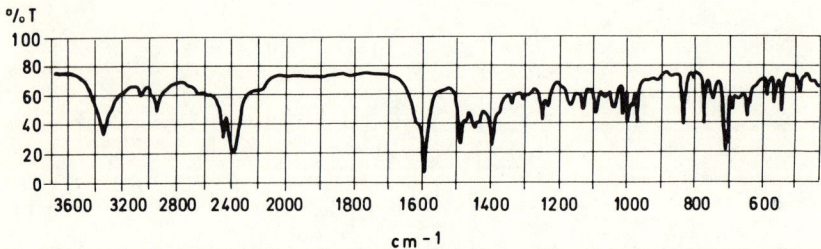

Fig. 7. IR spectrum of loperamide hydrochloride (KBr pellet).

2.3.3. IR Absorption

Figure 7 shows the IR absorption spectrum of a potassium bromide dispersion of R 18 553 recorded with a Perkin-Elmer 421 grating spectrometer. Strong absorption bands occur at 2500-2300 ($^+$NH stretching), 1600 (carbonyl stretching), and 700 cm^{-1} (monosubstituted benzene rings). A medium absorption band at 3315 cm^{-1} is attributed to OH stretching of associated OH groups.

2.3.4. Nuclear magnetic resonance spectrum

Figure 8 shows the nmr spectrum of R 18 553 in CDCl$_3$ and TMS as internal standard recorded with a Bruker HX60. The NMR assignments are given in Table 8.

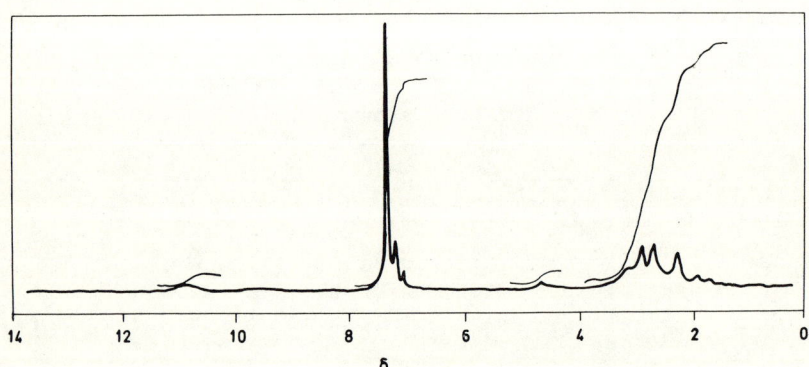

Fig. 8. NMR spectrum of loperamide hydrochloride in CDCl$_3$.

TABLE 8

NMR Assignments for Loperamide Hydrochloride

Protons	δ (ppm)	Relative surface	Multiplicity	J (Hz)
(a)	7.39		Doublet	8.8
(b)	7.14	14	Doublet	8.8
(f)	7.34		Broad singlet	—
(c)	4.7	1	Broad signal	—
(d) (e)	1.5–3.65	18	Broad multiplet	—
(g)	10.95	1	Broad singlet	—

2.3.5. Mass Spectrum

Figure 9 shows the mass spectrum recorded with a Varian MAT spectrometer (70 eV, source pressure 10^{-5} Torr, filament current 300 µA, sample rod temperature), m/e (%): 266(12), 240(39), 239(75), 238(100), 226(21), 224(53), 206(19), 72(40), 42(63), 36(22), and 32(73).

2.3.6. Quantitative analysis

Weigh accurately about 75 mg R 18 553, dissolve in 25 ml glacial acetic acid, add 2 ml of a 3% mercuric acetate solution in the same solvent, and titrate with 0.02 N acetous perchloric acid, either potentiometrically (glass-calomel electrodes) or visually (α-naphtolbenzeine). Each ml 0.02 N HClO$_4$ corresponds to 10.2698 mg R 18 553.

2.3.7. Purity tests

   a. Color and clarity of the solution: Dissolve 1 g R 18 553 in 10 ml methanol. The solution is clear and colorless to faintly yellow.

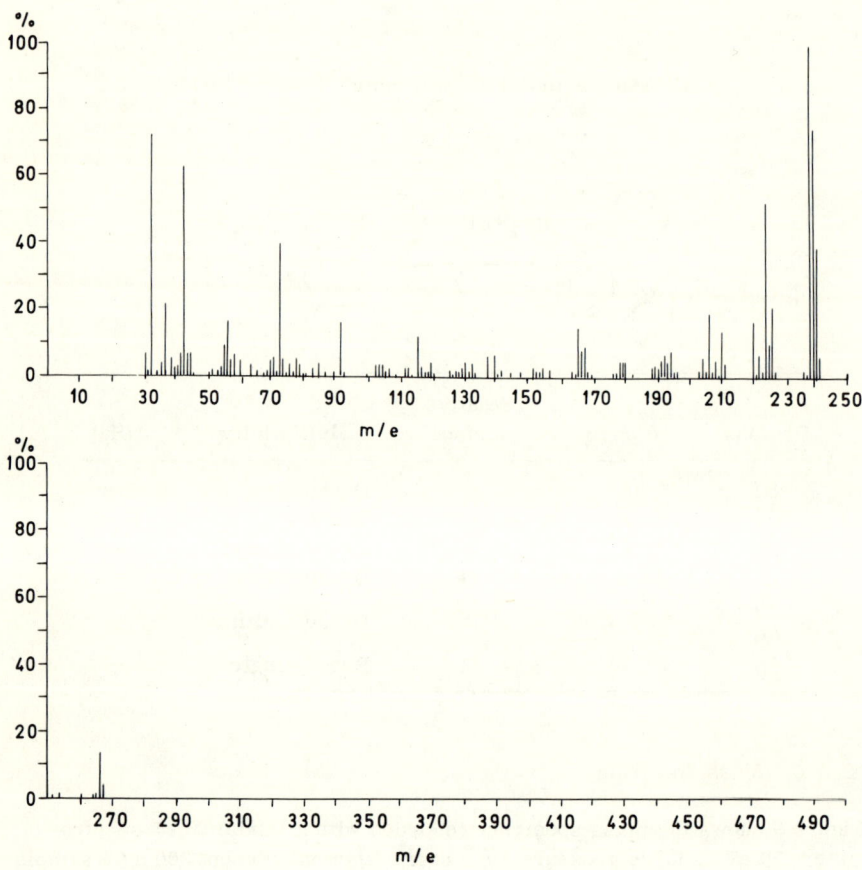

Fig. 9. Mass spectrum of loperamide hydrochloride.

Filter and measure the transmittance in a 1 cm cell at 400 nm; limit 70%.

b. Thin-layer chromatography: Dissolve 300 mg R 18 553 in 3 ml chloroform and spot 5 µl on a silica-gel plate HF254 (Merck). Develop with a mixture of 90 ml ethyl acetate, 10 ml ethanol, and 1 ml concentrated ammonia water. After drying the plate, develop with iodine vapor. R 18 553 has an Rf-value of approximately 0.42.

c. Loss on drying: After 4 hr at $100°C$, the product loses no more than 0.5% of its weight.

d. Sulfated ash: R 18 553 yields no more than 0.5% of its weight.

e. Chlorine: 13.81%. Weigh accurately about 13 mg R 18 553 on an ashless filter paper and burn according to Schöniger. Let absorb in a mixture of 10 ml 0.02 N sodium hydroxide and 2 drops of 30% hydrogen peroxide. After cooling, rinse the stopper and the inner walls of the flask with 20 ml isopropanol, add 4 ml of 0.1 N nitric acid, and dilute with 30 ml isopropanol. Titrate with 0.01 N mercuric nitrate in the presence of diphenylcarbazone as indicator. Each ml 0.01 N $Hg(NO_3)_2$ corresponds to 0.35457 mg chlorine.

III.3. STRUCTURE-ACTIVITY RELATIONSHIPS

Willem Van Bever, Karel Schellekens, and Carlos Niemegeers

Oral antidiarrheal activity in rats was assessed by measuring the protection from diarrhea caused by castor oil (Niemegeers et al., 1972). ED_{50} values for 1- and 8-hr protection against castor-oil-induced diarrhea were graphically estimated. The ratio of the ED_{50} value for 8 hr over the ED_{50} value for 1 hr gives an index for the duration of antidiarrheal activity. Oral analgesic activity in rats was assessed by measuring the inhibition of the warm-water-induced tail-withdrawal response TWR (Janssen et al., 1963), the criterion of activity being a reaction time greater than 10 sec (Janssen et al., 1971). The ratio of the ED_{50} value in the tail-withdrawal test over the ED_{50} value for 1 hr protection in the castor-oil test was used as an index of the dissociation of antidiarrheal activity from analgesic activity and was called relative antidiarrheal specificity (RAS).

Data for diphenoxylate, its active metabolite difenoxin (van Wijngaarden and Soudijn, 1972), and related esters of 1-(3-cyano-3,3-diphenylpropyl)-4-phenyl-4-piperidinecarboxylic acid (Janssen et al., 1959) are summarized in Table 9. Tables 11-13 contain similar data for loperamide and related 4-aryl-4-hydroxy-α, α-diphenyl-1-piperidinebutanamides (Stokbroekx et al., 1973). Table 10 contains comparative data on oral antidiarrheal activity based upon the charcoal test in mice (Janssen et al., 1959) for compounds related to diphenoxylate, but for which no castor-oil-test data are available.

Useful antidiarrheal activity, based upon high oral potency (ED_{50} 1 hr/castor oil < 0.2 mg/kg), long duration of action (ED_{50} 8 hr/ED_{50} 1 hr castor oil < 20), and high relative antidiarrheal specificity (ED_{50} tail withdrawal po/ED_{50} 1 hr castor oil > 100), is essentially limited to compounds structurally closely related to diphenoxylate [2a], difenoxin [2b], and loperamide [3a]. All these compounds have the same structural skeleton [1] in common, in which X is a nitrile or amide function and Y either a carboxyl group or an ester derivative thereof, or an hydroxyl group. Moreover X and Y are interdependent. When X is a cyano group, Y should be a carboxyl

TABLE 9

Antidiarrheal Activity of Diphenoxylate, Difenoxin, and Related Compounds (Castor-Oil Test)

Serial number or generic name	R	ED$_{50}$ castor oil[a]			ED$_{50}$,[b] TWR	RAS
		1 hr	8 hr	8 hr/1 hr		
Diphenoxylate	CH_2CH_3	0.15	4.77	32	12.8	85
R 1260	$CH_2CH_2CH_3$	0.152	4.75	31	14.2	93
Butoxylate	$(CH_2)_3CH_3$	0.13	3.95	30	13.6	105
R 1355	$(CH_2)_4CH_3$	0.255	4.30	17	10.8	42
R 1397	$CH_2-C_6H_5$	0.31	4.6	15	19.2	61
R 1375	$CH_2CH_2-C_6H_5$	0.36	9.0	25	19.2	53
R 12405	$CH_2CH_2-C_4H_3S$[d]	0.345	9.0	26	91	263
Fetoxylate	$CH_2CH_2OC_6H_5$	0.425	16.8	40	>160	>376
Difenoxin	H	0.040	0.91	23	4.06	102
Morphine hydrochloride	—	1.52	60.70	40	33.6	22
Codeine phosphate	—	2.85	70.00	25	56.6	20

[a]Milligram/kg po at stated hr after castor oil.
[b]Milligram/kg po, reaction time >10 sec.
[c]ED$_{50}$ TWR/ED$_{50}$ castor oil (1 hr).
[d]C_4H_3S: 2-thienyl.

Chemistry: Structure-Activity Relationships

TABLE 10

Antidiarrheal Activity of Diphenoxylate
and Related Compounds in the Charcoal Test

Serial number or generic name	R	ED_{50},[a] charcoal mice
Diphenoxylate	OCH_2CH_3	0.80
R 1326	OCH_3	2.21
R 1260	$OCH_2CH_2CH_3$	0.43
R 1261	$OCH(CH_3)_2$	3.52
R 1416	OCH_2CHOCH_2	0.16
Butoxylate	$O(CH_2)_3CH_3$	0.20
R 1355	$O(CH_2)_4CH_3$	0.43
R 1493	$O(CH_2)_5CH_3$	0.46
R 1357	OC_6H_{11}[b]	0.95
R 1500	$O(CH_2)_6CH_3$	0.60
R 1375	$O(CH_2)_2C_6H_5$	0.17
R 1301	CH_2CH_3	17.4
R 1302	$CH_2CH_2CH_3$	23.4
Morphine hydrochloride	—	9.0
Codeine phosphate	—	32.5
Loperamide	—	0.35

[a] Milligram/kg po influence on the rate of gastrointestinal propulsion of a charcoal meal in mice (Janssen et al., 1959b).

[b] C_6H_{11}: cyclohexyl.

group or ester and the 4-phenyl group on the piperidine ring should be unsubstituted. Diphenoxylate [2a] and difenoxin [2b], fulfill these requirements. On the other hand, when X is an amide, Y should be a hydroxyl group and the 4-phenyl group on the piperidine ring should be substituted, for example, with a 4-chloro substituent in the case of loperamide [3a] or a 4-chloro-3-trifluoromethyl substituent in the case of fluperamide [3b]. Deviation from these rules to date has invariably led to less specific or inactive compounds. 4-Hydroxy-4-phenyl-α, α-diphenyl-1-piperidine-butanenitrile [4] (X = CN, Y = OH), for instance, is a strong morphinelike

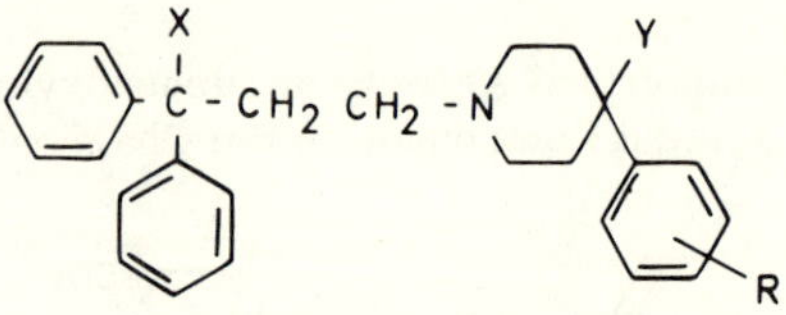

[Structure [1]: Ph₂C(X)-CH₂CH₂-N(piperidine with Y at 4-position and phenyl-R)]

[1]

agent, while the reverse combination [5] (X = CONMe₂, Y = COOCH₂CH₃) shows antidiarrheal activity of very short duration and low relative antidiarrheal specificity.

Structural modification of basic skeleton [1] mostly leads to inactive compounds or to other types of activity. Lengthening the side chain results in significantly decreased antidiarrheal activity, i.e., ethyl 1-(4-cyano-4,4-diphenylbutyl)-4-phenyl-4-piperidinecarboxylate [6], n = 3, is approximately 10 times less active than diphenoxylate [6], n = 2, while the corresponding pentyl derivative [6], n = 4, is 100 times less active than the diphenoxylate (Janssen et al., 1959). Replacement of the 4-phenylpiperidine moiety of [1]

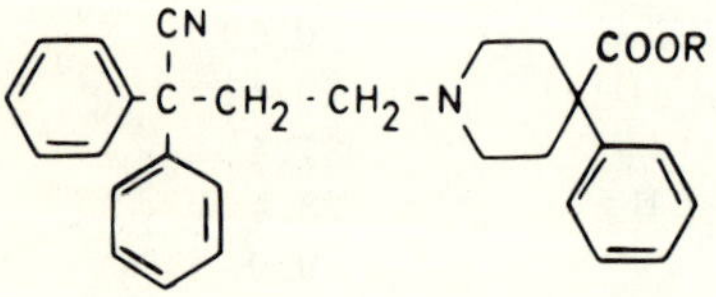

[2a] R = CH₂CH₃
[2b] R = H

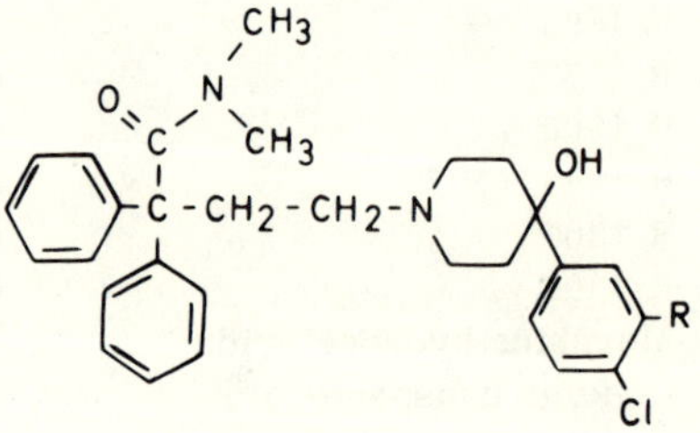

[3a] R = H
[3b] R = CF₃

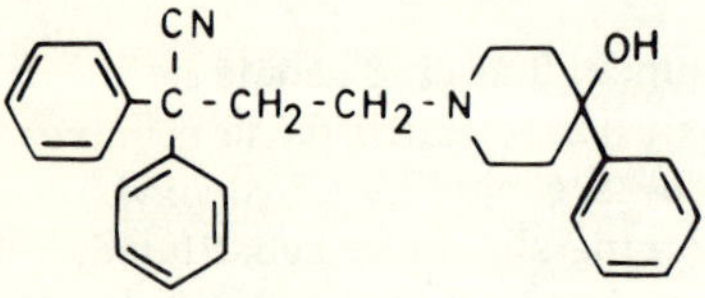

[4]

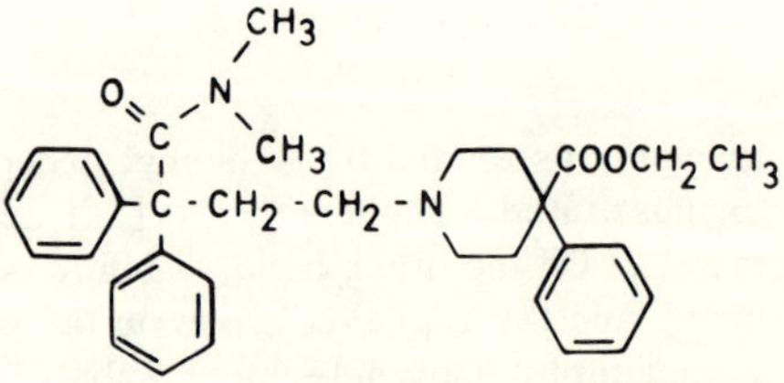

[5]

Chemistry: Structure-Activity Relationships 53

by small amine groups, such as dimethylamino, diethylamino, piperidine, pyrrolidine, or morpholine, i.e., compounds of type [7], leads to either anticholinergic or analgesic activity. The amines of type [7] where X is cyano, are typical atropine-like substances, whose potency is enhanced by

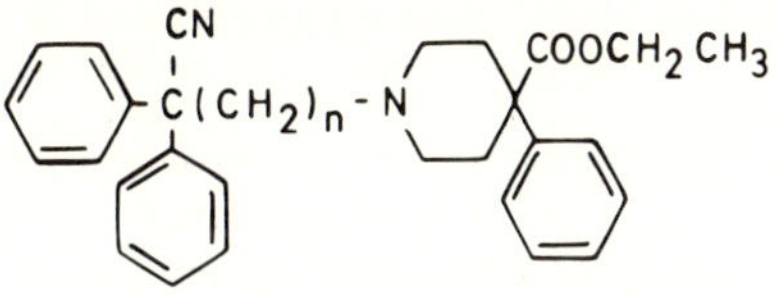

[6] 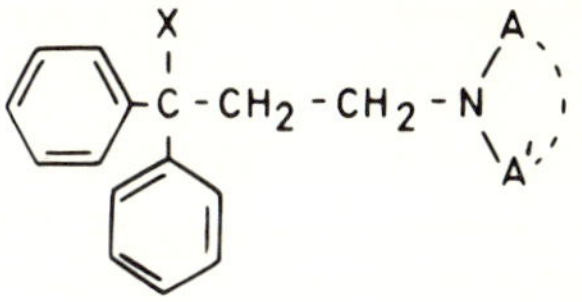   [7]

quaternization. Compounds of type [7], where X is a primary amide function, are mostly strong anticholinergic agents. A typical representative of this group is isopropamide iodide [8] (de Jongh et al., 1955). Compounds of type [7], where X is a secondary amide function, are generally parasympaticolytics of low potency when the side chain is unbranched; compounds branched in the β-position with regard to the secondary amide are active analgesics (Janssen, 1960). The tertiary amides of type [7] are very potent analgesics, especially when the side chain is branched with a methyl

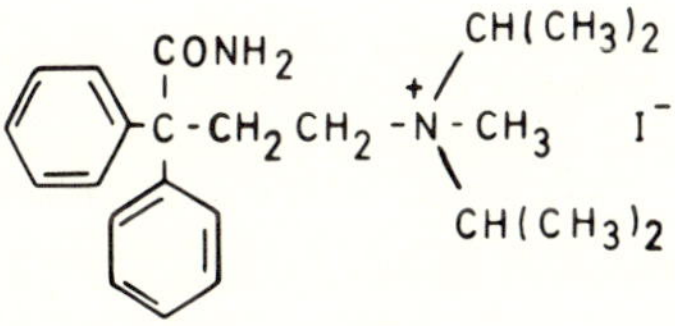

[8] 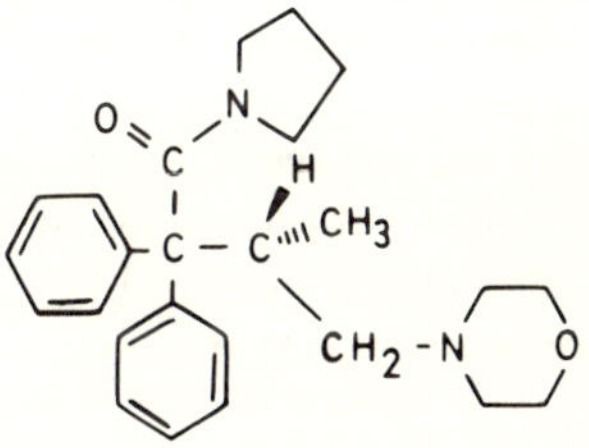   [9]

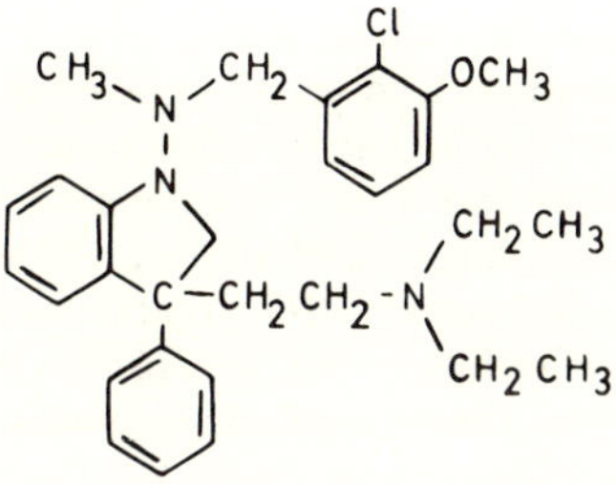

[10]

group in the β-position and when the amine moiety is morpholine. A typical representative of this group is the potent analgesic dextromoramide [9] (Janssen and Jageneau, 1957). One exception to these rules is perhaps CI-750 [10] (Bass et al., 1973). Its oral antidiarrheal activity evaluated by measuring faecal output was reported to be comparable to that of diphenoxylate. However, CI-750 is four times less potent than diphenoxylate in the castor-oil test.

All the ester derivatives of difenoxin (Table 9) have approximately the same potency in the castor-oil test. This is not surprising since they all have the same active metabolite, difenoxin, which is five times more potent than diphenoxylate. Difenoxin has a longer duration of activity and a higher relative antidiarrheal specificity. Diphenoxylate, butoxylate, R12405, and fetoxylate have the best relative antidiarrheal specificity of the ester derivatives of difenoxin. For comparative purposes ED_{50} values (mg/kg po) in the castor-oil test and the tail-withdrawal test for morphine and codeine are included. Diphenoxylate is approximately 10 times more potent than morphine, has a longer duration of action and four times the relative antidiarrheal specificity. Difenoxin is approximately 50 times more potent than morphine; it has a much longer duration of action and five times the relative antidiarrheal specificity. Comparative data on the antidiarrheal activity of diphenoxylate and related compounds in the charcoal test in mice (Janssen et al., 1959) are summarized in Table 10. Parallel to the results in the castor-oil test, diphenoxylate is again about 10 times more potent than morphine. Except for R 1326 (R = OCH_3) and R 1261 (R = $OCH(CH_3)_2$) the ED_{50} values are of the same order of magnitude, indicating that the antidiarrheal activity of the ester derivatives of difenoxin is largely independent of the actual length of the ester group. However, the corresponding ketones, R 1301 and R 1302, both deviating from the rules described for structure [1], are approximately 25 times less potent than diphenoxylate.

Comparative data on the antidiarrheal activity of loperamide and related compounds are summarized in Tables 11-13. The effect of the nature of the amide function and substitution of the 4-phenyl group of the piperidine ring on antidiarrheal activity, can be seen in Table 11. The primary amide R 21 345 is only four times less potent than loperamide, but has a low RAS. Its antidiarrheal activity may be partly anticholinergic in nature. The secondary amides R 21 531 and R 20 905 have also a low RAS. R 21 531 is very potent but has a short duration of action, while R 20 905 is about three times less active than loperamide. The combination of potent antidiarrheal activity and high relative antidiarrheal specificity is optimal when the amide function is tertiary, bearing two small alkyl groups, such as dimethylamino (loperamide) or ethylmethylamino (R 19 398). The diethylamino derivatives are generally equipotent to the corresponding dimethylamino compounds, but an approximately twofold increase of analgesic activity leaves them with a lower relative antidiarrheal specificity. The pyrrolidino derivatives (R 18 894-R 18 899) are generally two to three times less active than the corresponding dimethylamino compounds but retain mostly high RAS. Corresponding piperidino, morpholino, methylbenzylamino, methylpropylamino, isopropylmethylamino, and dipropylamino derivatives show a large decrease in antidiarrheal potency and duration of action, with the exception of piperidino derivative R 18 861, which is only two times less potent than loperamide and which has a long duration of action and a high RAS.

Substitution of the 4-phenyl ring of the piperidinol moiety is optimal for 4-chloro (loperamide), 4-bromo (R 18 937), and 4-chloro-3-trifluoromethyl substitution (fluperamide). In fact, loperamide is about 10 times more active than morphine for 1 hr protection in the castor-oil test and 34 times more potent for 8 hr protection from diarrhea. Its relative antidiarrheal specificity is at least 50 times higher than that of morphine. Fluperamide is only slightly less potent than loperamide, but has a considerably longer duration of activity and about the same relative antidiarrheal specificity. 4-Fluoro substituted compounds are very potent antidiarrheals, but also strong analgesics mostly with a short duration of action. The corresponding 3-trifluoromethyl compounds are also very potent antidiarrheals but are strong analgesics as well with a long duration of activity. 4-Methyl substitution results in a tenfold decrease in potency, while 2,4-dimethyl or 3,4-dichloro substitutions were only slightly less active. 2,4-Dimethyl substitution gives a low RAS, while 3,4-dichloro substitution results in long duration of action and high specificity (RAS). Other substitution patterns were less interesting.

The effect of 3-methyl substitution of the piperidine ring is given in Table 12. These compounds are less active than their respective parent compounds, except for R 19 451, which is a very potent antidiarrheal but has an unfavorable RAS in comparison with loperamide. The results of β- or γ-branching of the side chain are summarized in Table 13. γ-Branching of the dimethylbutanamides tends to increase analgesic potency rather than the antidiarrheal activity, resulting in derivatives with lower RAS. γ-Branching of loperamide results in a twofold increase of antidiarrheal potency but a tremendous increase of the analgesic activity gives a compound with RAS at least four times lower.

γ-Branching of the pyrrolidinobutanamide has various effects. The unsubstituted compound R 18 940 is far less active than its unbranched counterpart R 18 894, while the 4-chlorosubstituted compound R 18 948 shows an increased analgesic potency. γ-Branching of the 4-fluoro and 3-trifluoromethyl substituted compounds results in a ten- and fortyfold loss, respectively, of antidiarrheal activity.

β-Branching results, as would be expected, in increased antidiarrheal potency but also in an even larger increase of analgesic potency. Compounds R 21 108, R 21 615, and R 21 624 are, in fact, strong orally active analgesics.

TABLE 11

Antidiarrheal Activity of Loperamide and Related Compounds

Serial number or generic name	−N⟨	R	ED$_{50}$ castor oil			ED$_{50}$, TWR	RAS
			1 hr	8 hr	8 hr/1 hr		
R 21 345	NH$_2$	4-Cl	0.71	5.0	7	>40	>56
R 21 531	NHCH$_3$	H	0.025	1.50	60	5.0	200
R 20 905	NHCH$_3$	4-Cl	0.31	4.00	13	>40.0	129
R 18 936	N(CH$_3$)$_2$	H	0.0115	0.532	46	4.3	374
R 18 976	N(CH$_3$)$_2$	4-F	0.04	3.10	78	22.5	563
Loperamide	N(CH$_3$)$_2$	4-Cl	0.15	1.81	12	>160	>1067
R 18 937	N(CH$_3$)$_2$	4-Br	0.101	2.01	20	92.5	916
R 18 907	N(CH$_3$)$_2$	3,4-Cl$_2$	0.267	1.76	7	>160	>599
Fluperamide	N(CH$_3$)$_2$	3-CF$_3$, 4-Cl	0.152	0.73	5	>80	>526
R 18 946	N(CH$_3$)$_2$	3-CF$_3$	0.02	0.31	16	5.6	280
R 18 818	N(CH$_3$)$_2$	4-CH$_3$	1.25	8.18	7	160	128
R 19 391	N(CH$_3$)$_2$	2,4-(CH$_3$)$_2$	0.16	2.76	17	20.0	125
R 9 423	N(CH$_3$)$_2$	3,4,5-(CH$_3$)$_3$	0.88	5.00	6	93.0	106
R 19 685	N(CH$_3$)$_2$	2,5-CH$_3$O$_2$	0.63	2.76	4	>160	>254

Chemistry: Structure-Activity Relationships

Code	R	R'					
R 18 898	N(CH$_2$CH$_3$)$_2$	H	0.025	0.63	25	2.7	108
R 18 885	N(CH$_2$CH$_3$)$_2$	4-F	0.044	0.70	16	16.2	368
R 18 892	N(CH$_2$CH$_3$)$_2$	4-Cl	0.17	1.85	11	44.0	259
R 18 938	N(CH$_2$CH$_3$)$_2$	4-Br	0.33	3.1	9	50.0	152
R 18 887	N(CH$_2$CH$_3$)$_2$	3,4-Cl$_2$	0.31	1.4	5	12.1	39
R 18 860	N(CH$_2$CH$_3$)$_2$	3-CF$_3$,4-Cl	0.08	0.87	11	55.0	688
R 18 900	N(CH$_2$CH$_3$)$_2$	3-CF$_3$	0.017	0.16	9	1.4	82
R 18 894	NC$_4$H$_8$[a]	H	0.017	1.85	109	7.1	418
R 18 895	NC$_4$H$_8$[a]	4-F	0.16	5.4	34	91.5	572
R 18 356	NC$_4$H$_8$[a]	4-Cl	0.27	3.85	14	>160	>593
R 18 939	NC$_4$H$_8$[a]	3,4-Cl$_2$	0.56	3.2	6	>320	>571
R 18 906	NC$_4$H$_8$[a]	3-CF$_3$,4-Cl	0.46	2.5	5	>160	>348
R 18 947	NC$_4$H$_8$[a]	3-CF$_3$	0.114	0.76	7	12.7	111
R 18 899	NC$_4$H$_8$[a]	4-Me	2.05	>10	>5	>160	>78
R 18 861	NC$_5$H$_{10}$[b]	H	0.256	3.46	14	>320	>1250
R 18 580	NC$_5$H$_{10}$[b]	4-Cl	1.77	>10	>6	>160	>90
R 18 819	NC$_5$H$_{10}$[b]	3,4-Cl$_2$	3.1	>10	>3	>160	>52
R 18 812	NC$_5$H$_{10}$[c]	3-CF$_3$,4-Cl	5.0	>10	>2	>160	>32
R 18 848	NC$_5$H$_{10}$[c]	3-CF$_3$	0.53	2.4	5	>160	>302
R 18 798	NC$_5$H$_{10}$[c]	4-CH$_3$	10.0	>10	>1	>160	>16
R 18 897	NC$_4$H$_8$O[d]	H	0.63	>10	16	>160	>254
R 18 491	NC$_4$H$_8$O[d]	4-Cl	10.0	>10	>1	>160	>16
R 18 875	NC$_4$H$_8$O[d]	3,4-Cl$_2$	8.18	>10	>1	>160	>20
R 18 869	NC$_4$H$_8$O[d]	3-CF$_3$,4-Cl	1.25	8.18	7	>160	>128
R 18 837	NC$_4$H$_8$O[d]	3-CF$_3$	0.63	7.68	12	>160	>254
R 19 380	NC$_6$H$_{12}$O[e]	4-Cl	10.0	>10	>1	>160	>16
R 19 395	NC$_6$H$_{12}$[f]	4-Cl	10.0	>10	>1	>160	>16
R 19 424	NC$_6$H$_{12}$[g]	4-Cl	10.0	>10	>1	>160	>16
R 19 398	N(CH$_3$)CH$_2$CH$_3$	4-Cl	0.13	1.56	12	>160	>1231
R 19 426	N(CH$_3$)CH$_2$C$_6$H$_5$	4-Cl	1.25	>10	>8	>160	>128

TABLE 11 (Continued)

Serial number or generic name	-N⟨ ⟩	R	ED$_{50}$ castor oil			ED$_{50}$, TWR	RAS
			1 hr	8 hr	8 hr/1 hr		
R 19 442	N(CH$_2$CHCH$_2$)$_2$	4-Cl	10.0	>10	>1	>160	>16
R 19 450	N(CH$_3$)CH$_2$CH$_2$CH$_3$	4-Cl	0.63	>10	>16	>160	>254
R 19 469	N(CH$_3$)CH(CH$_2$)$_3$	4-Cl	0.63	>10	>16	>160	>254
R 19 207	N(CH$_2$CH$_2$CH$_3$)$_2$	4-Cl	10.0	>10	>1	>160	>16

[a]NC$_4$H$_8$: 1-(pyrrolidinyl).
[b]NC$_5$H$_{10}$: 1-(piperidinyl).
[c]NC$_5$H$_{10}$: 1-(piperidinyl).
[d]NC$_4$H$_8$O: 4(-morpholinyl).
[e]NC$_6$H$_{12}$O: 4-(2,6-dimethylmorphoninyl).
[f]NC$_6$H$_{12}$: 1-(4-methylpiperidinyl).
[g]NC$_6$H$_{12}$: 1-(3-methylpiperidinyl).

TABLE 12

Antidiarrheal Activity of 4-Aryl-4-hydroxy-α,α-diphenyl-N,N,3-trimethyl-1-piperidinebutanamides

Serial number	R	ED$_{50}$ castor oil			ED$_{50}$, TWR	RAS
		1 hr	8 hr	8 hr/1 hr		
R 19 470	H	0.069	3.75	54	57.0	826
R 19 510	4-Cl	0.345	4.15	12	>160	>464
R 19 451	3-CF$_3$, 4-Cl	0.092	1.35	15	59.0	641
R 19 427	3-CF$_3$	0.48	2.85	6	>160	>333

TABLE 13

Antidiarrheal Activity of 4-Aryl-4-hydroxy-α,α-diphenyl-$\beta(\gamma)$-methyl-1-piperidinebutanamides

Serial number	$-\overset{\frown}{N}$	R_1	R_2	R_3	ED_{50} castor oil				ED_{50}, TWR	RAS
					1 hr	8 hr	8 hr/1 hr			
R 18 921	$N(CH_3)_2$	H	CH_3	H	0.057	1.87	33		17.0	298
R 18 920	$N(CH_3)_2$	H	CH_3	4-F	0.032	0.60	19		28.5	891
R 18 874	$N(CH_3)_2$	H	CH_3	4-Cl	0.074	0.58	8		26.0	351
R 19 029	$N(CH_3)_2$	H	CH_3	3-CF_3, 4-Cl	0.058	0.10	2		2.3	40
R 18 955	$N(CH_3)_2$	H	CH_3	3-CF_3	0.022	0.071	3		3.0	136
R 18 940	NC_4H_8[a]	H	CH_3	H	1.25	5.0	4		80.0	45
R 19 001	NC_4H_8[a]	H	CH_3	4-F	1.28	7.10	6		69.5	63
R 18 948	NC_4H_8[a]	H	CH_3	4-Cl	0.42	3.55	8		69.5	165
R 19 014	NC_4H_8[a]	H	CH_3	3-CF_3	2.05	5.0	2		>160	>78
R 21 108	$N(CH_3)_2$	CH_3	H	4-Cl	0.0054	0.22	41		0.97	180
R 21 605	$N(CH_3)_2$	CH_3	H	3-CF_3, 4-Cl	0.028	0.08	3		1.25	45
R 21 624	$N(CH_3)_2$	CH_3	H	3-CF_3	0.0059	0.026	4		1.25	212

[a]NC_4H_8: 1-pyrrolidinyl.

It can be concluded that 3-methyl substitution of the piperidine ring and β- or γ-branching of the side chain, which are structural deviations from formula [1], are indeed unfavorable for antidiarrheal activity.

REFERENCES

Attenburrow, J., Elks, J., Hems, B. A., and Spencer, K. N. (1949). Analgesics. II. The synthesis of amidone and some of its analogues. J. Chem. Soc., 510-518.

Bass, P., Kennedy, J. A., Wiley, J. N., Villareal, J., and Butler, D. E. (1973). CI-750, a novel antidairrheal agent. J. Pharm. Exp. Ther. 186, 183-198.

Briggs, F. B. (1972). Nouveaux N-[N-(cyano-3-diphenyl-3,3-propyl)-phenyl-4-piperidinecarbonyloxy-4-amides] utiles notamment comme agents antidiarrhétiques et leur procédé de preparation. Belg. Pat. 776.644.

Bockmühl, M. and Ehrhart, G. (1948). Über eine neue Klasse von spasmolytisch and analgetisch wirkenden Verbindungen, I. Anal. Chem., 561-585.

Butler, D. E., Meyer, R. F., Alexander, S. M., Bass, P., and Kennedy J. A. (1973). Synthetic Antidiarrheal agents. I. An approach to the separation of antidiarrheal activity from narcotic analgesic activity. J. Med. Chem. 16, 49-54.

Carabateas, P. M. (1972). N-[1-Substituted-4-(or 3)]piperidylacylanilides. U.S. Pat. 3655675; Chem. Abstr. 77, 34349a.

Claude, C. L. C., Jullien, A. F., and Manoury, P. M. J. (1972). Pharmaceutical 4-aryl-1-(3,3-diphenylpropyl)piperidine derivatives. Ger. Offen., 2158077; Chem. Abstr. 77, 88328 m (1972).

Craig, P. N. (1952). Cyclic quarternary immonium compounds derived from 2,2-diphenyl-4-pentenoic acid. J. Amer. Chem. Soc. 74, 129-131.

Dupre, D. J., Elks, J., Hems, B. A., Spencer, K. N., and Evans, R. M. (1949). Analgesics. I. Esters and ketones derived from -α-amino-ω-cyano-ω,ω-diarylalkanes. J. Chem. Soc., 500-510.

Eisleb, O. and Schaumann, O. (1939). Dolantein, a new antispasmodic and analgesic. Deut. Med. Wochschr. 65, 967-968.

Eisleb, O. (1941). New synthesis with sodium amide. Ber. Deut. Med. Ges. 74, 1433-1450.

Hermans, B., Verhoeven, H., and Janssen, P. (1970). 4-Substituted piperidines. V. Local anesthetic 4-aminoalkoxy-4-arylpiperidines. J. Med. Chem. 13, 835-838.

Janssen, P. A. J. and Jageneau, A. H. (1957). A new series of potent analgesics: dextro 2,2-diphenyl-3-methyl-4-morpholinobutyryl pyrrolidine and related amides. I. Chemical structure and pharmacological activity. J. Pharm. Pharmacol. 9, 381-400.

Janssen, P. A. J. (1959a). 2,2-Diaryl-ω-(4'-phenyl-1'-piperidino)alkanonitriles. U.S. Pat. 2898340.

Janssen, P. A. J., Jageneau, A. H., and Huygens, J. (1959b). Synthetic antidiarrheal agents. I. Some pharmacological properties of R 1132 and related compounds. J. Med. Pharm. Chem. 1, 299-308.

Janssen, P. A. J. (1960). Synthetic Analgesics. Part I. Diphenylpropylamines. Pergamon Press, London.

Janssen, P. A. J., Niemegeers, C. J. E., and Dony, J. G. H. (1963). The inhibitory effect of fentanyl and other morphine-like analgesics on the warm water induced tail withdrawal reflex in rats. Arzneimittel-Forsch. 13, 502-507.

Janssen, P. A. J. (1970). Thienyl-alkyl esters of 1-(3-cyano-3,3-diphenylpropyl)-4-phenyl-piperidine-4-carboxylic acid. U.S. Pat. 3497519.

Janssen, P. A. J., Niemegeers, C. J. E., Schellekens, H. K. L., Marsboom, H. H. M., Herin, V. V., Amery, W. K. P., Admiraal, P. V., Bosker, J. T., Crul, J. F., Pearce, C., and Zegveld, C. (1971). Bezitramide (R 4845), a new potent and orally long-acting analgesic compound. Arzneimittel-Forsch. 21, 862-867.

Janssen, P. A. J., Niemegeers, C. J. E., Stokbroekx, R. A., and Vandenberk, J. (1973). 2,2-Diaryl-4-(4'-aryl-4-hydroxy-piperidino)-butyramides. U.S. Pat. 3714159.

de Jongh, D. K., van Proozdy-Hartzema, E. G., and Janssen, P. (1955). Substituted phenylpropylamines. II. Pharmacological properties of basic butyronitriles and butyramides. Arch. Intern. Pharmacodyn. 103, 100-119.

Kennedy, J. A., Wiley, J. N., and Bass, P. (1972). Measurement of fecal output in rats. Am. J. Digest Diseases 10, 925-928.

Lands, A. M. (1951). An investigation of the molecular configuration favorable for stimulation or blockade of the acetylcholine-sensitive receptors of visceral organs. J. Pharmacol. Exp. Therap. 102, 219-236.

Makosza, M. and Serafin, B. (1965). Reactions of organic anions. IV. Alkylation of diphenylacetonitrile in aqueous medium. Rocznicki Chem. 39, 1799-1803.

Mervyn, J. M. and Fothergill, G. A. (1972). 2-[3-Aryl-3-hydroxy (or acyloxy)propyl]6,7-dimethoxy-1-methyl-1,2,3,4-tetrahydroisoquinoline hydrochlorides. Ger. Offen., 2156069; (1972). Chem. Abstr. 77, 88342.

Niemegeers, C. J. E., Lenaerts, F. M., and Janssen, P. A. J. (1972). Difenoxine (R 15 403), the active metabolite of diphenoxylate (R 1132). 2. Difenoxine, a potent, orally active and safe antidiarrheal agent in rats. Arzneimittel-Forsch. 22, 516-518.

Pagliarini, G., Cignarella, G., and Testa, E. (1966). I. Synthesis of α-phenyl-γ-aminobutyric acid and 3-phenylpyrrolidin-2-one from α-phenyl-γ butyrolactone. New synthesis of 1-aminopyrrolidin-2-ones. Farmaco (Pavia) Ed. Sci. 21, 355-369.

Salmon-Legagneur F. and Neveu C. (1959). Recherces dans la série des diacides α, α-disubstués et de leurs dérivés. XI. Les acides α,α-diphenyl-α'-alkylsucciniques et leurs dérivés. Bull. Soc. Chim. France, 1958-1963.

Soudijn, W. and Van Wijngaarden, I. (1972). Pharmaceutical compositions. U.S. Pat. 3646207.

Stokbroekx, R. A., Vandenberk, J., Van Heertum, A. H. M. T., van Laar, G. M. L. W., Van der Aa, M. J. M. C., Van Bever, W. F. M., and Janssen, P. A. J. (1973). Synthetic antidiarrheal agents. 2,2-Diphenyl-4-(4'-aryl-4'-hydroxypiperidino)butyramides. J. Med. Chem. 16, 782-786.

van Wijngaarden, I. and Soudijn, W. (1972). Difenoxine (R 15 403), the active metabolite or diphenoxylate (R 1132). 1. The excretion and metabolism in rats of difenoxine, the pharmacologically active metabolite of the antidiarrheal agent diphenoxylate. Arzneimittel-Forsch. 22, 513-516.

CHAPTER IV

PRECLINICAL ANIMAL STUDIES
OF MODERN ANTIDIARRHEALS

IV.1. IN VIVO PHARMACOLOGY
Carlos Niemegeers, Fred Lenaerts, and Frans Awouters

1.1. SELECTION OF AN APPROPRIATE METHOD FOR TESTING ANTIDIARRHEAL ACTIVITY

1.1.1. General Considerations

An appropriate in vivo procedure in laboratory animals is the obvious means by which antidiarrheal activity can be assessed. Several methods of measuring gastrointestinal propulsion and of inducing diarrhea in a number of animal species have been described. Among the existing methods, the ideal test in the study of new antidiarrheal drugs should possess the following general characteristics:

a. The test should be one that calls for a commonly available animal species and a minimum of equipment. The measurement of antidiarrheal activity should be very objective, so that it can be recorded without any human bias. There should be a minimal need for training of technicians to perform the test and to record the results. The usual models of statistical analysis should be directly applicable to the readings obtained from the test. A built-in safety system should exclude errors in large-scale testing.

b. With a minimum effort, the test should yield a maximum of relevant data, and the essential information should be available in the shortest period of time. Thus the selected procedure should induce diarrhea in all test animals within a very short and predictable period, so that all animals in which no diarrhea occurs within the predetermined period can be considered as being protected by the antidiarrheal drug.

Known antidiarrheal drugs should be effective at low doses and produce a dose- and time-related effect. The experimental design should be such, that only a small number of animals is needed to reveal significant drug effects and that the reliability of the collected data is maximal. These data should directly predict the active dose, the time of onset, and the duration of activity.

c. The test should indicate the potency of antidiarrheal activity and differentiate between antidiarrheal effects and constipating side effects. If possible, the test should predict efficacy in clinical diarrhea of various etiology.

d. Assuming that the factors determining the experimental results are known and are adequately controlled, it is essential that the test gives reproducible results. Replications of the test using the same drug and dosage should produce similar results so that the data recorded from each replication fall within a narrow range.

In short, an adequate experimental design for detecting and evaluating antidiarrheal activity in laboratory animals is characterized by its simplicity, efficacy, and reproducibility; its degree of specificity is known, the data are efficiently processed, and the results are summarized in statistically meaningful figures, predicting various aspects of the drug's biological activity.

1.1.2. Different Experimental Methods

In general, the experimental in vivo methods consist either of the measurement of gastrointestinal transit for detecting cathartic or constipating effects of the investigated compounds, or of the blocking of experimentally induced diarrhea with potential antidiarrheal drugs.

To the best of our knowledge the earliest experimental studies in this field were carried out by Magnus (1906, 1908) in cats. Milk-induced diarrhea was blocked with morphine and the progress of digestion was assessed using a duodenal fistula or the X-ray technique introduced by Cannon. Subsequently, a number of bioassay methods in various animal species was described. Early reviews on this subject (Krueger et al., 1941; Collier et al., 1948; Lou, 1949), however, reveal that, up to 1950, most studies were concerned with the effects of laxatives and cathartics.

In more recent years, inhibition of gastrointestinal motility was studied in different animal species, using several methods of measurement. The "charcoal-meal test" in the rat, introduced by Macht and Barba-Gose (1931), was adapted to mice by Loewe (1939) and used by Janssen and Jageneau (1957), Janssen et al. (1958, 1959a, b, and c), Lee et al. (1972), McCarty et al. (1965) and, after further modification, by Schmid (1952), and Niemegeers et al. (1974d). In this test, constipating effects are measured either as an "all-or-none" response (e.g. presence or absence of charcoal in the caecum), or as an inhibition percentage of the rate of passage of the charcoal meal (i.e., as compared with the total length of the intestinal tract).

Using this same principle, Bass et al. (1973) and Purdon and Bass (1973) evaluated the inhibition of gastrointestinal transit in rats by means of a radioactive test meal ($Ba^{133}SO_4$); in dogs, inhibition of gastrointestinal contractions was measured by means of cannulated Thiry-Vella loops of the intestine (Williams and Streeten, 1950) and of implanted extraluminal strain-gauge-force transducers (Bass et al., 1973).

Reduction of faecal output, a method introduced by Green et al. (1936) in guinea-pigs, and by Geiger (1940) in mice, is currently used in rats by Bass et al. (1972, 1973), Butler et al. (1973), Janssen (1961a,b), Janssen et al. (1958, 1959b, 1963b, 1968, 1970a,b), Niemegeers et al. (1974a,b). In monkeys, reduction of faecal output as described by Loewe (1939) was also used by Bass et al. (1973). In pigs, Marsboom et al. (1973) evaluated the intestinal motility by counting the excretion of colored plastic pellets mixed with the food. In sheep, gastrointestinal transit was assessed either by measuring faecal output or by recording ruminal motility, using Teflon catheters implanted in the dorsal sacs of the rumen (Marsboom and Van Ravestyn, 1971).

Diarrhea has been described as occuring in mice following the administration of 5-hydroxytryptophan, prostaglandins (Lee et al., 1972; Marrazzi-Uberti and Turba, 1966; Sanner, 1972), rhubarb, calomel, magnesium sulfate, and castor oil, but not following phenolphthaleine or its analogs (Tsurumi et al., 1969).

In rats, diarrhea has been induced with castor oil (Lee et al., 1972; Niemegeers et al., 1972, 1974c) and with Salomella typhimurium (Maenza et al., 1970; Powell et al., 1971a,b,c). Iwao and Terada (1962) studied castor-oil-induced diarrhea in guinea pigs. In rabbits toxin-induced experimental cholera was described by Finkelstein et al. (1964) and Dutta et al. (1972), but a more detailed survey of bacterial enterotoxigenic diarrhea in different animal species can be found in Banwell and Sherr (1973). In dogs, Janssen et al. (1971a) used magnesium sulfate to induce diarrhea. Lin et al. (1967) induced diarrhea in monkeys with castor oil, magnesium sulfate, and Staphylococcus-aureus toxins. Finally, Marsboom (1974) induced experimental diarrhea in pigs by mixing magnesium sulfate, magnesium citrate, castor oil and milk-powder with their food.

In selecting a routine test for antidiarrheal studies, our aim was not only to induce diarrhea in an easily available laboratory animal within a short time after administration of the agonist, but also to be able to antagonize this diarrhea with a low oral dose of diphenoxylate,* a well-known and widely used antidiarrheal drug.

---

*Diphenoxylate: ethyl 1-(3-cyano-3,3-diphenylpropyl)-4-phenyl-4-piperidine-carboxylate hydrochloride.

In mice, oral doses of polyethyleneglycol 200, paraffin oil, croton oil and castor oil in amounts of 0.1, 0.2, 0.3, and 0.5 ml were tested. None of these substances induced diarrhea within 1 hr. PEG 200 and paraffin oil were ineffective whereas croton oil was toxic at all doses tested. Castor oil induced diarrhea within 1 hr in only 50% of the mice; diarrhea within 3 hr after administration was obtained in 100% of the mice with 0.2 and 0.3 ml.

Prostaglandin E_2, 0.025 mg/ml injected intraperitoneally at a volume of 0.25 ml induced diarrhea within 30 min in all mice. Lee et al. (1972) showed that prostaglandin-induced diarrhea can only be blocked with very high doses of diphenoxylate (16.7 mg/kg).

In rats, phenolphthaleine, magnesium sulfate, croton oil, castor oil, and glycerine were tested. Magnesium sulfate did not induce diarrhea, except at toxic doses (1 g/kg). Phenolphthalein up to 1.280 mg/kg and glycerine up to 1 mg/100 g rat were rather ineffective cathartics. Croton oil and castor oil both induced diarrhea within 1 hr in all rats treated. Croton oil however was rejected because of its toxicity.

In dogs, castor oil failed to produce diarrhea consistently. Magnesium sulfate, however, induced a delayed diarrhea, easily blocked with anticholinergics (Janssen et al., 1971a).

As a result of these findings, we selected the rat and castor oil-induced diarrhea for further experimental studies. Preliminary tests showed that oral administration of 1, 2, and 3 ml castor oil induced profuse diarrhea within 1 hr in all rats. Diarrhea induced with 1 ml was blocked with lower doses of diphenoxylate and for a longer period of time, than diarrhea induced with 3 ml. Furthermore, diarrhea was found to occur more regularly in rats starved overnight than in rats fed ad libitum. Since, in addition, overnight starvation results in more regular resorption of orally administered compounds, we decided to select for our test rats starved overnight and treated with 1 ml of castor oil.

1.1.3. The Castor-oil Test in Rats

Castor oil is an extract from the seeds of Ricinus communis and is primarily composed of the triglyceride of the fatty acid, ricinoleic acid (12-hydroxy-cis-9-octadecenoic acid). About 90% of the fatty acid residue of castor oil is made up of ricinoleic acid, which differs from the much more common oleic acid only by the presence of the hydroxy group. According to Masri et al. (1962) this group on C_{12} and the double bond between C_9 and C_{10} are considered essential for the cathartic action of the ricinoleic acid moiety of castor oil. The configuration of the double bond seems to be secondary since both the trans- and the naturally occurring cis-isomer possess cathartic activity.

Following oral administration, castor oil is treated by the organism in essentially the same way as other triglycerides (Watson and Gordon, 1962). Intestinal lipase is capable of hydrolyzing the oil liberating the free ricinoleate at least as rapidly as a common vegetable oil. However, the first resorptive step, i.e., activation of the free ricinoleate to a coenzyme-A derivative, is slow. Nevertheless, the delay between administration of the oil and the appearance of ricinoleic acid as a constituent of circulating chylomicrons is less than 1 hr. Continuous feeding of the oil results in the incorporation of ricinoleic acid into depot fat. Thus, as far as can be judged from studies to date, the metabolism of castor oil is similar to that of normal dietary triglyceride and no species difference between rat and man is apparent (Watson et al., 1963).

After administration of a purgative dose, histological changes in the rat intestine are localized in the lower ileum, where an inflammatory swelling of the villi is observed with sloughing of their tips in severe cases and an increase in the number of goblet cells. No definite changes are found elsewhere in the gastrointestinal tract (Reynell and Spray, 1958). The increase in the number of goblet cells as described by these authors is probably a consequence of the depletion of secretory granules in the existing cells (Binder, 1973).

Numerous studies have contributed to the understanding of the mechanism by which castor oil induces diarrhea. As long ago as 1890, Meyer had already drawn attention to the fact that its purgative action is not due to the oil as such, but to its ricinoleic acid component. When this is set free by intestinal lipase, irritation of the gastrointestinal tract is provoked (Bonnycastle, 1965; Fingl, 1970). In the classical concept this chemically induced gastroenteritis alters intestinal motor activity and mucus secretion into the lumen is increased. Further gastric emptying is delayed and, to a lesser extent, transit through the upper intestine is slowed down (Reynell and Spray, 1958). On the other hand, transit through the lower intestine is increased and the partially digested fluid bowel contents are moving so fast that contact time with the mucosal cells is too short for normal absorption of water and electrolytes; this leads to the passage of watery unformed stools (Schmid, 1952, Iwao and Terada, 1962; Lin et al., 1967).

Some details of this process, including contractions of isolated intestinal segments upon the application of castor-oil components, are described in the studies referred to above.

So far, there is no doubt that liberation of ricinoleic acid is the first step towards increased peristalsis and mucus secretion; the previously discussed metabolism of castor oil indicates that an effective concentration of ricinoleic acid may rapidly be built up in the intestinal lumen and be maintained for some time. However, the classical concept of castor-oil-induced diarrhea does imply that the malabsorption of water and electrolytes are a consequence of increased peristalsis, with mucus and residual oil possibly facilitating the expulsion of fecal matter. More recent studies (Phillips et al., 1965; Forth et al., 1966) propose the idea that stimulant cathartics may also act more directly on electrolyte transport and, in general, on secretory and absorptive processes in the intestine. A decrease in the net transport of electrolytes, especially of Na^+ and water from the intestinal lumen, would increase the bulk of the intestinal contents, and part of the motor effect might arise reflexly as a result of distention of the bowel. In this context, Bright-Asare and Binder (1973) compared the effects of ricinoleic and oleic acid on the rat colon. Continuous perfusion in vivo of the organ, especially with ricinoleic acid, resulted in net secretion of water, sodium, and chloride, and was accompanied by a marked increase in mucosal permeability and a decrease of the electrical potential difference. Many aspects of gastrointestinal function are apparently affected by the relatively mild irritant ricinoleic acid and at present it is rather difficult to evaluate the contribution of every single process to the overall efficient cathartic activity. It is also premature to claim that there are definite links between ricinoleic acid irritation and prostaglandins, which are known to induce diarrhea in several animal species, including man. The effects of cholera enterotoxin and of other bacterial enterotoxins (Kimberg et al., 1971; Banwell and Sherr, 1973) may be at least partly ascribed to endogenous prostaglandins, which would then, by stimulation of intestinal adenyl cyclase, lead to higher levels of cyclic AMP in the mucosal cells. In this area, too, research has progressed rapidly and a much clearer picture of the regulation of gastrointestinal motility may be acquired in the next few years.

For the time being, the advantage of castor-oil-induced diarrhea as a test method lies in its polyvalent but always rather mild stimulation of gastrointestinal functions and from the parallelism which can frequently be drawn between a particular aspect and an etiological factor of human diarrhea.

Functional disorders causing diarrhea in man can be classified in three major categories: those causing osmotic retardation of water absorption, those which give rise to abnormal electrolyte and water transport, and those provoking disorders of transit (Phillips, 1972). The osmotic mechanism, typical in diarrhea induced by magnesium salts, may be partially operative in castor-oil-induced diarrhea, with free ricinoleate playing a role analogous to nonresorbed carbohydrates in sugar malabsorption diarrhea of man. Abnormal electrolyte and water transport, known to be particularly prominent in cholera enterotoxin diarrhea, may be more important in the castor-oil model than hitherto recognized, especially since bacterially produced hydroxy fatty acid may be causally related to human diarrhea (Binder, 1973). Finally, in castor-oil-induced diarrhea, gastrointestinal motor activity is increased, but apparently confined to peristalsis without manifest cramps, and no toxic reactions are associated with the accelerated propulsion.

Preclinical studies: In Vivo Pharmacology

In our standardized procedure the experimental animals are inbred Wistar rats of 230 ± 20 g body weight. They are transferred from their rearing quarters to the air-conditioned laboratories (21 ± 1°C; 65 ± 5 R.H.) 24 hr before the start of the experiments. After being starved overnight, but with ad libitum access to tap water, they are treated orally with the compounds under investigation. The compounds are given in aqueous solutions (1 ml per 100 g body weight) or, if insoluble, in aqueous suspensions freshly prepared with an ultrasonic sonifier and containing 1% polysorbate 80. A standard dose is administered first and in each single experiment all rats receive a different compound, one of them being treated with water, and one with a selected dose of diphenoxylate, our reference antidiarrheal preparation. This procedure is repeated several times and for further investigation of a potentially interesting new antidiarrheal agent different doses are given to five or ten animals per dose level in as many different experimental sessions, so that a particular drug treatment is given only once daily. The following considerations prompted the choice of this procedure: it randomizes day-to-day variability, it reduces systematic errors to a minimum, and it provides a means of comparing the intensity of effect and duration of activity with our reference compound diphenoxylate. Each animal is challenged with 1 ml of castor oil orally 1 hr after treatment and is then placed in a small individual makrolon cage (11 × 17 × 12 cm). At intervals of 1, 2,

TABLE 1

Castor-oil Test in Rats: Control Results[a]

Number of rats	Hours after castor oil					
	1	2	3	4	6	8
1-100	2	0	0	0	0	0
101-200	4	0	0	0	0	0
201-300	6	0	0	0	0	0
301-400	6	3	3	3	3	2
401-500	5	0	0	0	0	0
501-600	5	2	1	1	1	1
601-700	6	1	1	1	0	0
701-800	3	0	0	0	0	0
801-900	3	2	2	2	1	1
901-1000	6	3	1	1	1	1
% positives	4.6	1.1	0.8	0.8	0.6	0.5

[a] Number of rats protected from diarrhea at stated hours.

TABLE 2

Castor-oil Test in Rats: Number of Rats Protected from Diarrhea after Treatment with Diphenoxylate at Stated Hours after Castor Oil[a]

Dose, mg/kg	1st group[b] (Hours)						2nd group[b] (Hours)						3rd group[b] (Hours)						4th group[b] (Hours)						Total[c] (Hours)					
	1	2	3	4	6	8	1	2	3	4	6	8	1	2	3	4	6	8	1	2	3	4	6	8	1	2	3	4	6	8
0.04	0						0						1	0					0						1	0				
0.08	1	1	0				2	0					1	0					1	0					6	1	0			
0.16	2	1	0				2	0					2	1	0				2	0					8	2	0			
0.31	3	1	1	1	0		3	1	1	0			2	1	0				4	1	0				12	4	2	1	0	
0.63	5	2	0				5	3	3	1	0		5	2	2	2	2	1	5	3	2	1	0		20	10	7	4	2	1
1.25	5	3	2	0			5	5	3	3	2	0	5	4	2	2	2	0	5	5	3	2	0		20	19	11	9	4	0
2.50	5	4	3	2	2		5	4	3	3	2	1	5	5	4	2	1	0	5	5	4	4	3	2	20	18	15	12	8	5
5.00	5	5	4	4	2	2	5	5	5	5	5	3	5	5	5	5	5	2	5	5	5	5	4	2	20	20	20	20	18	9
10.0	5	5	5	5	4	4	5	5	5	5	3	3	5	5	5	5	5	4	5	5	5	5	5	5	20	20	20	20	17	16
20.0	5	5	5	5	5	5	5	5	5	5	4	4	5	5	5	5	5	4	5	5	5	5	5	4	20	20	20	20	19	17
40.0	5	5	5	5	5	5	5	5	5	5	5	5	5	5	5	5	5	5	5	5	5	5	5	5	20	20	20	20	20	20

Hours	ED_{50} values, mg/kg and fiducial limits				
1	0.20 (0.12–0.34)	0.18 (0.06–0.55)	0.20 (0.10–0.41)	0.18 (0.10–0.32)	0.19 (0.13–0.27)
2	0.55 (0.29–1.05)	0.58 (0.30–1.11)	0.63 (0.27–1.47)	0.51 (0.31–0.84)	0.56 (0.40–0.79)
3	1.15 (0.34–3.95)	0.85 (0.37–1.95)	1.25 (0.71–2.21)	1.00 (0.47–2.12)	1.06 (0.75–1.49)
4	1.57 (0.21–11.7)	1.25 (0.74–2.13)	1.63 (0.58–4.60)	1.37 (0.73–2.57)	1.43 (1.02–2.00)
6	3.10 (2.03–4.74)	3.08 (1.41–6.75)	2.88 (1.23–6.75)	2.50 (1.09–5.76)	2.90 (2.02–4.17)
8	5.00 (2.48–10.1)	5.80 (2.83–11.9)	6.15 (2.80–13.5)	5.00 (2.81–8.90)	5.39 (3.68–7.89)

[a] Four groups of five rats were selected at random but with one to two year intervals in the period 1968 to 1974.
[b] Five rats per dose.
[c] Twenty rats per dose.

3, 4, 6, 8, and 24 hr after castor-oil administration the easily removable floor underneath the stainless grid (bars 0.2 cm in diameter, 1.5 cm apart) of the cage is examined for the presence or absence of diarrhea. Diarrhea is defined as watery unformed stools, splashed on the tray and very different from normal fecal excretion in the rat, which consists of well formed boluses, firm and relatively dry. If diarrhea occurs at one of these intervals, the animal is removed. Absence of diarrhea is the criterion for drug effectiveness and ED_{50} values with 5% fiducial limits are computed by Finney's (1962) iterative method at indicated time intervals after the intake of castor oil.

Table 1 shows the results obtained over a period of 6 yr in 1000 control rats who received the solvent 1 hr before the castor-oil challenge, Table 2 shows the antidiarrheal effect of diphenoxylate in four successive groups of five rats treated between 1968 and 1974. From these results it is evident that our standard procedure of castor-oil-induced diarrhea in rats fulfils most of the requirements outlined in the general considerations as already described.

1.2. THE SEARCH FOR SPECIFIC ANTIDIARRHEAL AGENTS

1.2.1. Introduction

Diarrhea is one of the most common disorders and yet is frequently considered to be more of a nuisance than a major health problem. In many parts of the world, however, diarrhea produces more illness and kills more infants and children than all other diseases combined (Gordon, 1968). Effective treatment of diarrhea may therefore save more lives and relieve more disability than is generally realized.

Progress in the study of gastrointestinal function, especially that of secretory and absorptive processes, has certainly contributed to a better understanding of the different pathological mechanisms which may lead to diarrhea (Dupont and Hornick, 1969; Eichenwald and McCracken, 1970; Low-Beer and Read, 1971). These studies offer also new therapeutic approaches. A well-known case is cholera with its extremely profuse diarrheal water loss. This is almost entirely due to stimulation of intestinal secretion and not to deficient absorptive processes. Oral administration of electrolyte and glucose solution which, upon active resorption by the ileum, also promote water flow out of the intestine, give rapid improvement of the acidosis and dehydration of cholera (Cash et al., 1970). In the next few years other improvements in replacement measures and in the treatment of causal factors may be forthcoming, but the extent of their applicability remains questionable. This may be illustrated by the progress in the etiology of diarrhoea caused by intestinal infections. As a matter of fact, antibiotic treatment may be effective in controlling diarrhea known to be of bacterial origin. However, the type of pathological organism, the risks of promoting resistant strains, and the imbalance of the natural intestinal flora, which results from systemic antibiotic therapy and is, in itself, sufficient to induce diarrhea, are all factors restricting the use of the any particular preparation to a small field (Dupont and Hornick, 1969; McMurdoch, 1971).

On the other hand, the use of opium alkaloids effectively controls diarrhea and remains a standard form of therapy (Rakatansky and Kirsner, 1974; Read, 1971). Certain restrictions are made with respect to the use of the traditional alkaloids and also with respect to the use of newer agents with similar activity on the gastrointestinal tract.

One of the considerations is that their use is frequently seen as a symptomatic approach as opposed to a much more attractive treatment of the underlying causes. Apart from such practical questions as whether the cause can definitely be established and whether time and specific treatment are available to follow this second approach, a question also arises as to the extent to which newer agents, in fact, accomplish only an increase in transit time (However valuable this increase may be in itself) by allowing a longer period of contact between the intestinal contents and the absorptive surfaces. Part of the activity of the newer agents may be a more fundamental and direct improvement of abnormal secretory and absorptive processes.

Also to be considered are problems of tolerance and habituation and well-known risks of morphine treatment, especially important when compounds are used for the treatment of chronic diarrhea; in the same context greater sensitivity of children to the side effects of morphine-like drugs is a serious risk. The lack of difference between effects on the gastrointestinal tract and CNS effects is indeed disadvantageous for the natural opium alkaloids but this has been considerably improved with the introduction of diphenoxylate. Further exploration of compounds with a pronounced antidiarrheal effect should certainly be directed towards improving safety and making a direct impact on disturbed motor and fluid balances.

1.2.2. The Dissociation Between Antidiarrheal and Analgesic Drug Activity in Rats

Thus everything indicated the need for synthetic antidiarrheal agents with a greater dissociation between antidiarrheal activity and central effects. Janssen and Jageneau (1957) found that in mice there was a poor correlation between "analgesic" effect, as measured in the hot-plate test, and "constipating" effect, as measured in the charcoal test, in a series of active meperidine derivatives. To the best of our knowledge the parallelism between the narcotic and antidiarrheal properties of the known analgesics has never been systematically explored. However, it is apparent that morphine and methadone, which have similar narcotic properties, do not appear to have similar constipating effects (Goodman and Gilman, 1965) and that morphine and codeine which have similar constipating effects do not have the same degree of addiction liability. In fact, we must distinguish between narcotics which have, in our view, useful constipating side effects and between antidiarrheals which may possibly have central side effects when given in excessive doses.

In the present section we are reporting in detail on the antidiarrheal activity of 18 known compounds as compared with their analgesic activity (Table 3). The antidiarrheal activity was measured in the castor-oil test, as described by Niemegeers et al. (1972, 1974c) and in this chapter. The analgesic activity was measured in the "tail-withdrawal" test (Janssen et al., 1963a, 1971b). All compounds were given orally by gavage to rats starved overnight.

In the castor-oil (CO) test the rats received 1 ml of castor oil 1 hr after treatment with the different compounds under investigation. At intervals of 1, 2, 3, 4, 6, and 8 hr after castor-oil administration, the rats with diarrhea were removed, the remaining rats being considered protected against diarrhea; ED_{50} values for each time interval were calculated using Finney's iterative method (Niemegeers et al., 1972, 1974).

In the tail-withdrawal-reaction test (TWR) the tail-withdrawal reaction was measured 1, 2, 3, 4, 6, and 8 hr after treatment and the results were analyzed according to the following criteria (Janssen et al., 1963, 1971; Niemegeers et al., 1974):

Moderate effect: tail-withdrawal reaction time more than 6 sec (TWR > 6).

Pronounced effect: no tail-withdrawal response within 10 sec (cutoff time) (TWR > 10).

For each of these criteria ED_{50} values were calculated at the different times of measurement using Finney's iterative method.

For all compounds a geometrical series of doses 0.005, 0.01, 0.02, ... 40.0, 80.0, 160 mg/kg was given to at least 10 rats per dose level.

The results obtained for all compounds tested are shown in Tables 4 and 5. Figures 1 to 18 are graphical representations of the time-effect curves of the compounds in the castor-oil test and in the tail-withdrawal test using the criterion of pronounced effect (TWR > 10 sec). The results show that there is a clear dissociation between "analgesic" and "antidiarrheal" activity. All the compounds studied have antidiarrheal properties as measured in the castor-oil test but, in view of the lowest ED_{50} values for pronounced analgesia (TWR > 10) and for anticastor oil activity (CO), it is evident that in morphine-like analgesics the relative antidiarrheal specificity (RAS) is less than 10 for phenazocine, dextromoramide, anileridine, propoxyphene, phenoperidine, bezitramide, pethidine, fentanyl, and methadone, less than 20 for piritramide and codeine, and is 22 for morphine.

TABLE 3

Comparative Antidiarrheal and Analgesic Activity of 18 Compounds

Compound	Dose range, mg/kg	
	CO	TWR
Analgesics		
Anileridine	2.50-40.0	1.25-40.0
Bezitramide	0.08-10.0	0.08-5.00
Codeine	0.31-320	5.00-320
Dextromoramide	0.63-20.0	0.08-10.0
Fentanyl	0.08-2.50	0.01-5.00
Methadone	0.63-40.0	0.63-40.0
Morphine	0.31-160	1.25-320
Pethidine	5.00-160	2.50-160
Phenazocine	2.50-40.0	2.50-40.0
Phenoperidine	2.50-80.0	0.63-80.0
Piritramide	0.31-80.0	0.16-80.0
Propoxyphene	5.00-160	5.00-160
Antidiarrheals		
Butoxylate	0.04-20.0	2.50-160
Difenoxin	0.005-40.0	0.04-40.0
Diphenoxylate	0.04-160	0.31-160
Fetoxylate	0.08-160	2.50-160
Fluperamide	0.04-40.0	5.00-160
Loperamide	0.04-40.0	5.00-160

For the antidiarrheal drugs tested, the RAS is approximately 100 for diphenoxylate, difenoxin, and butoxylate, more than 372 for fetoxylate, and more than 1000 for fluperamide and loperamide.

As far as antidiarrheal activity is concerned the most potent antidiarrheal drug is difenoxin (lowest ED_{50} = 0.043 mg/kg). Butoxylate, diphenoxylate, loperamide, and fluperamide are equipotent (lowest $ED_{50} \simeq$ 0.15 mg/kg), while fetoxylate is somewhat less potent (lowest ED_{50} = 0.43 mg/kg).

The differences in ED_{50} values obtained 1 and 8 hr after castor-oil administration are indicative of the duration of action of the antidiarrheal activity. Fetoxylate is the antidiarrheal compound with the shortest period of activity (ED_{50} 8 hr/ED_{50} 1 hr = 40). Thus, to obtain protection against diarrhea for 8 hr the dose of fetoxylate must be 40 times higher than the dose required to protect for 1 hr. A comparable duration of action is obtained with

TABLE 4

ED_{50} Values and Fiducial Limits (LL and UL) in mg/kg Obtained in the TWR and CO Tests After Oral Administration of Various Analgesic Agents

Compounds	Criteria		Hours					
			1	2	3	4	6	8
Bezitramide	TWR > 6"	ED_{50}	0.38	0.56	0.73	0.92	1.29	1.60
		LL	0.25	0.39	0.51	0.62	0.87	1.03
		UL	0.58	0.79	1.05	1.36	1.92	2.49
	TWR > 10"	ED_{50}	0.88	0.97	1.08	1.37	2.64	3.00
		LL	0.64	0.74	0.77	0.91	1.51	1.66
		UL	1.23	1.29	1.52	2.07	4.64	5.44
	CO	ED_{50}	0.26	0.89	1.02	1.20	1.37	1.61
		LL	0.16	0.62	0.76	0.76	0.89	1.05
		UL	0.41	1.30	1.37	1.91	2.12	2.47
Fentanyl	TWR > 6"	ED_{50}	0.42	0.83	1.01	1.71	2.90	3.09
		LL	0.28	0.55	0.70	1.23	2.18	2.37
		UL	0.64	1.25	1.45	2.37	3.87	4.02
	TWR > 10"	ED_{50}	1.14	1.62	1.99	2.51	2.98	≥ 5
		LL	0.82	1.19	1.50	1.89	2.11	—
		UL	1.58	2.21	2.64	3.33	4.20	—
	CO	ED_{50}	0.19	0.49	0.76	0.96	1.19	1.60
		LL	0.12	0.30	0.44	0.60	0.80	0.97
		UL	0.31	0.79	1.30	1.54	1.76	2.63
Dextromoramide	TWR > 6"	ED_{50}	1.98	2.91	4.28	5.76	5.77	7.92
		LL	1.52	2.18	3.03	4.32	4.16	5.94
		UL	2.57	3.89	6.05	7.67	8.00	10.6
	TWR > 10"	ED_{50}	3.29	4.38	5.35	6.90	7.65	>10
		LL	2.65	3.32	4.34	5.73	6.03	—
		UL	4.08	5.78	6.59	8.30	9.70	—
	CO	ED_{50}	1.80	2.83	4.42	5.58	5.58	8.25
		LL	1.13	1.92	3.27	4.21	4.21	5.48
		UL	2.86	4.18	5.98	7.40	7.40	12.4

TABLE 4 (Continued)

Compounds	Criteria		Hours					
			1	2	3	4	6	8
Phenazocine	TWR > 6"	ED_{50}	6.45	10.5	12.8	20.6	36.0	>40
		LL	3.94	6.61	7.65	14.1	20.8	—
		UL	10.6	16.5	21.3	30.1	62.2	—
	TWR > 10"	ED_{50}	8.90	13.4	17.8	24.7	≥40	>40
		LL	5.69	8.91	12.2	17.0	—	—
		UL	13.9	20.0	26.0	35.8	—	—
	CO	ED_{50}	6.65	15.3	19.2	23.0	36.9	≥40
		LL	4.28	9.63	12.8	14.7	29.2	—
		UL	10.3	24.3	28.9	36.0	46.6	—
Anileridine	TWR > 6"	ED_{50}	9.70	13.0	13.7	19.4	25.9	≥40
		LL	6.61	10.2	10.9	12.8	20.8	—
		UL	14.2	16.6	17.3	29.4	32.3	—
	TWR > 10"	ED_{50}	11.6	13.7	18.6	21.8	37.6	≥40
		LL	7.90	9.98	11.4	14.4	22.9	—
		UL	17.0	18.8	30.4	33.1	61.7	—
	CO	ED_{50}	4.42	8.05	14.1	17.8	22.2	33.0
		LL	3.36	5.61	11.2	14.2	17.7	25.1
		UL	5.81	11.6	17.8	22.3	27.8	43.5
Methadone	TWR > 6"	ED_{50}	11.6	13.6	16.5	19.7	25.7	32.9
		LL	8.16	10.9	12.9	16.0	19.7	27.2
		UL	16.5	17.0	21.1	24.3	33.4	39.8
	TWR > 10"	ED_{50}	16.9	17.2	20.5	24.2	28.6	38.0
		LL	13.3	13.5	16.4	19.1	23.7	30.1
		UL	21.5	21.9	25.7	30.6	34.5	48.0
	CO	ED_{50}	2.19	6.38	10.3	12.6	14.0	16.9
		LL	1.50	4.82	8.07	10.3	10.4	14.2
		UL	3.21	8.44	13.1	15.4	18.8	20.2
Phenoperidine	TWR > 6"	ED_{50}	21.6	26.2	31.6	42.8	48.0	≤80
		LL	14.9	18.3	21.4	26.5	40.4	—
		UL	31.3	37.4	46.7	69.2	57.1	—

TABLE 4 (Continued)

Compounds	Criteria		Hours					
			1	2	3	4	6	8
(Phenoperidine)	TWR > 10"	ED_{50}	26.9	37.5	42.2	47.9	56.5	80.0
		LL	20.1	23.6	27.3	35.9	42.8	48.9
		UL	36.0	59.6	65.3	63.8	74.5	131
	CO	ED_{50}	8.70	21.2	22.2	23.7	38.2	44.8
		LL	5.55	14.8	17.0	18.5	26.0	33.6
		UL	13.6	30.3	29.0	30.3	56.1	59.8
Piritramide	TWR > 6"	ED_{50}	12.9	19.1	24.9	27.1	36.9	45.6
		LL	7.69	12.1	16.1	17.2	23.6	30.5
		UL	21.6	30.1	38.3	42.7	57.6	68.2
	TWR > 10"	ED_{50}	32.9	47.6	47.6	47.2	54.0	59.8
		LL	20.4	37.4	37.4	31.1	40.3	41.8
		UL	53.0	60.6	60.6	71.6	72.3	85.5
	CO	ED_{50}	1.97	6.61	12.6	14.0	17.9	21.1
		LL	1.16	4.82	10.3	10.4	14.0	16.4
		UL	3.35	9.07	15.4	18.9	22.9	27.1
Morphine	TWR > 6"	ED_{50}	13.5	14.3	21.8	32.5	66.2	102
		LL	8.58	9.11	13.6	19.3	36.0	44.7
		UL	21.2	22.6	35.0	54.6	122	234
	TWR > 10"	ED_{50}	33.6	33.6	38.2	52.7	100	168
		LL	22.6	23.1	26.1	39.6	69.9	120
		UL	49.8	48.7	56.1	70.1	143	235
	CO	ED_{50}	1.52	5.21	14.5	30.9	50.6	60.7
		LL	1.01	4.04	10.0	20.8	32.6	46.7
		UL	2.27	6.70	21.1	45.9	78.6	78.9
Codeine	TWR > 6"	ED_{50}	19.0	20.9	37.8	75.8	112	164
		LL	13.3	15.0	26.1	52.0	73.0	94.5
		UL	27.7	29.3	54.5	110	173	284
	TWR > 10"	ED_{50}	56.6	59.1	84.2	124	162	213
		LL	40.0	41.6	62.7	96.3	139	157
		UL	80.1	84.0	113	159	189	290

TABLE 4 (Continued)

Compounds	Criteria		Hours					
			1	2	3	4	6	8
(Codeine)	CO	ED_{50}	2.85	10.8	20.0	28.8	52.4	70.0
		LL	1.87	8.71	15.0	21.5	37.6	50.1
		UL	4.35	13.5	26.6	38.6	72.9	97.7
Pethidine	TWR > 6"	ED_{50}	33.0	51.7	83.2	111	≥160	>160
		LL	22.9	38.5	60.9	79.8	—	—
		UL	47.5	69.3	114	153	—	—
	TWR > 10"	ED_{50}	63.5	90.5	113	142	>160	>160
		LL	48.8	67.7	86.8	104	—	—
		UL	82.6	121	147	194	—	—
	CO	ED_{50}	16.3	30.2	38.9	52.5	80.0	87.0
		LL	11.9	22.0	25.0	39.2	52.7	62.8
		UL	22.3	41.4	60.6	70.2	122	121
Propoxyphene	TWR > 6"	ED_{50}	65.0	78.2	≥160	≥160	>160	>160
		LL	47.1	55.3	—	—	—	—
		UL	89.7	111	—	—	—	—
	TWR > 10"	ED_{50}	65.0	139	≥160	>160	>160	>160
		LL	47.1	92.7	—	—	—	—
		UL	89.7	209	—	—	—	—
	CO	ED_{50}	25.0	50.1	76.0	90.0	101	101
		LL	20.0	40.9	58.7	74.2	81.6	81.6
		UL	31.3	61.3	98.4	109	125	125

TABLE 5

ED_{50} Values and Fiducial Limits in mg/kg Obtained in the TWR and CO Tests after Oral Administration of Various Antidiarrheal Agents

Compounds	Criteria		Hours					
			1	2	3	4	6	8
Difenoxin	TWR > 6"	ED_{50}	2.57	1.73	1.65	2.44	3.52	3.75
		LL	1.57	1.16	1.10	1.63	2.27	2.69
		UL	4.21	2.57	2.47	3.66	5.45	5.23
	TWR > 10"	ED_{50}	16.6	4.06	4.58	6.52	7.60	7.02
		LL	11.1	2.82	3.02	4.37	5.12	4.70
		UL	24.9	5.86	6.95	9.72	11.3	10.5
	CO	ED_{50}	0.04	0.16	0.22	0.31	0.60	0.91
		LL	0.03	0.11	0.16	0.21	0.40	0.59
		UL	0.07	0.22	0.31	0.45	0.89	1.38
Butoxylate	TWR > 6"	ED_{50}	9.50	10.7	10.6	14.3	14.6	25.2
		LL	6.19	6.35	7.20	8.63	8.28	14.9
		UL	14.6	18.0	15.6	23.7	25.7	42.6
	TWR > 10"	ED_{50}	25.0	13.6	19.1	32.2	31.8	71.0
		LL	14.4	7.52	11.3	19.2	18.3	43.8
		UL	43.4	24.6	32.4	54.1	55.4	115
	CO	ED_{50}	0.13	0.42	0.71	1.02	1.91	3.95
		LL	0.09	0.25	0.48	0.67	1.14	2.03
		UL	0.19	0.71	1.05	1.56	3.20	7.69
Diphenoxylate	TWR > 6"	ED_{50}	6.93	5.10	6.27	6.27	10.5	14.2
		LL	3.34	3.20	3.92	3.94	6.52	8.78
		UL	14.4	8.12	10.0	9.96	17.0	23.1
	TWR > 10"	ED_{50}	27.4	13.5	12.8	15.6	18.2	26.2
		LL	13.6	8.35	7.99	9.82	11.5	15.3
		UL	55.1	21.8	20.4	24.9	28.7	44.8
	CO	ED_{50}	0.15	0.54	1.05	1.41	2.70	4.77
		LL	0.11	0.40	0.79	1.07	1.99	3.44
		UL	0.22	0.72	1.40	1.87	3.68	6.61

TABLE 5 (Continued)

Compounds	Criteria		Hours					
			1	2	3	4	6	8
Fluperamide[a]	TWR > 6"	ED_{50}	≥80.0	≥80.0	>80.0	>80.0	>80.0	>80.0
		LL	—	—	—	—	—	—
		UL	—	—	—	—	—	—
	TWR > 10"	ED_{50}	>80.0	>80.0	>80.0	>80.0	>80.0	>80.0
		LL	—	—	—	—	—	—
		UL	—	—	—	—	—	—
	CO	ED_{50}	0.15	0.21	0.31	0.31	0.53	0.73
		LL	0.10	0.15	0.18	0.18	0.35	0.40
		UL	0.24	0.31	0.54	0.54	0.80	1.32
Loperamide[b]	TWR > 6"	ED_{50}	≥160	>160	>160	>160	>160	>160
		LL	—	—	—	—	—	—
		UL	—	—	—	—	—	—
	TWR > 10"	ED_{50}	>160	>160	>160	>160	>160	>160
		LL	—	—	—	—	—	—
		UL	—	—	—	—	—	—
	CO	ED_{50}	0.15	0.29	0.43	0.61	1.07	1.81
		LL	0.11	0.23	0.34	0.45	0.77	1.25
		UL	0.20	0.38	0.56	0.83	1.51	2.63
Fetoxylate	TWR > 6"	ED_{50}	>160	>160	>160	>160	>160	>160
		LL	—	—	—	—	—	—
		UL	—	—	—	—	—	—
	TWR > 10"	ED_{50}	>160	>160	>160	>160	>160	>160
		LL	—	—	—	—	—	—
		UL	—	—	—	—	—	—
	CO	ED_{50}	0.43	1.08	1.76	2.50	3.72	16.9
		LL	0.25	0.73	1.10	1.74	2.53	9.23
		UL	0.76	1.60	2.82	3.60	5.48	30.9

[a] Out of ten rats three died at 80.0 mg/kg.
[b] Out of ten rats four died at 160 mg/kg.

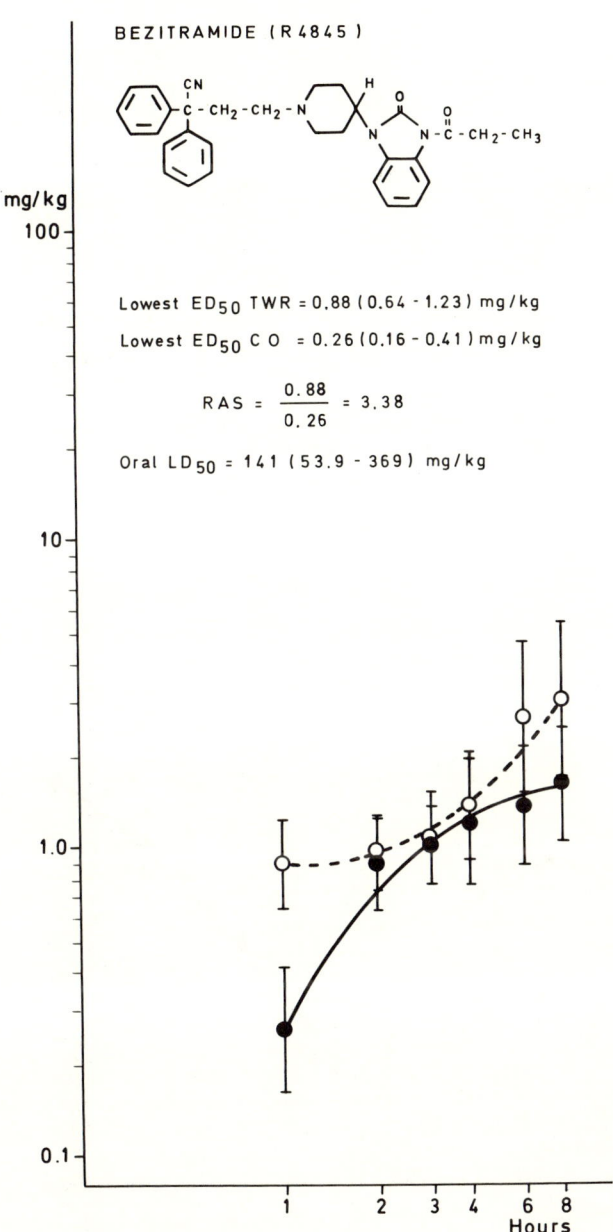

Fig. 1. ED_{50} values with fiducial limits at indicated hours after castor oil (●) and in the tail-withdrawal test (o), reaction time more than 10 sec with bezitramide.

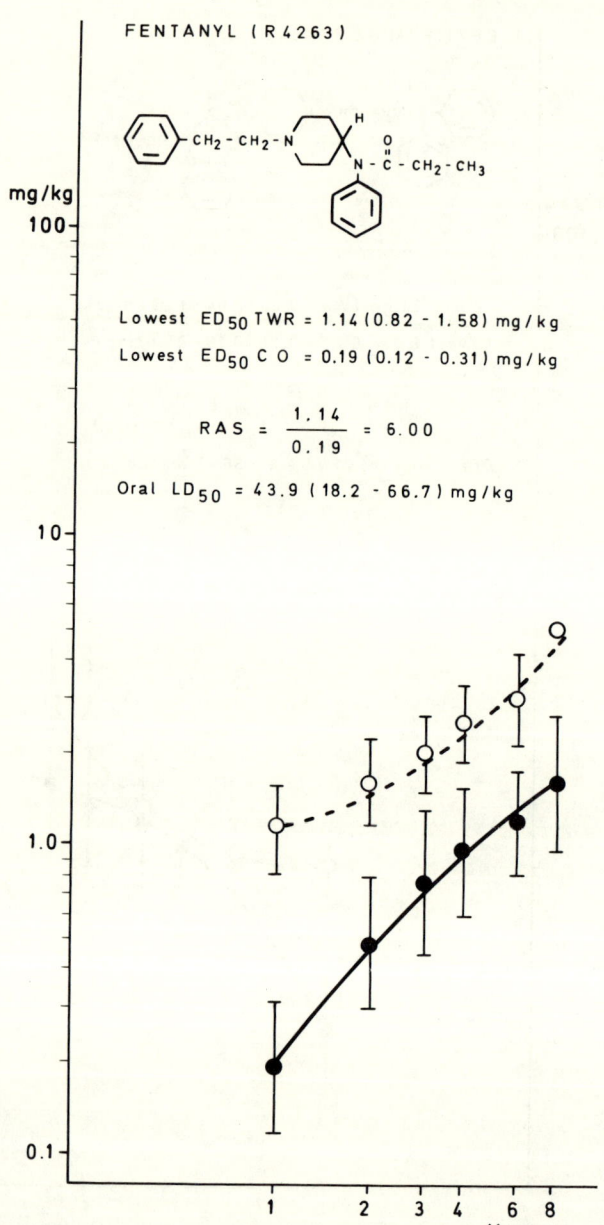

Fig. 2. ED_{50} values with fiducial limits at indicated hours after castor oil (●) and in the tail-withdrawal test (o), reaction time more than 10 sec with fentanyl.

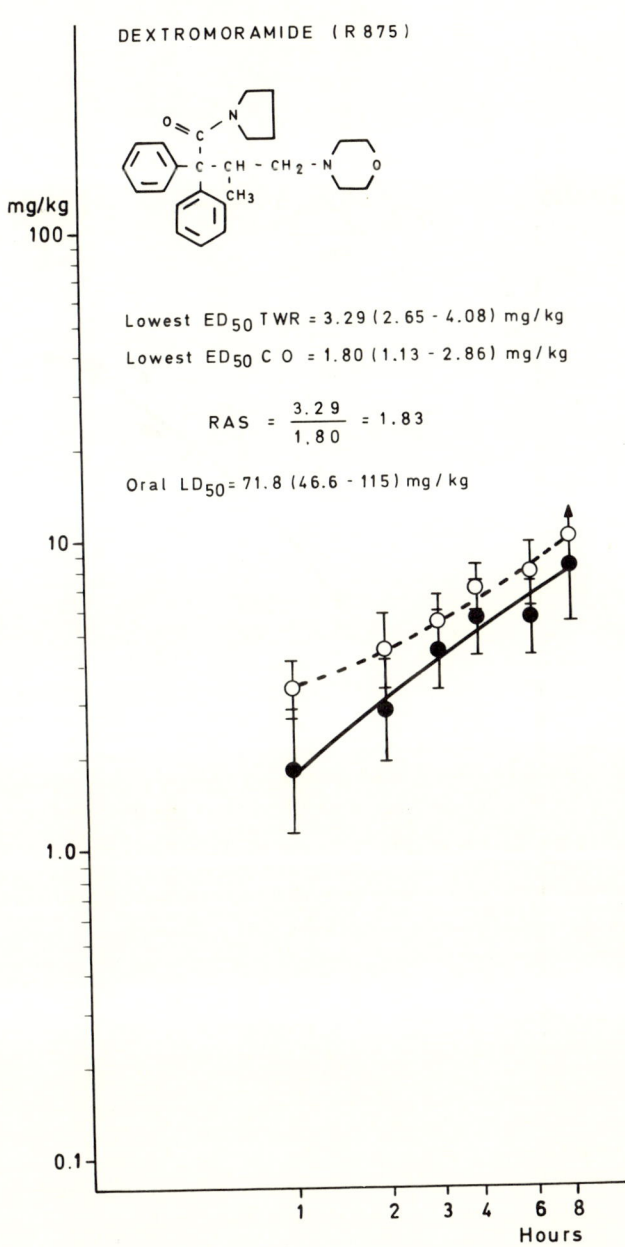

Fig. 3. ED_{50} values with fiducial limits at indicated hours after castor oil (●) and in the tail-withdrawal test (o), reaction time more than 10 sec with dextromoramide.

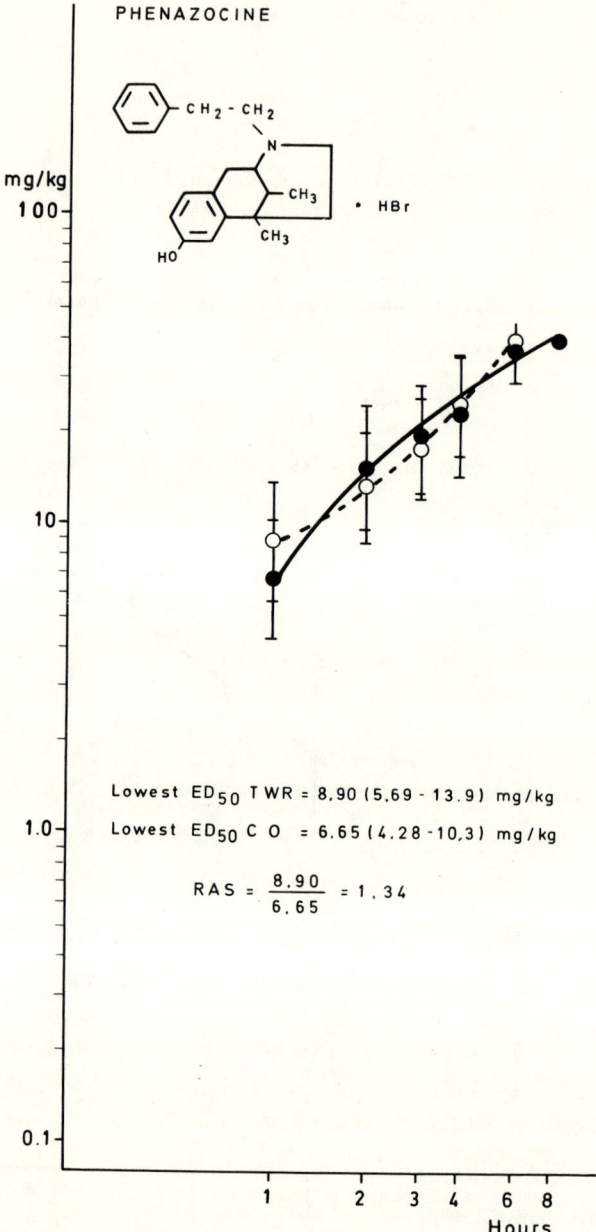

Fig. 4. ED_{50} values with fiducial limits at indicated hours after castor oil (●) and in the tail-withdrawal test (o), reaction time more than 10 sec with phenazocine.

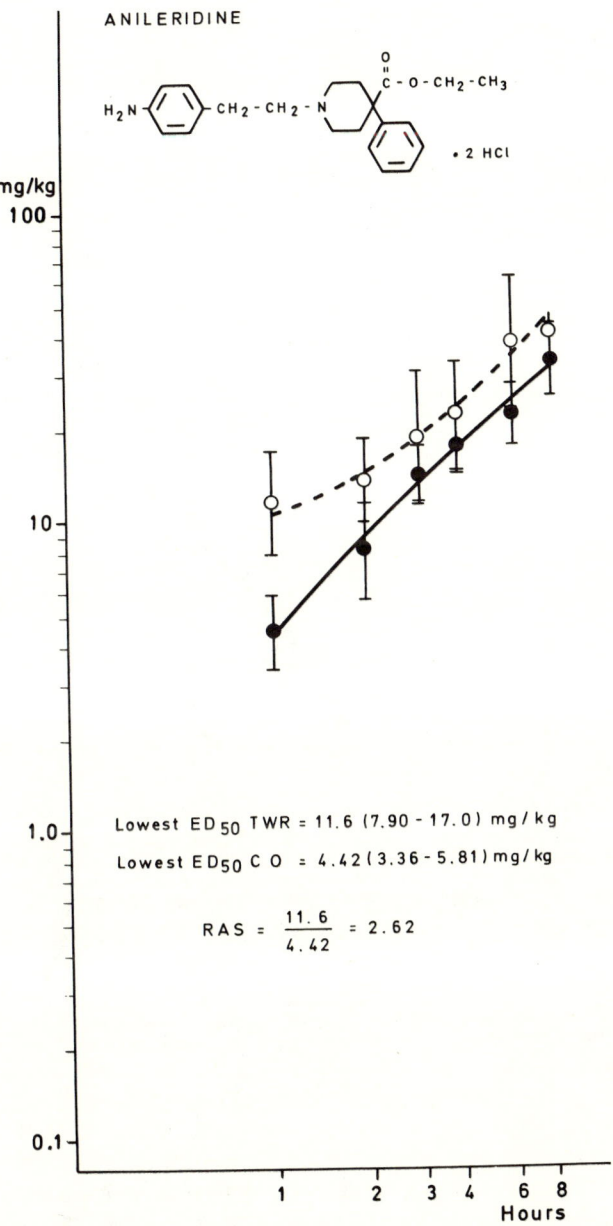

Fig. 5. ED$_{50}$ values with fiducial limits at indicated hours after castor oil (●) and in the tail-withdrawal test (o), reaction time more than 10 sec with anileridine.

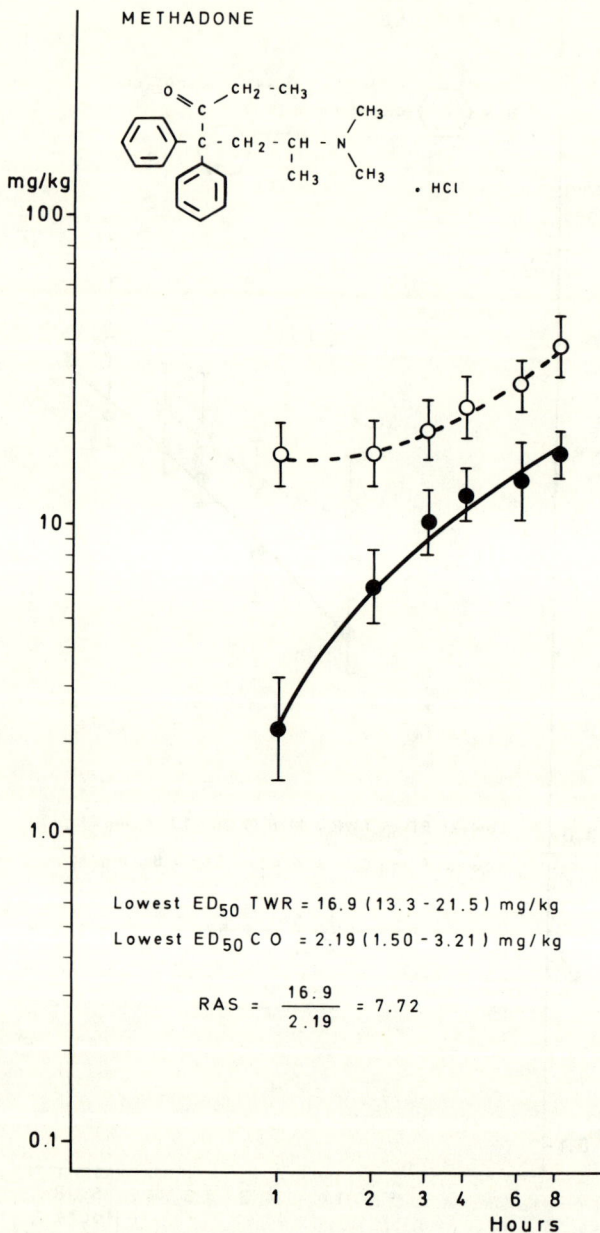

Fig 6. ED_{50} values with fiducial limits at indicated hours after castor oil (●) and in the tail-withdrawal test (o), reaction time more than 10 sec with methadone.

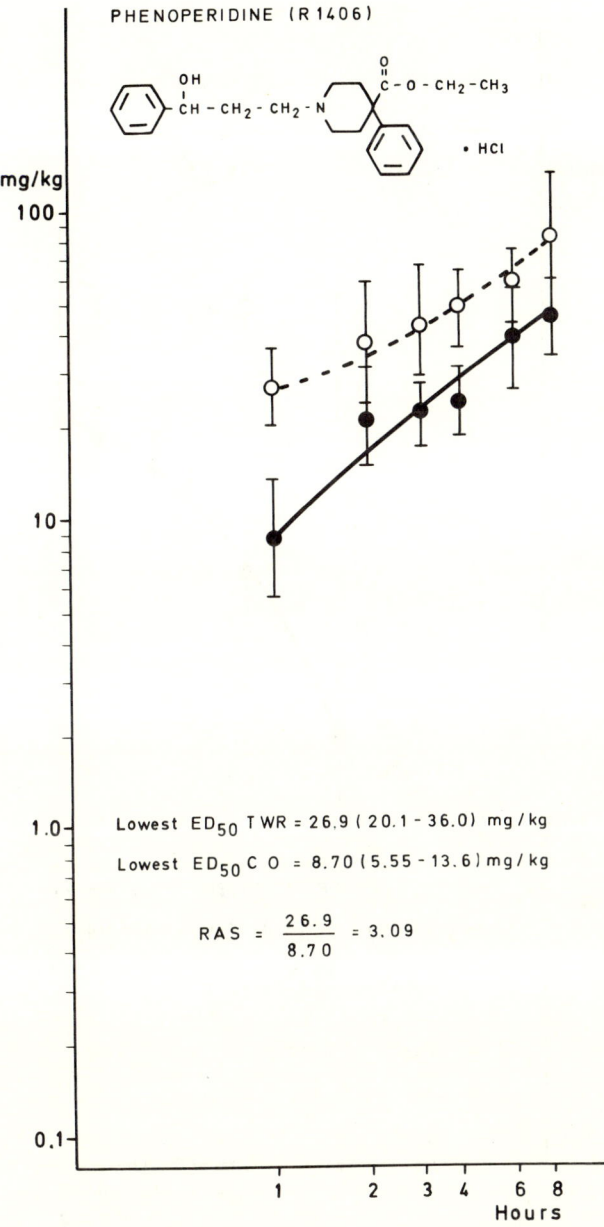

Fig. 7. ED_{50} values with fiducial limits at indicated hours after castor oil (●) and in the tail-withdrawal test (o), reaction time more than 10 sec with phenoperidine.

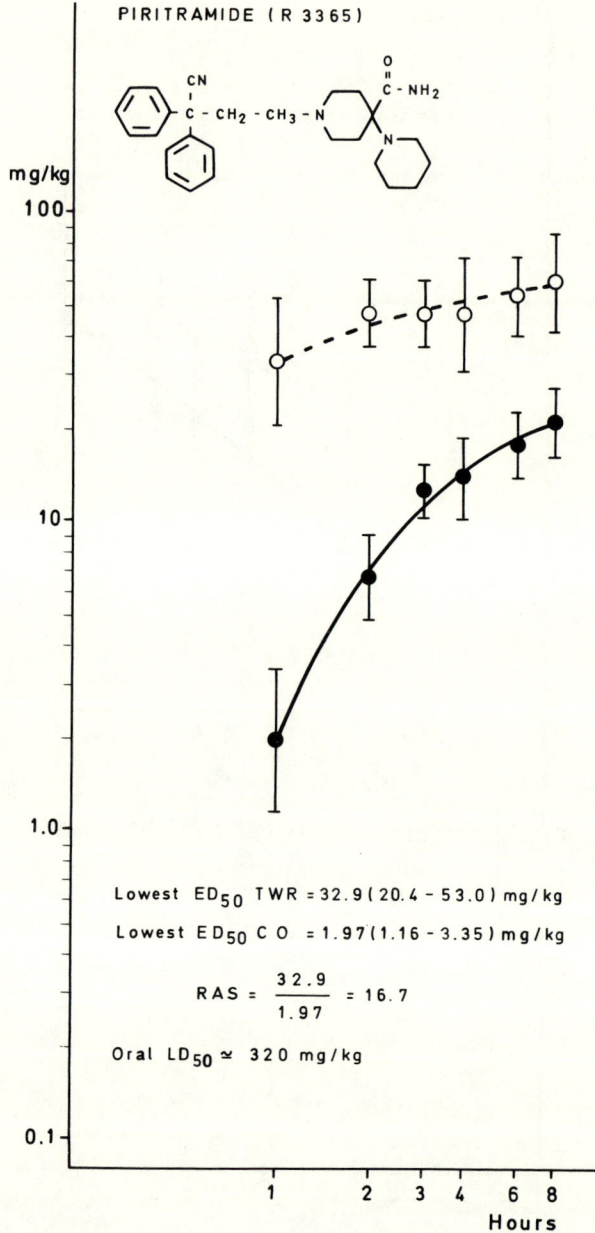

Fig. 8. ED_{50} values with fiducial limits at indicated hours after castor oil (●) and in the tail-withdrawal test (o), reaction time more than 10 sec with piritramide.

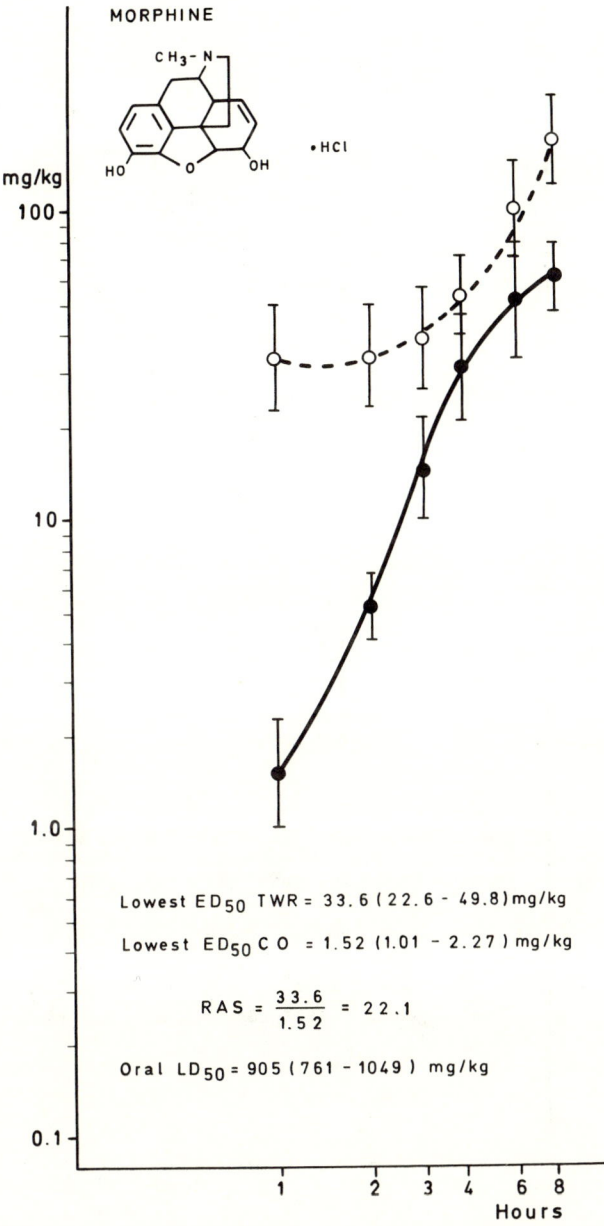

Fig. 9. ED_{50} values with fiducial limits at indicated hours after castor oil (●) and in the tail-withdrawal test (o), reaction time more than 10 sec with morphine.

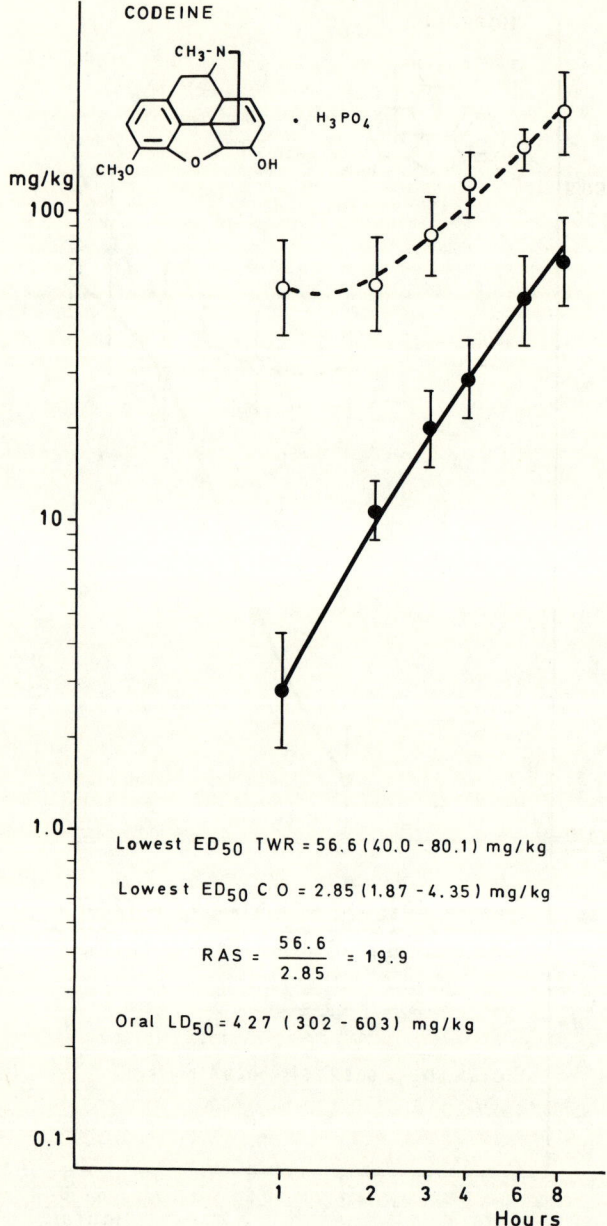

Fig. 10. ED_{50} values with fiducial limits at indicated hours after castor oil (●) and in the tail-withdrawal test (o), reaction time more than 10 sec with codeine.

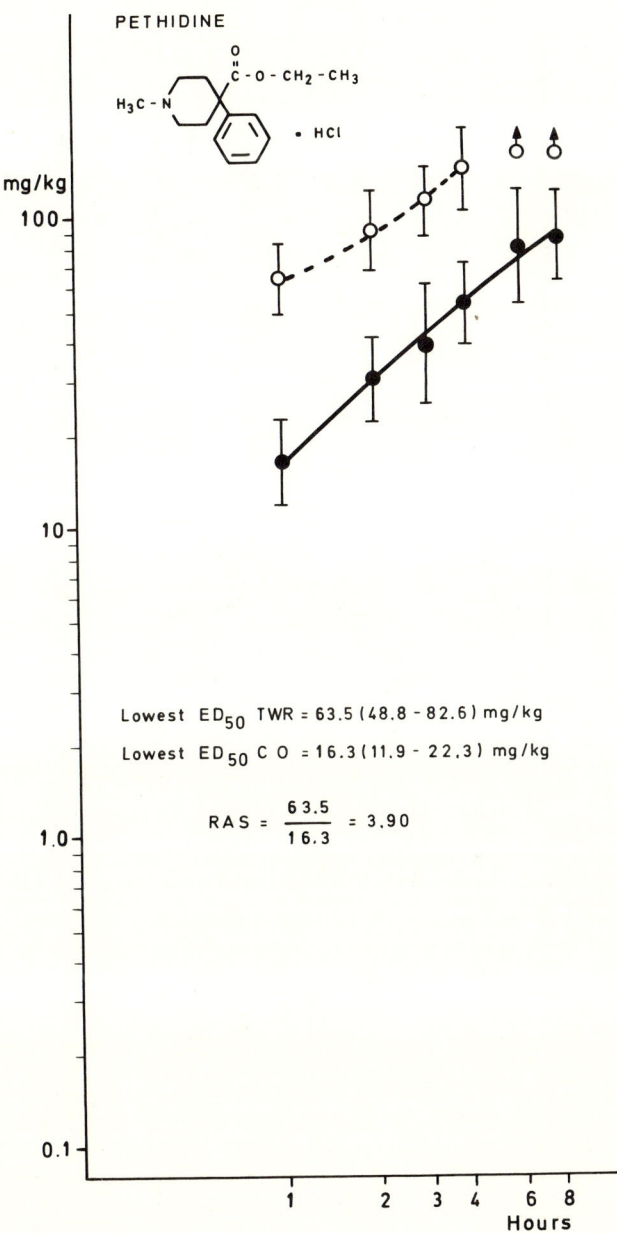

Fig. 11. ED$_{50}$ values with fiducial limits at indicated hours after castor oil (●) and in the tail-withdrawal test (o), reaction time more than 10 sec with pethidine.

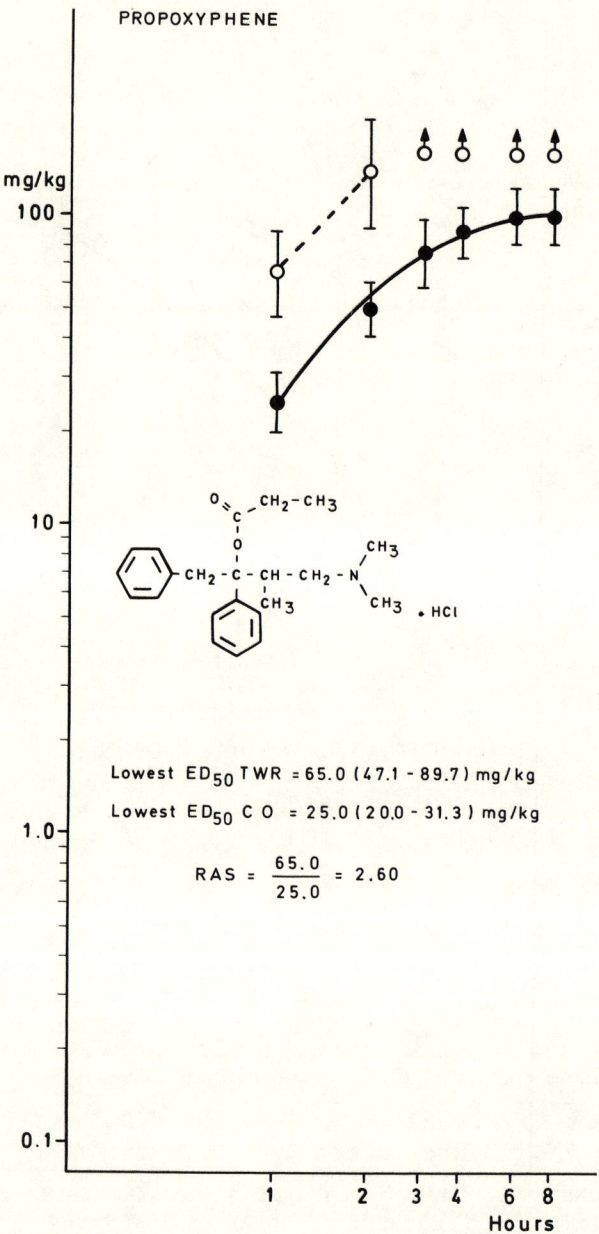

Fig. 12. ED_{50} values with fiducial limits at indicated hours after castor oil (●) and in the tail-withdrawal test (o), reaction time more than 10 sec with propoxyphene.

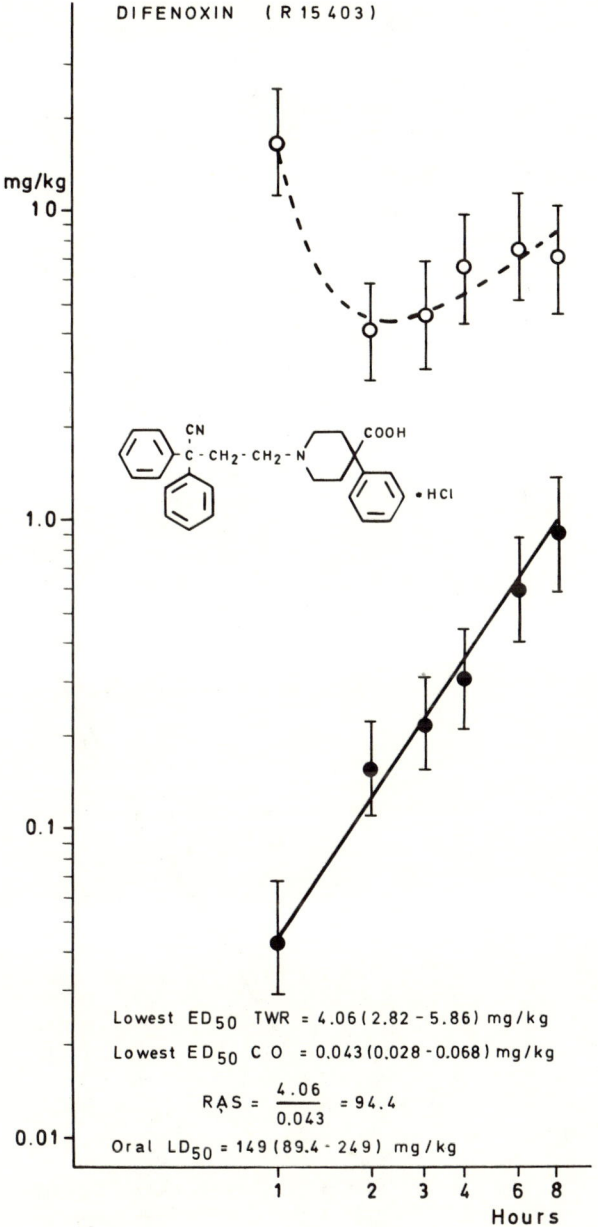

Fig. 13. ED_{50} values with fiducial limits at indicated hours after castor oil (●) and in the tail-withdrawal test (o), reaction time more than 10 sec with difenoxin.

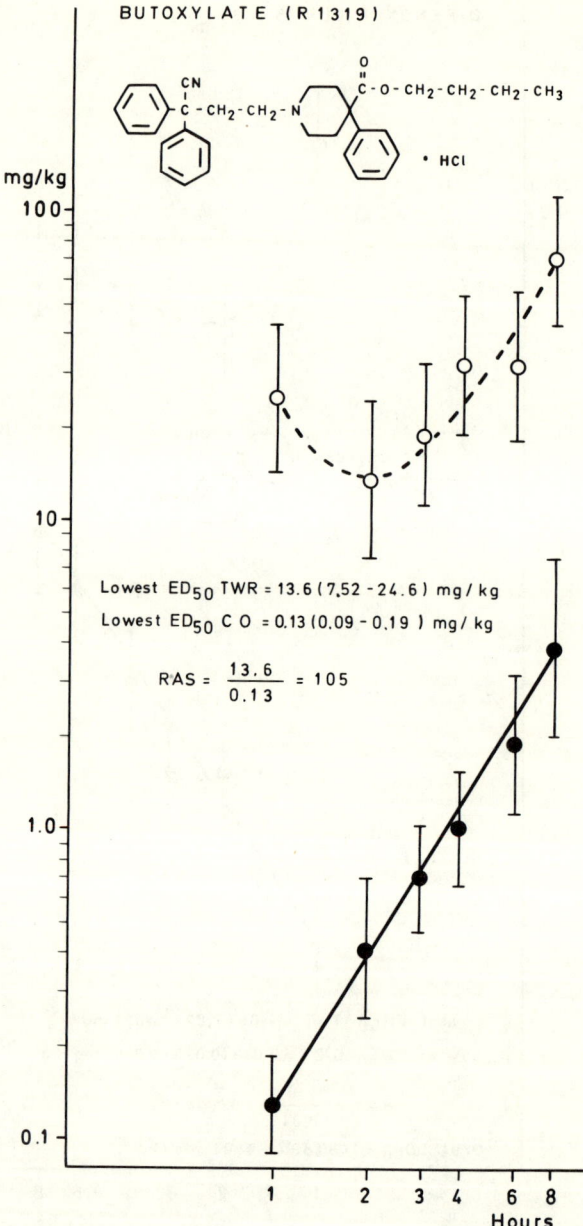

Fig. 14. ED_{50} values with fiducial limits at indicated hours after castor oil (●) and in the tail-withdrawal test (o), reaction time more than 10 sec with butoxylate.

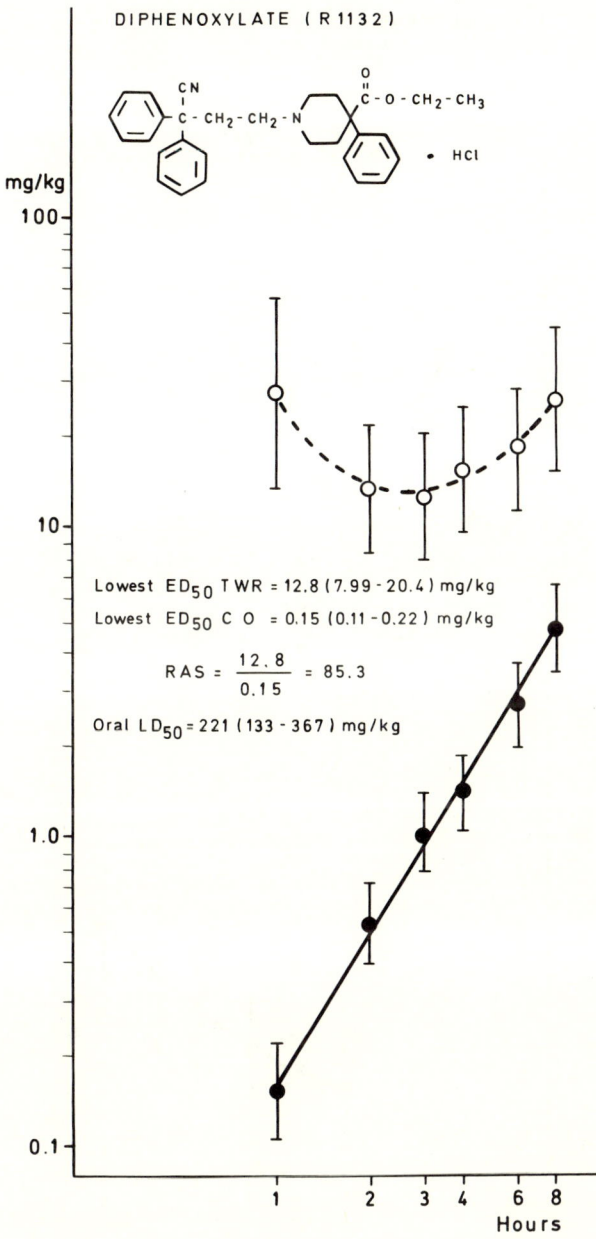

Fig. 15. ED_{50} values with fiducial limits at indicated hours after castor oil (●) and in the tail-withdrawal test (o), reaction time more than 10 sec with diphenoxylate.

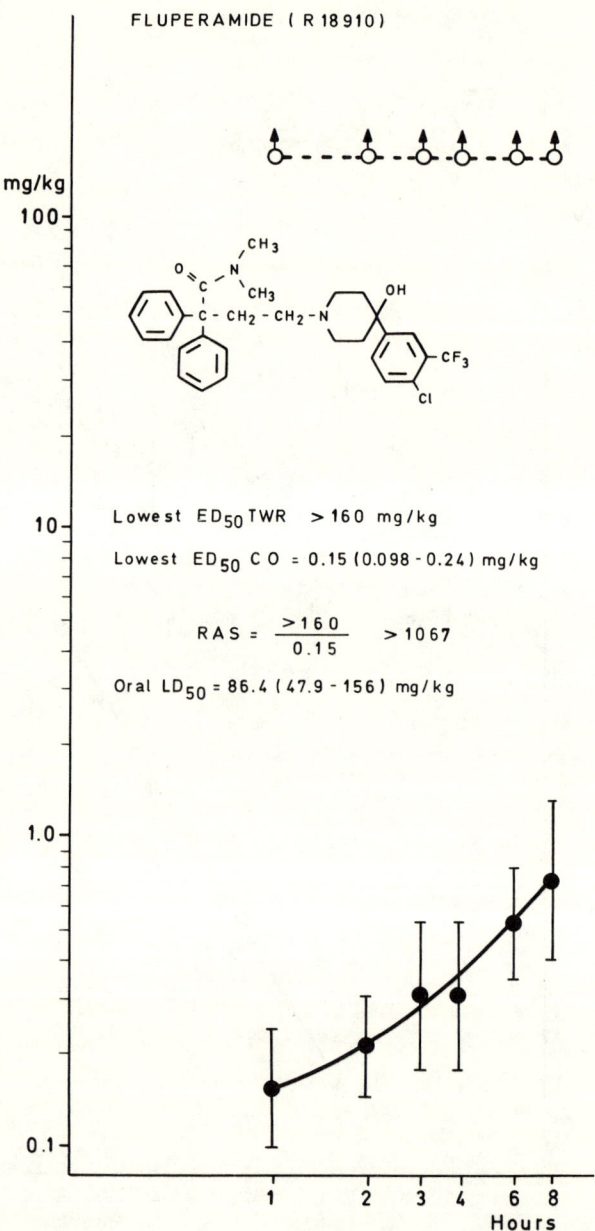

Fig. 16. ED_{50} values with fiducial limits at indicated hours after castor oil (●) and in the tail-withdrawal test (o), reaction time more than 10 sec with fluperamide.

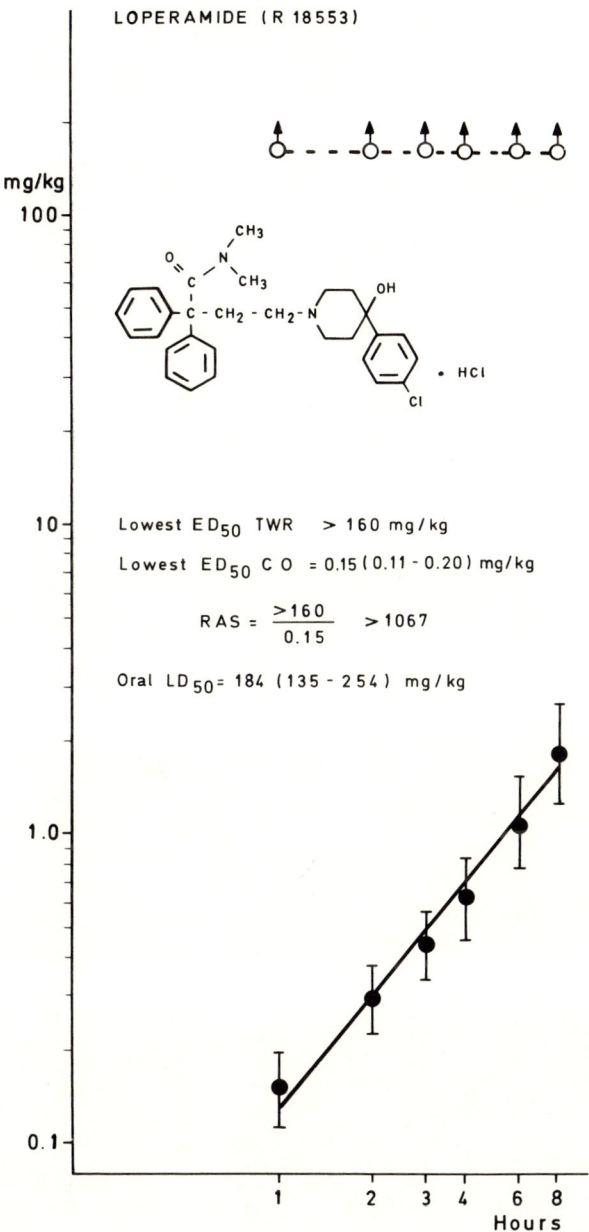

Fig. 17. ED_{50} values with fiducial limits at indicated hours after castor oil (●) and in the tail-withdrawal test (o), reaction time more than 10 sec with loperamide.

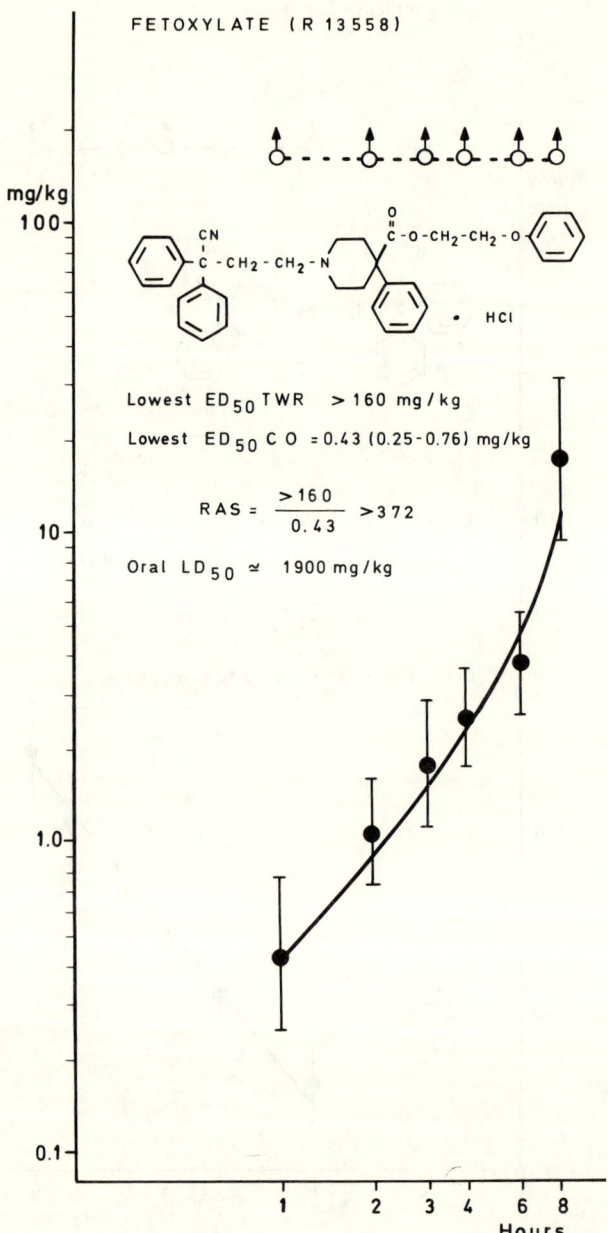

Fig. 18. ED_{50} values with fiducial limits at indicated hours after castor oil (●) and in the tail-withdrawal test (o), reaction time more than 10 sec with fetoxylate.

butoxylate and diphenoxylate (ED_{50} 8 hr/ED_{50} 1 hr = 31). Difenoxin has a longer duration of action (ED_{50} 8 hr/ED_{50} 1 hr = 21), while loperamide and fluperamide are antidiarrheal drugs with extremely prolonged action (ED_{50} 8 hr/ED_{50} 1 hr being 12 and 5, respectively).

The data presented most clearly demonstrate the considerable discrepancy between the relative capacity of drugs to antagonize castor-oil-induced diarrhea and to produce analgesia. The concept of RAS provides an operational means of comparing this relative discrepancy from drug to drug. Of the large number of drugs studied all appear to lie on RAS continuum. Drugs commonly regarded as narcotic analgesics are on the left side of this continuum, antidiarrheal drugs are on its right side. Difenoxin, butoxylate, and diphenoxylate were found to have a large RAS, indicating that they are very specific antidiarrheal agents. Fetoxylate up to 160 mg/kg was found to be devoid of central effects; the same holds true for fluperamide and loperamide up to toxic dose levels. These findings indicate that these three compounds are the most specific antidiarrheals of all the compounds tested.

The next section, which describes some other data in mice, in which morphine, codeine, diphenoxylate, and loperamide were submitted to tests for the inhibition of gastrointestinal propulsion and narcotic drug properties, provides further confirmation of this general conclusion.

1.2.3. The Dissociation Between Constipating and Central Drug Effects in Mice

The search for specific antidiarrheal agents has led us to investigate the relative capacity of drugs to antagonize (castor-oil-induced) diarrhea and to produce analgesia in rats. Contrary to what is generally held true, it appears from this study that antidiarrheal activity and specific narcotic effects such as analgesia are not necessarily closely related.

Analgesia, as well as a number of gross behavioral effects, is most typical for all drugs belonging to the narcotic class. In mice, increased locomotion and Straub-tail on arched back reliably occur following the administration of any narcotic (Krueger et al., 1941). The present section describes the occurrence of these behavioral phenomena on the one hand, and the inhibition of gastrointestinal motility on the other, as they have been studied following parenteral administration of morphine, codeine, diphenoxylate, and loperamide. Male white mice of Swiss substrain, starved overnight, and weighing 23 ± 3 g were used.

The compounds studied were morphine, codeine, diphenoxylate, and loperamide given subcutaneously and intraperitoneally at dose levels selected from the following geometrical series: 1280, 640, 320, ... 1.25, 0.63, 0.31 ... mg/kg. All compounds were given in aqueous solutions (0.1 ml per 10 g body weight). To the loperamide concentrations of 2 mg/ml and higher (20 mg/kg and above) 10% propylene glycol was added. At concentrations of 2 mg/ml and higher, diphenoxylate was given in aqueous suspensions micronized with an ultrasonic sonifier. The highest concentration of morphine given was 64 mg/ml of which 0.2 ml per 10 g body weight was injected in order to obtain 1280 mg/kg. For each group of treated mice, a series of control mice was injected with either saline or with an aqueous solution, containing 10% propylene glycol.

All control and treated mice received orally, by gavage, 0.3 ml of a 10% charcoal suspension in 5% gum arabic immediately (t = 0), 1(t = 1), or 2(t = 2) hr after the parenteral treatment.

Immediately after injection of the investigated compounds each mouse was put into a glass beaker (diameter 14 cm), the bottom of which was divided into four equal parts by two perpendicular red lines, which crossed in the middle of the beaker.

Motor rotary movement was recorded by counting the number of line crossings during a two-minute observation period, 1/2, 1, 1 1/2, 2, 2 1/2 and 3 hr after injection of the compounds. During the same periods, and without disturbing the animals, the presence or absence of Straub tail on arched back was noted.

The mice were killed with chloroform 3 hr after the charcoal administration. The intestines were immediately removed from stomach to caecum and carefully laid out on a clean white "formica" covered table. The inhibition of the gastrointestinal motility was evaluated by measuring the progression in cm of the charcoal suspension from stomach to caecum.

Based on the results obtained in the control mice, ED_{50}'s and 95% fiducial limits (Litchfield and Wilcoxon, 1949) were calculated, according to the following "all-or-none" criteria:

a. For inhibition of gastrointestinal motility: absence of the charcoal in caecum, which occurred in 3% of the control mice.

b. For morphine-like behavioral effects: presence of Straub tail on arched back. These typical morphine-like effects were never observed in control mice.

c. Mortality within the period of 3 to 5 hr after injection for calculating the acute LD_{50}'s.

In preliminary experiments the standardized charcoal suspension was given to different groups of starved mice, and gastrointestinal propulsion of the charcoal was measured 1, 2, 3, and 4 hr later. Table 6 shows the number of mice in each group and those in which the charcoal reached the caecum (black caecum). The mean distance from stomach to caecum, measured in 70 control mice was 49.5 ± 0.47 cm.

Preclinical Studies: In Vivo Pharmacology

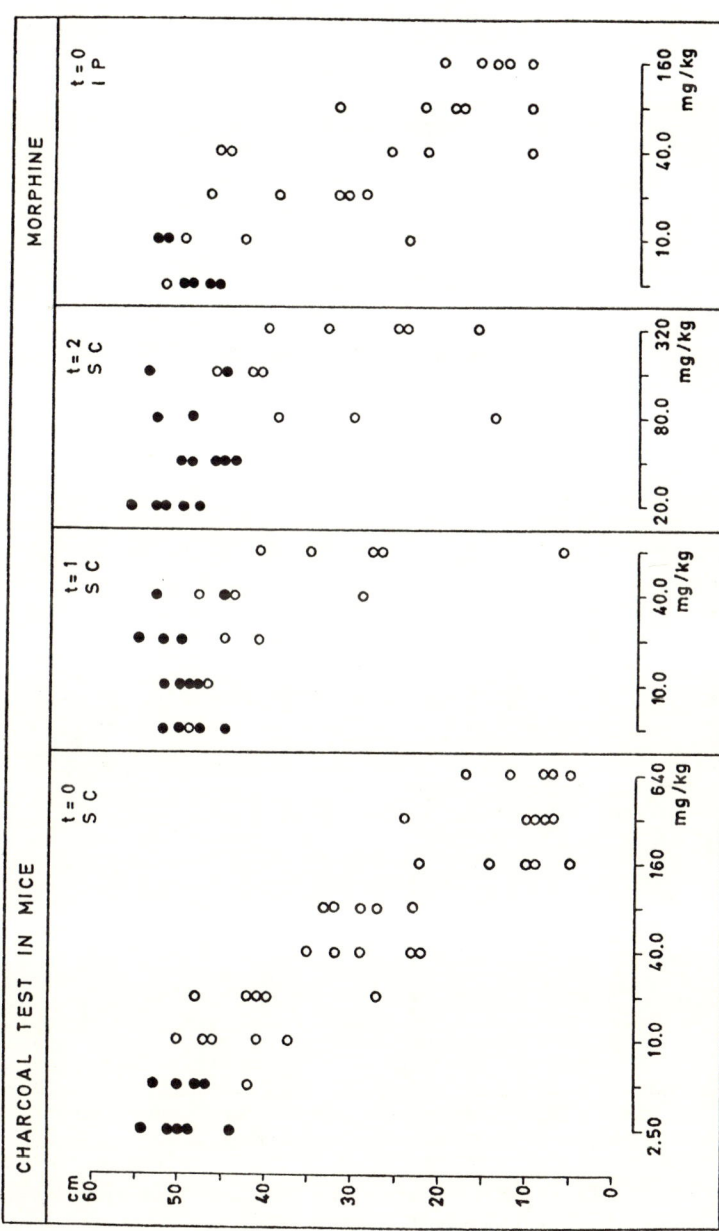

Fig. 19. Charcoal test. Progression in cm of charcoal suspension from stomach to caecum after treatment with different SC and IP doses of morphine, immediately (t = 0), 1 hr (t = 1), and 2 hr (t = 2) before charcoal. Black circles: charcoal present in caecum, open circles: caecum protected from charcoal. Each point represents one mouse. Source: Arzneimittel-Forsch. 24, 1637 (1974), permission granted.

TABLE 6

Charcoal Test in Mice[a]

Hours after charcoal	Ratio of number of mice with black caecum to number of mice treated	Mice with black caecum
1	6/40	15
2	32/40	80
3	323/332	97
4	20/20	100

[a]Number of mice with "black" caecum at different time intervals after administration of the charcoal suspension.

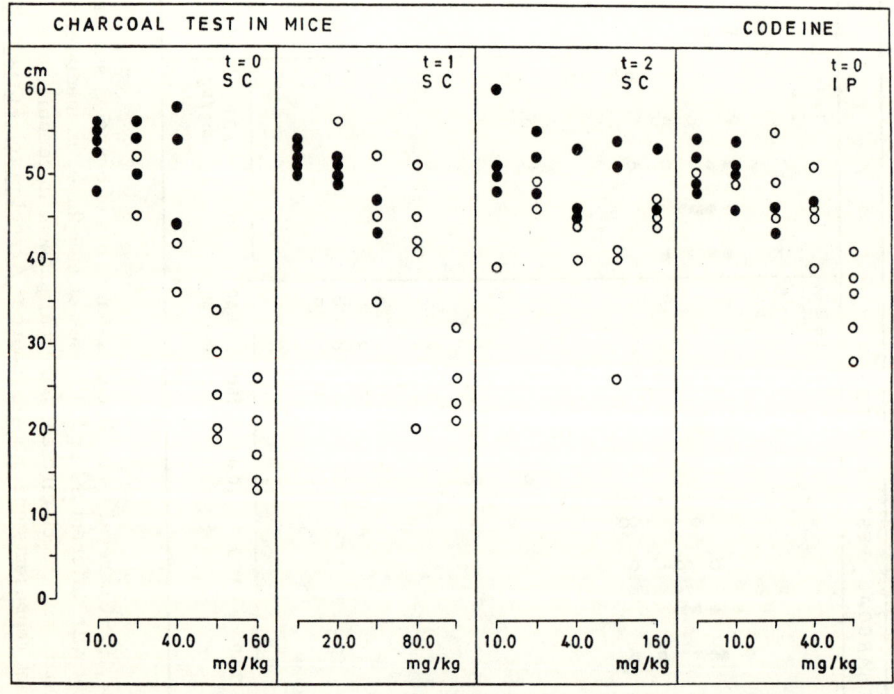

Fig. 20. Charcoal test. Progression in cm of charcoal suspension from stomach to caecum after treatment with different SC and IP doses of codeine, immediately (t = 0), 1 hr (t = 1), and 2 hr (t = 2) before charcoal. Black circles: charcoal present in caecum, open circles: caecum protected from charcoal. Each point represents one mouse. Source: Arzneimittel-Forsch. 24, 1637 (1974), permission granted.

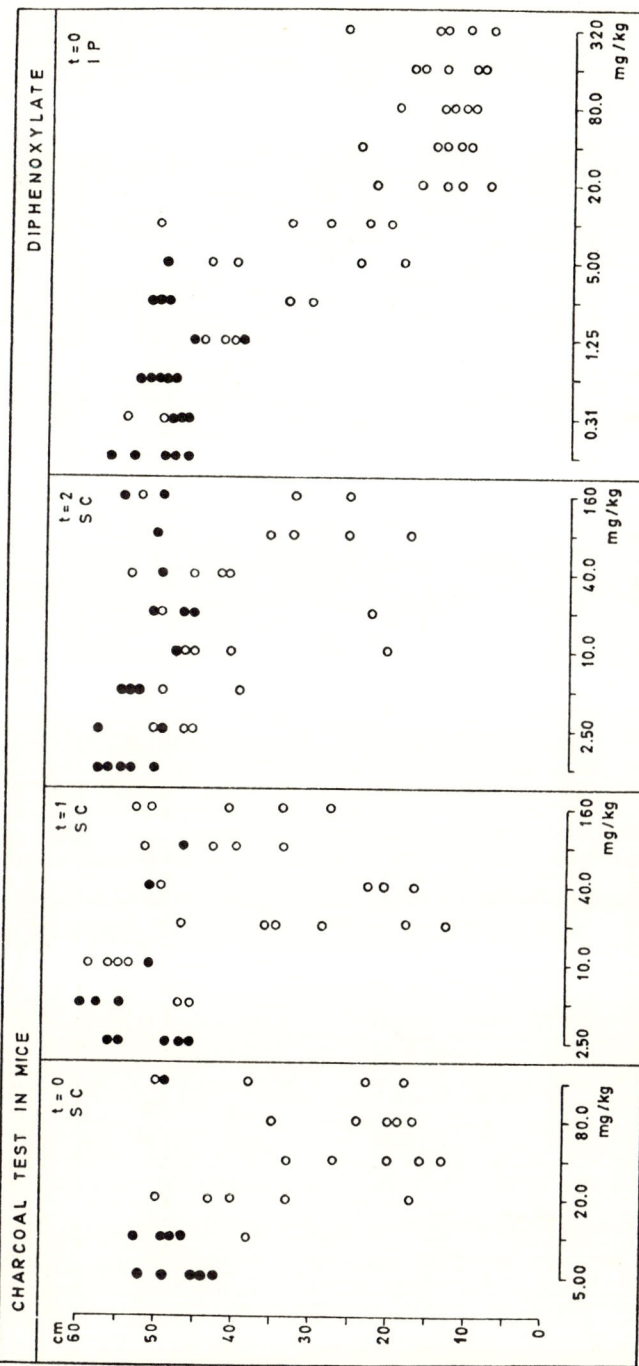

Fig. 21. Charcoal test. Progression in cm of charcoal suspension from stomach to caecum after treatment with different SC and IP doses of diphenoxylate, immediately (t = 0), 1 hr (t = 1) and 2 hr (t = 2) before charcoal. Black circles: charcoal present in caecum, open circles: caecum protected from charcoal. Each point represents one mouse. Source: Arzneimittel-Forsch. 24, 1637 (1974), permission granted.

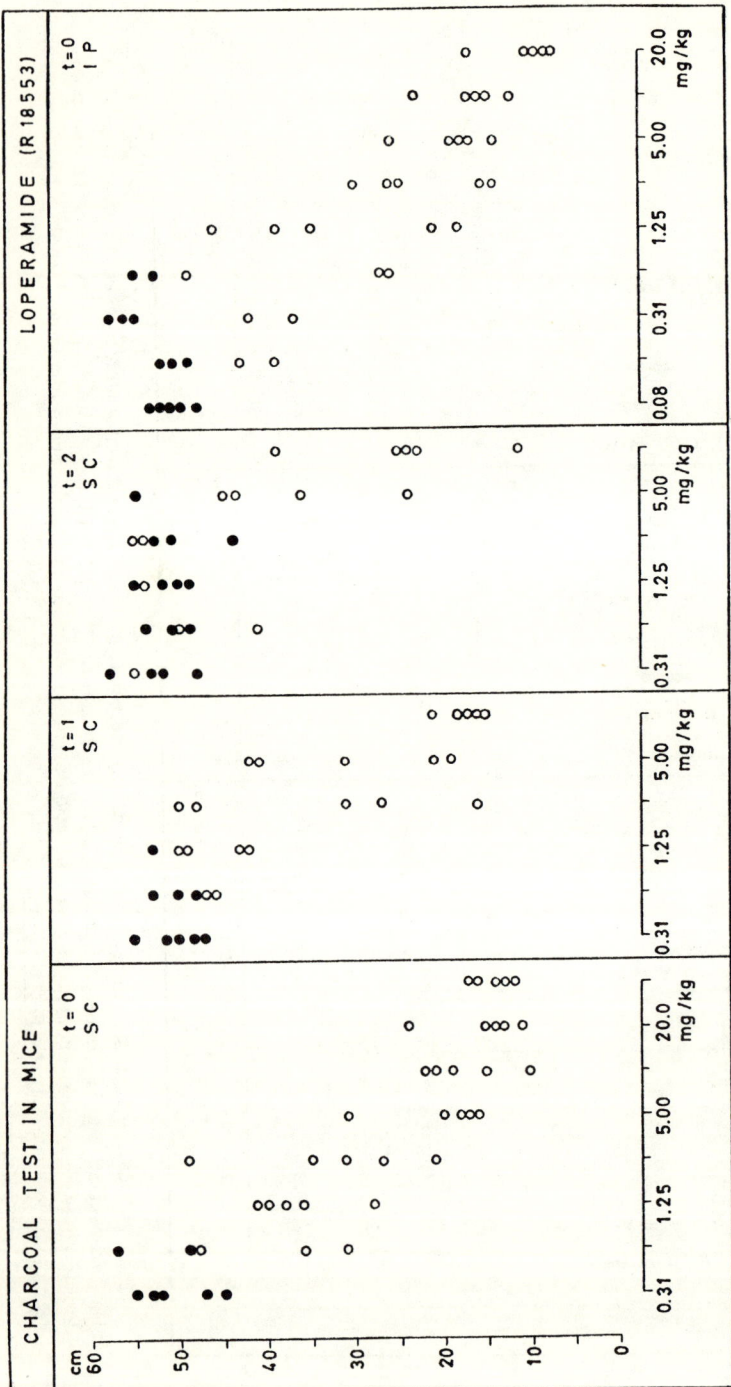

Fig. 22. Charcoal test. Progression in cm of charcoal suspension from stomach to caecum after treatment with different SC and IP doses of loperamide, immediately (t = 0), 1 hr (t = 1), and 2 hr (t = 2) before charcoal. Black circles: charcoal present in caecum, open circles: caecum protected from charcoal. Each point represents one mouse. Source: Arzneimittel-Forsch. 24, 1638 (1974), permission granted.

TABLE 7
Inhibition of Gastrointestinal Motility in Mice after Parenteral Administration of Morphine, Codeine, Diphenoxylate, and Loperamide[a]

Dose, mg/kg	Morphine					Codeine					Diphenoxylate					Loperamide				
	SC			IP		SC			IP		SC			IP		SC			IP	
	t=0	t=1	t=2	t=0		t=0	t=1	t=2	t=0		t=0	t=1	t=2	t=0		t=0	t=1	t=2	t=0	
0.08	—	—	—	—		—	—	—	—		—	—	—	—		—	—	—	—	
0.16	—	—	—	—		—	—	—	—		—	—	—	0		—	—	—	2	
0.31	—	—	—	—		—	—	—	—		—	—	—	2		0	0	1	2	
0.63	—	—	—	—		—	—	—	—		—	—	0	0		3	2	2	3	
1.25	0	0	—	—		—	—	—	—		—	—	3	3		5	4	1	5	
2.50	1	1	—	1		—	—	—	1		—	0	2	2		5	5	2	5	
5.00	5	1	—	3		0	0	1	1		2	2	2	4		5	5	4	5	
10.0	5	2	0	5		2	1	2	3		1[b]	4	4[b]	5[b]		5	5	5	5	
20.0	5	3	0	5		2	3	2	4		5[b]	5[b]	2[b]	5[b]		5	5	—	5	
40.0	5	5	3	5		5	5	3	5		5[b]	4[b]	4[b]	5[b]		5	5	—	5	
80.0	5	—	3	5		5	5	3	—		5[b]	4[b]	4[b]	5[b]		5[c]	—	—	—	
160	5	—	5	5		5	—	3	—		4	5	3	5[b]		2[c]	—	—	—	
320	5	—	—	—		—	—	—	—		—	—	—	5		—	—	—	—	
640	5	—	—	—		—	—	—	—		—	—	—	—		—	—	—	—	
1280	—	—	—	—		—	—	—	—		—	—	—	—		—	—	—	—	
ED_{50}	5.95	22.0	92.5	8.10		34.2	32.5	50.0	16.4		14.1	6.15	4.50	1.49		0.59	0.77	1.93	0.35	
LL	4.32	11.2	45.5	5.16		20.3	18.5	20.9	8.95		10.6	3.82	2.58	0.63		0.39	0.44	0.94	0.17	
UL	8.19	43.5	188	12.7		57.5	57.2	120	30.1		18.8	9.87	7.85	3.46		0.89	1.34	3.98	0.71	

Source: Arzneimittel-Forsch. 24, 1638 (1974); permission granted.

[a] Number of mice, out of five, protected from charcoal in the caecum.
[b] Aqueous suspension not included for calculating the ED_{50}'s, except 20 mg/kg SC for t = 0.
[c] Three mice died.

Figures 19-22 show the detailed results obtained with different subcutaneous (SC) and intraperitoneal (IP) doses of morphine, codeine, diphenoxylate, and loperamide at different time intervals after injection. Charcoal progression in the intestine allows a comparative evaluation of the degree of inhibition of gastrointestinal motility for the different compounds.

For the different dose of each compound Table 7 shows the number of mice protected from charcoal in the caecum and the calculated ED_{50}'s with fiducial limits.

In a preliminary experiment on behavioral morphine-like effects, 10 narcotic analgesics were subcutaneously injected at a selected dose, each to three mice; 1/2, 1, 1 1/2, 2, 2 1/2, and 3 hr thereafter the mice were observed during a 2-min period. Table 8 shows, for each compound, the number of line crossings counted during the 2-min observation period with the highest motility and the presence (+) or absence (-) of Straub tail or arched back.

In 70 control mice, injected with saline or 10% aqueous propylene glycol, the mean number of line crossings obtained during the 2-min period with the highest motility was 4.43 ± 0.59. The highest number ever reached in control mice, during a 2-min period was 32. Straub tail on arched back were never observed.

TABLE 8

Behavioral Morphine-like Effects with 10 Selected Morphine-like Compounds[a]

Compound	Dose, SC mg/kg	Number of line crossings			Presence of Straub tail on arched back		
		1	2	3	1	2	3
Fentanyl (R 4263)	0.63	95	93	106	+	+	+
Dextromoramide (R 875)	2.50	80	89	92	+	+	+
Phenazocine	2.50	78	65	70	+	+	+
Phenoperidine (R 1406)	2.50	76	68	108	+	+	+
Methadone	10.0	25	88	87	+	+	+
Anileridine	40.0	122	83	114	+	+	+
Morphine	40.0	110	77	75	+	+	+
Pethidine	40.0	42	11	90	+	+	+
Piritramide (R 3365)	40.0	60	51	60	+	+	+
Codeine	160	76	32	83	+	+	+
Solvent	0.2 ml	7	2	9	−	−	−

Source: Arzneimittel-Forsch. 24, 1639 (1974); permission granted.

[a] Three mice per compound.

[b] In 2-min period with highest motility.

TABLE 9

Mean Number of Line Crossings[a] and Standard Errors Obtained during a 2-min Observation Period with the Highest Motility after Parenteral Administration of Morphine, Codeine, Diphenoxylate, and Loperamide

Dose, mg/kg	Morphine		Codeine		Diphenoxylate		Loperamide	
	SC	IP	SC	IP	SC	IP	SC	IP
0.08	—	—	—	—	—	—	—	3.60 ± 0.75
0.16	—	—	—	—	—	—	—	3.20 ± 0.92
0.31	—	—	—	—	—	4.90 ± 0.97	8.87 ± 2.06	3.40 ± 1.03
0.63	—	—	—	—	—	6.70 ± 1.37	7.00 ± 1.51	3.00 ± 1.34
1.25	—	—	—	—	—	5.70 ± 1.50	8.40 ± 2.00	4.20 ± 1.28
2.50	5.40 ± 1.21	—	—	—	—	4.10 ± 0.75	4.80 ± 1.64	3.00 ± 0.95
5.00	15.6 ± 2.60	14.6 ± 4.65	—	4.80 ± 1.59	—	4.10 ± 1.07	3.13 ± 0.82	5.40 ± 1.66
10.0	20.0 ± 3.20	7.80 ± 2.25	6.70 ± 0.91	2.00 ± 0.55	2.40 ± 0.68	5.70 ± 1.44	4.40 ± 1.15	2.20 ± 1.96
20.0	57.7 ± 7.73	39.2 ± 18.8	10.7 ± 3.19	1.80 ± 0.80	5.60 ± 1.75	6.90 ± 1.46	3.20 ± 1.24	3.00 ± 2.51
40.0	124 ± 12.2	34.2 ± 13.3	8.53 ± 2.52	3.60 ± 1.17	6.80 ± 1.20	13.2 ± 6.59	1.00 ± 0.77	—
80.0	95.7 ± 8.76	99.6 ± 30.0	12.9 ± 2.88	11.4 ± 6.52	7.00 ± 1.00	18.0 ± 8.00	—	—
160	117 ± 10.5	117 ± 16.4	53.8 ± 10.2	35.0	7.40 ± 1.72	37.2 ± 11.6	2.50	—
320	95.3 ± 4.19	72.0 ± 18.1	—	—	6.40 ± 2.60	75.1 ± 14.7	—	—
640	53.4 ± 14.4	80.0	—	—	11.6 ± 3.37	25.9 ± 8.26	—	—

Source: Arzneim-Forsch. 24, 1639 (1974); permission granted.
[a]The number of treated mice per dose level are given in Table 6.

The results obtained with different SC and IP doses of morphine, codeine, diphenoxylate, and loperamide are shown in Table 9. The mean number of line crossings allows a comparative evaluation of the degree of rotary-motor excitement induced by the different compounds. Table 10 shows, for different doses of each compound, the number of mice with "Straub tail on arched back" and the calculated ED_{50}'s with fiducial limits.

Table 11 shows the comparative ED_{50} values with fiducial limits of morphine, codeine, diphenoxylate, and loperamide for inhibition of gastrointestinal motility (caecum protected from charcoal) and for morphine-like

TABLE 10

Morphine-like Behavioral Effects after Parenteral Administration in Mice of Morphine, Codeine, Diphenoxylate, and Loperamide[a]

Dose, mg/kg	Morphine		Codeine		Diphenoxylate		Loperamide	
	SC	IP	SC	IP	SC	IP	SC	IP
0.08	–	–	–	–	–	–	–	0/5
0.16	–	–	–	–	–	0/10	–	0/5
0.31	–	–	–	–	–	0/10	0/15	0/5
0.63	–	–	–	–	–	0/10	0/15	0/5
1.25	–	–	–	–	0/5	0/10	0/15	0/5
2.50	0/5	–	–	–	0/10	0/10	0/15	0/5
5.00	1/10	1/5	–	0/5	0/15	0/10	0/15	0/5
10.0	7/10	0/5	0/15	0/5	0/15	0/10	0/15	0/5
20.0	15/15	3/5	1/15	0/5	1/15[b]	2/10[b]	0/5	0/5
40.0	15/15	5/5	3/15	0/5	1/15[b]	2/10[b]	0/5	–
80.0	15/15	5/5	7/15	2/5	0/15[b]	7/10[b]	0/2	–
160	10/10	5/5	11/14	1/1	1/15[b]	9/10[b]	–	–
320	10/10	3/3	–	–	–	5/10[c]	–	–
640	5/5	1/1	–	–	–	–	–	–
ED_{50}	8.10	16.5	81.0	≈80.0	>160	57.5	Inactive at	
LL	6.66	8.65	56.9			36.0	80.0	20.0
UL	9.85	31.5	115			92.0		

Source: Arzneimittel-Forsch. 24, 1639 (1974), permission granted.

[a] Ratio of "Straub on arched back" to number of mice treated.
[b] Micronized suspension
[c] Not included for calculating the ED_{50}.

TABLE 11

Comparative ED_{50} Values with Fiducial Limits of Morphine, Codeine, Diphenoxylate, and Loperamide for Inhibition of Gastrointestinal Motility[a] and for Morphine-like Behavior;[b] LD_{50} Values with Fiducial Limits[c]

Experimental procedures			Morphine	Codeine	Diphenoxylate	Loperamide
Gastrointestinal motility	SC	t = 0	5.95 (4.32–8.19)	34.2 (20.3–57.5)	14.1 (10.6–18.8)	0.59 (0.39–0.89)
		t = 1	22.0 (11.1–43.5)	32.5 (18.5–57.2)	6.15 (3.83–9.87)	0.77 (0.44–1.34)
		t = 2	92.5 (45.5–188)	50.0 (20.9–120)	4.50 (2.58–7.85)	1.93 (0.94–3.98)
	IP	t = 0	8.10 (5.16–12.7)	16.4 (8.95–30.1)	1.49 (0.64–3.46)	0.35 (0.17–0.71)
Morphine-like behavior	SC		8.10 (6.66–9.85)	81.0 (56.9–115)	>160	Inactive at 80.0[d]
	IP		16.5 (8.65–31.5)	≃80.0	57.5 (36.0–92.0)	Inactive at 20.0[e]
Acute toxicity	SC		900 (726–1116)	205 (172–244)	Atoxic at 160	75.0 (55.8–109)
	IP		390 (221–960)	135 (92.6–197)	Atoxic at 320	28.0 (20.7–37.9)

Source: Arzneimittel-Forsch. 24, 1640 (1974), permission granted.

[a]Caecum protected from charcoal.
[b]Straub on arched back.
[c]Mortality within 3–5 hr after injection of the compound.
[d]Toxic dose.
[e]Highest atoxic dose.

behavior (Straub on arched back). In the same table the LD_{50} values with fiducial limits (mortality within 3 to 5 hr) of the compounds are compared.

Morphine hydrochloride: the lowest ED_{50} blocking gastrointestinal motility is 5.95 (4.32-8.19) mg/kg SC and 8.10 (6.66-9.85) mg/kg IP. Characteristic morphine-like behavior was observed in 50% of the mice at 8.10 (6.66-9.85) mg/kg SC and at 16.5 (8.65-31.5) mg/kg IP. Morphine is somewhat more toxic IP [LD_{50} = 390 (221-960) mg/kg] than SC [LD_{50} = 900 (726-1116) mg/kg]. Thus, morphine has no specific gastrointestinal blocking activity in mice, the difference between the inhibition of the gastrointestinal motility and the central effects being 1 : 1.4 SC and 1 : 2.0 IP. The safety ratios (lowest ED_{50}/LD_{50}) for morphine are 1 : 151 SC and 1 : 48 IP.

Codeine phosphate: the lowest ED_{50} affecting gastrointestinal motility is 32.5 (18.5-57.2) mg/kg SC and 16.4 (8.95-30.1) mg/kg IP. In the same mice the ED_{50} values obtained for characteristic morphine-like behavior were 81.0 (56.9-115) mg/kg SC and ≃80.0 mg/kg IP. The LD_{50}'s for codeine were 205 (92.6-197) mg/kg SC and 135 (92.6-197) mg/kg IP. The difference between the gastrointestinal-inhibiting properties and the central effects of codeine is somewhat more pronounced than that obtained with morphine, i.e., 1 : 2.5 SC and 1 : 4.9 IP. Codeine in mice is much more toxic than morphine, the safety ratios being 1 : 6.3 SC and 1 : 8.2 IP.

Diphenoxylate hydrochloride: the lowest ED_{50}'s inhibiting gastrointestinal motility are 4.50 (2.58-7.85) mg/kg SC and 1.49 (0.64-3.46) mg IP. In the same mice the ED_{50}'s obtained for characteristic morphine-like behavior were >160 mg/kg SC and 57.5 (36.0-92.0) mg/kg IP. Mortality was not observed within the dose range tested (highest doses 160 SC and 320 IP). The slow resorption of the diphenoxylate suspensions could be responsible for the lack of typical morphine-like behavioral effects after SC administration. Diphenoxylate can be considered as a specific inhibitor of gastrointestinal motility, the dissociation between the inhibition of gastrointestinal motility and the eliciting of morphinelike behavioral effects being 1 : 71 IP and more than 1 : 39 SC. Furthermore, diphenoxylate is atoxic in mice SC and IP, as far as immediate toxicity is concerned.

Loperamide hydrochloride: the lowest ED_{50} inhibiting gastrointestinal motility is 0.59 (0.39-0.89) mg/kg SC and 0.35 (0.17-0.71) mg/kg IP. Typical morphine-like behavior could not be induced with loperamide. Neither a SC toxic dose of 80.0 mg/kg (three mice out of five died), i.e., 136 times the ED_{50} for inhibition of gastrointestinal motility, nor the highest atoxic IP dose of 20 mg/kg (57 times the ED_{50} dose for inhibiting gastrointestinal motility) was able to induce morphine-like behavioral effects. Moreover, in mice loperamide is relatively atoxic with a safety margin of 1 : 127 SC and 1 : 80 IP.

Inhibition of gastrointestinal motility using the "charcoal test" has been described previously (Janssen et al., 1959b). Morphine-like rotary motor excitement in mice (Krueger et al., 1941) is a very characteristic and well-known central effect induced by all morphine-like compounds, as is shown by the results summarized in Table 6. The tail is erected on the arched back in an S-shape (Straub tail) and excitement is characterized by a compulsive circling movement. The turning is either clockwise, counter clockwise, or alternates in both directions. The circling may be fast or slow, continuous or interrupted by short or long intervals of immobility during which the animal exhibits a typical crouched appearance which persists even when it is in motion.

Loperamide is found to be a potent inhibitor of gastrointestinal motility in mice via both the SC and IP route. Subcutaneously, loperamide is 7.6 times more potent than diphenoxylate, 10 times more potent than morphine, and 55 times more potent than codeine. Intraperitoneally, loperamide is 4.3 times more potent than diphenoxylate, 23 times more potent than morphine, and 47 times more potent than codeine. As shown in Table 7, loperamide in mice has a fast onset and a long duration of action (ED_{50} charcoal SCT = 0 : 0.59 mg/kg; ED_{50} charcoal SCT = 2 : 1.93 mg/kg). Loperamide in mice is devoid of morphine-like behavioral effects. Induction of morphine-like behavior could not be obtained even at toxic dose levels. These findings indicate that loperamide differs considerably from all known potent antidiarrheals. With reference to the conclusion reached in the previous section, it is suggested that loperamide represents a novel type of antidiarrheal drug.

1.3. SUMMARY

An attempt was made to select the most appropriate method for the reliable detection of antidiarrheal drug activity in laboratory animals. The castor-oil test in rats appeared to be an adequate method which made it possible to study antidiarrheal activity for large numbers of compounds

The RAS concept expresses the dissociation between antidiarrheal and analgesic drug effects in rats. Subsequent investigations in mice, conducted as a comparative study of the inhibition of gastrointestinal motility and narcotic behavioral effects, confirmed that loperamide is the prototype of a novel class of antidiarrheal agents. The most essential characteristic of this class of drugs is their complete lack of narcotic-like central effects, even when tested up to subtoxic dose levels. Moreover loperamide and fluperamide possess, besides very pronounced antidiarrheal potency, a considerable longer duration of action as compared with diphenoxylate, difenoxin, and other compounds of this class.

IV.2. IN VITRO PHARMACOLOGY: STUDY OF THE PERISTALTIC REFLEX AND OTHER EXPERIMENTS ON ISOLATED TISSUES

Jan M. Van Nueten and Jeanine Fontaine

2.1. INTRODUCTION

As pointed out in Chapter II, diarrhea can be caused by abnormal intestinal motility. Increased propulsion of the intestinal content is one kind of disordered intestinal motility that results directly in diarrhea. Yet, as several factors may be involved in this phenomenon, the actual pathophysiology is not always entirely understood.

Questions concerning the mode of action of antidiarrheal drugs can only be answered if the patterns of intestinal motility are sufficiently known. It is necessary, therefore, to study these patterns using appropriate methods that give reliable and reproducible results. Propulsion of the intraluminal content of the gut is produced mainly by the peristaltic movements of the intestine, due to coordinated contractions of the longitudinal and circular muscle coat. Therefore our investigations should be focused on these peristaltic movements.

In 1899, Bayliss and Starling observed that peristalsis was elicited by local stimuli and controlled by local nervous mechanisms. In 1904, Magnus discovered the influence of intraluminal pressure on the intestinal movements and in 1917 Trendelenburg was the first to set up a systematic study of the peristaltic reflex on guinea-pig ileum.

Further in vitro methods have made it possible to standardize the experimental conditions and study the gut disconnected from the central nervous system. So far, studies have shown similarities in the patterns of peristalsis of the small intestines of different species such as dog, cat, guinea-pig, rabbit, and man.

In the course of the last 10 yr, the study of peristalsis has been intensified and numerous review articles and reports have been published (Kosterlitz and Lees, 1964; Kottegoda, 1970; Bortoff, 1972; Frigo et al., 1972; Bennett and Misiewicz, 1973; Daniel, 1973; and others).

Trendelenburg's method has been improved repeatedly and a number of phenomena occurring during induced peristaltic reflex are now measured quite accurately (Van Nueten et al., 1973; Fontaine and Van Nueten, 1976).

The coordinated reflex response of the gut to distension, called "peristalsis," is mediated by nervous mechanisms of the intestinal wall and results in the propulsion of the contents. Radial distension is the mechanical stimulus activating the sensory receptors located in the mucosa or the submucosa. The exact site is still unknown. When the intestinal lumen is distended slowly, the longitudinal muscle contracts first shortening the intestine (preparatory phase). Thereafter the circular muscle is activated. Its contraction travels like a wave in the aboral direction, expelling the contents of the gut (emptying phase). Meanwhile the longitudinal muscle relaxes. There is sufficient evidence to show that in the longitudinal reflex the neuromuscular transmission is only partially cholinergic and that the involvement of a noncholinergic synapse, or even the absence of a synapse, must be assumed. An important part of this reflex may be due to a noncholinergic transmitter of unknown structure. Prostaglandins seem to have a role in motility (Bennett et al., 1968a; 1968b). Recently, we observed that the prostaglandins E_1 and E_2 potentiate the noncholinergic part of the longitudinal reflex response of the guinea-pig ileum (Fontaine et al., 1976).

On the other hand, it appears that one or several cholinergic synapses are involved in the circular reflex response and in the propulsion of the intestinal content. Furthermore, intramural ganglia (Auerbach's plexus) seem to be important for the activity of the circular muscle layer. Here again an unknown inhibitory transmitter has been postulated so far. The physiological significance of the inhibition of circular muscle response observed with prostaglandins (Bennett et al., 1968b, Fontaine et al., 1976) remains an open question.

Our method makes it possible to study the mechanism of action of antidiarrheal compounds producing constipation by direct local effects on the gastrointestinal wall. The results obtained with diphenoxylate, difenoxin, and loperamide are reported here. In addition to the study on peristaltic reflex, the three compounds have been compared in miscellaneous experiments on isolated tissues.

Diphenoxylate, a well-known therapeutic agent in acute and chronic diarrhea (Winkelstein, 1961), is a potent inhibitor of the peristaltic reflex activity of the guinea-pig ileum in vitro (Van Nueten, 1968) and was shown to retard small-bowel propulsion in rats without influencing gastric evacuation (Nilsson and Johansson, 1973). Difenoxin was found to be a potent antidiarrheal agent in humans (Van Wijngaarden and Soudijn, 1972), more active than the parent diphenoxylate (Rubens et al., 1972) and was also a very potent inhibitor of peristaltic activity in vitro (Van Nueten and Janssen, 1972). Loperamide, is a new highly potent and orally long-acting antidiarrheal agent (Demeulenaere et al., 1974). As an inhibitor of peristaltic activity in vitro, loperamide acts rapidly with long-lasting effects (Van Nueten et al., 1974).

2.2. METHODS

2.2.1. The Induction and Inhibition of Peristaltic Activity

The experimental set-up is shown in Fig. 23. A nonterminal ileum segment (a), 7 cm in length, taken from a guinea-pig of 300-400 g weight is suspended in a Tyrode solution (b) at 37 °C. The guinea-pig is starved overnight before being killed. The open aboral end of the segment is connected to a glass tube (c) and the closed end to a Grass force transducer (f), allowing isometric recording of longitudinal muscle contractions. The glass tube is connected, via PVC (d)* and glass tubing (e), to a pressure bottle (l). Ileum segment, tubing, and pressure bottle are filled with a Tyrode solution. The glass bypass (h) is used to discard air and is closed afterwards with a stopcock. Pressure in the tubing and hence in the lumen of the ileum segment, is measured with a Statham pressure transducer (g). Gradual lifting of the pressure bottle with a servomotor (m) causes a linear increase in pressure in the lumen of the ileum and at the same time a filling of the ileum segment. The result is radial distension. By this mechanical stimulus, the sensory receptors are activated and this, in turn, results in coordinated contractions and relaxations of longitudinal and, after a few seconds, of circular muscle layers. The peristaltic movements are these repeated contractions and relaxations (cycles) which produce the expulsion of fluid from the ileum segment. Such induced peristaltic waves travel from the top to the aboral end of the segment and the resulting volume displacement ends up in the tubing, where it can be measured with an ultrasonic transit-time device (Geivers et al., 1974).

The measurement is made as follows: before the experiment, an air bubble (i), 2 cm in length, is introduced into the glass tubing (e) via the bypass with stopcock (j), as far as 3 cm from the crystal (k) of the transit-time device. The precise location of the air bubble is established by measuring the transit time of an ultrasonic wave travelling from the crystal to the air bubble and back. Volume displacement can be determined by measuring the distance which the air bubble travels in the tube. Flow rate is the volume displacement per unit of time determined with a differentiator.

In our experiments the pressure in the lumen of the segment was linearly increased from -5 to 20 mm H_2O in 50 sec. After the pressure had been maintained at this level for 100 sec, it was reduced linearly to -5 mm

---

*Polyvinylchloride (Tygon).

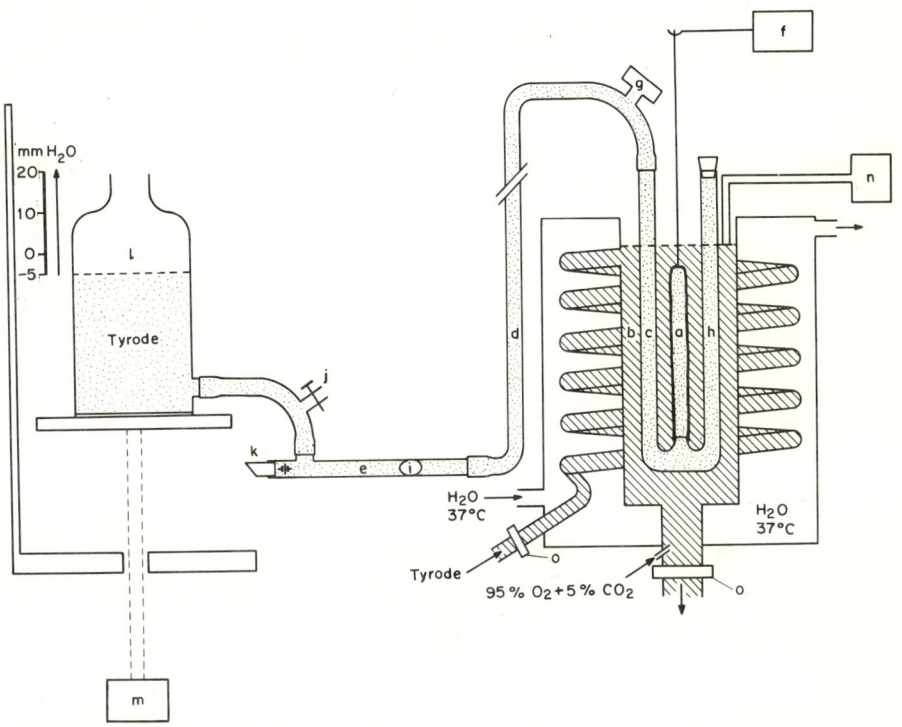

Fig. 23. Schematic diagram of the apparatus used in the study of peristaltic reflex: (a) guinea-pig ileum segment; (b) thermostatically controlled bath; (c) glass tube; (d) PVC tubing; (e) glass tubing; (f) force transducer; (g) pressure transducer; (h) glass bypass to discard air; (i) air bubble; (j) PVC bypass with stopcock; (k) crystal; (l) pressure bottle; (m) servo motor; (n) fluid level control; (o) electromagnetic valves.

H_2O and the bath fluid replaced. This sequence of pressure increase and pressure decrease is called a run. An experimental run consisted of a series of consecutive peristaltic cycles and was repeated seven times in one experiment at $7\frac{1}{2}$ min interval. One complete run is shown in Fig. 24. Runs 1-3 are control runs.

Inhibitory effects were studied in the presence of the drug during run 4 (3-min contact period) and, after removal of the substance, during runs 5 to 7 (up to 29 min).

The entire device was operated by a programmer designed especially for these experiments.

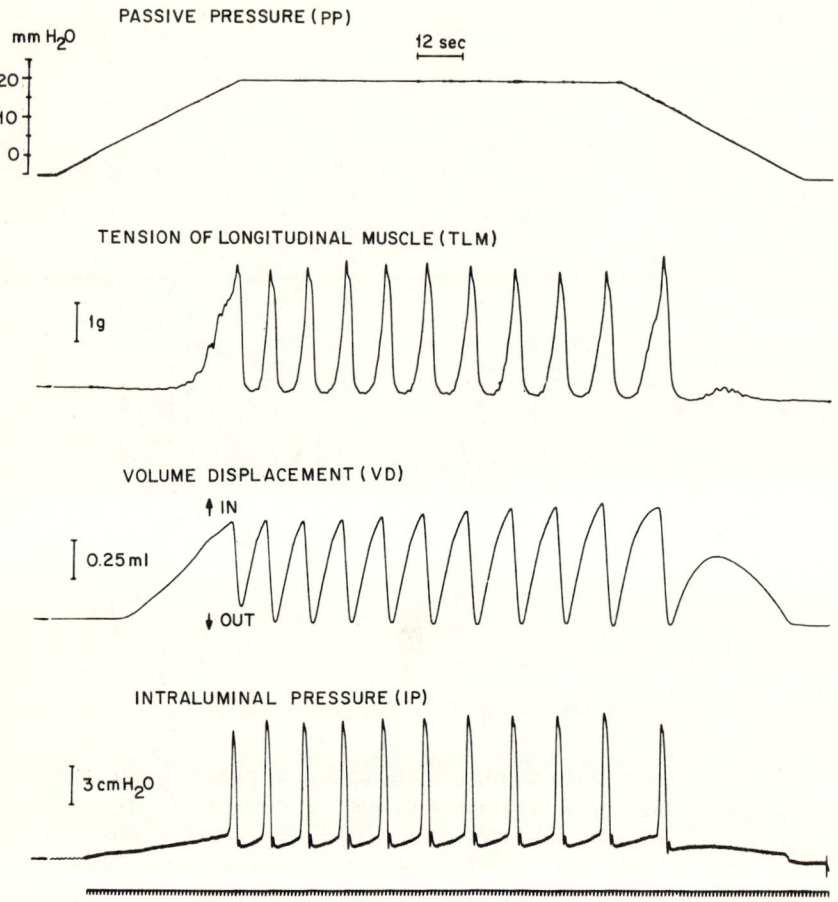

Fig. 24. Peristaltic reflex of guinea-pig ileum; one complete run.

2.2.2. Miscellaneous Experiments on Isolated Tissues

The interaction of drug (3-5 min contact time) and various agonists was studied on guinea-pig ileum, rabbit duodenum, rabbit spleen, and rat fundus, using single supramaximal doses of the agonists. Histamine antagonism was studied using cumulative doses, which produced dose-related contraction (Van Rossum, 1963; Janssen et al., 1968).

Isoprenaline induced a relaxation on the hen rectal caecum and on the guinea-pig trachea, the latter being in contraction in the presence of methacholine. Drug effects were studied after an incubation period of 30 min.

A possible direct effect on tonus could be observed on hen rectal caecum and on rabbit duodenum.

The influence on the response of guinea-pig ileum to coaxial stimulation was also studied. Strips 6 cm in length were cut from guinea-pig ileum and suspended in a 100-ml Krebs-Henseleit bath (37.5°C; pH 7.3) with an initial load of 1 g and gassed with a 95% O_2 and 5% CO_2 mixture.

Transmural excitation was applied over the whole length of the ileum strip by means of two platinum electrodes (0.5 mm diameter); the anode was threaded through the lumen of the ileum and the cathode dipped into the physiological solution parallel to the strip (Paton, 1955; Van Nueten et al., 1974).

The preparation was excited with single rectangular stimuli of 1 msec duration and submaximal intensity at a frequency of six per min, resulting in contractions.

The upper end of the ileum strip was connected to a strain-gauge transducer for isometric recording of contractions.

Drug effect was observed for 15 min and expressed in percent of the response before adding the compound.

In experiments on heart tissues, right ventricular papillary muscles from cat hearts, dissected under light ether anaesthesia, were suspended in oxygenated Tyrode (37°C) containing 2 mg/ml of glucose, with optimal preload, i.e., the preload at which the isometric force development is maximal for a given stimulus.

Muscles were excited with rectangular stimuli of supramaximal intensity and 5 msec duration at a frequency of 60/min. Tension development was measured isometrically with a Grass force transducer. The effect of three cumulative concentrations of the compounds was determined after a 30-min incubation period for each of the concentrations.

Chronotropic effects were determined on the spontaneously beating right atria of the guinea-pig, prepared as described by Black et al. (1965), during a 30-min incubation period with the three compounds. Following this period the effect on the increase in rate produced by linearly increased doses of isoprenaline or histamine were studied on the same preparation.

Drugs were studied at concentrations of the 0.00016, 0.00031 ... 5, 10 mg-per-liter series. The solvent was water (for loperamide and diphenoxylate), or water containing 10 mg per liter of sodium carboxymethylcellulose and 5 mg per liter of polysorbate 80 (for difenoxin).

The volume added to the organ bath was 0.25 ml (0.25%) in the study on peristaltic reflex and 1 ml (1%) in the other experiments.

Six experiments per dose and six or more control experiments were performed in all studies.

A 50% inhibition of the agonist-induced response was used as criterion for effectiveness and these ED_{50} values with confidence limits were determined by probit analysis. Analysis of the results, obtained using the cumulative-dose technique used for the study of histamine-antagonism, was performed according to Arunlakshana and Schild (1959). pA_{10} is the negative logarithm of the molar concentration of the antagonist, which produces a ten-fold shift to the right of the dose-responsive curve for the agonist. pA_h is the negative logarithm of the molar concentration of the antagonist which depressed the maximum of the dose-response curve for the agonist by 50%.

2.3. RESULTS

2.3.1. Inhibition of Peristaltic Activity

Diphenoxylate, difenoxin, and loperamide appear to be inhibitors of the peristaltic reflex activity on the guinea-pig ileum; this effect is dose-related.

The total amount of fluid expelled by the intestinal segment during the successive reflex waves of a given experimental run was selected as a quantitative measure for effectiveness. The ED_{50} value is the dose, in mg per liter, which produces a 50% decrease in this total expelled amount as compared with the quantity measured in the control run 3 recorded before adding the drug. It was calculated for the run in which peak effect was noted.

The calculated ED_{50} values with the 95% fiducial limits are listed in Table 12 in order of decreasing activity.

Unlike the slow-acting diphenoxylate, both difenoxin and loperamide were fast-acting. On the other hand, whereas difenoxin effects were readily reversed, both loperamide and diphenoxylate produced a long-lasting effect.

As shown in Table 13 and Fig. 25 diphenoxylate induced inhibition progressed in the course of time even after replacement of the bath fluid. This was

TABLE 12

Inhibition of Peristaltic Reflex

Compound	ED_{50} mg/liter	Lower and upper fiducial limits	Run
Difenoxin	0.0015	0.0008-0.0028	4
Loperamide	0.007	0.004-0.014	5
Diphenoxylate	0.097	0.059-0.160	7

TABLE 13

Inhibition of Peristaltic Reflex Activity on Guinea-pig Ileum by Diphenoxylate, Difenoxin, and Loperamide [a]

Dose, mg/liter	Diphenoxylate				Difenoxin				Loperamide			
	Run 4	Run 5	Run 6	Run 7	Run 4	Run 5	Run 6	Run 7	Run 4	Run 5	Run 6	Run 7
0	3.90	5.45	7.70	9.60	3.90	5.45	7.70	9.60	3.65	5.45	6.80	8.37
0.00016					10.70	15.10[b]	11.70	6.55				
0.00031					11.50[b]	16.55[b]	6.60	1.45				
0.00063					17.10[b]	12.85[b]	14.55	19.85				
0.00125					58.20[b]	9.65	5.60	2.55	1.90	0.50	5.65	6.90
0.0025					68.35[d]	34.20[c]	26.65[b]	21.05[b]	10.45	10.20	14.0	17.50
0.005					95.90[d]	75.10[d]	42.30[b]	23.85	40.80[d]	44.0[d]	41.0[d]	36.05[d]
0.01									59.80[d]	76.85[d]	67.90[d]	58.20[d]
0.02	2.95	5.85	16.25	15.90					97.95[d]	100[d]	100[d]	100[d]
0.04	11.95	9.90[b]	17.20	8.80[c]								
0.08	12.20	20.35[b]	42.75[c]	52.50[d]								
0.16	24.65[c]	60.10[c]	54.85[d]	61.20[d]								
0.31	41.75[d]	100[d]	100[d]	100[d]								
0.63	59.70[d]	98.40[d]	98.05[d]	100[d]								
1.25	80.40[d]	100[d]	96.35	100								

[a] Median (n = 6) percent reduction of volume expelled as compared with control run 3. Significant difference with control experiments was assessed using the Mann-Whitney U-test.

[b] $p \leq 0.05$.
[c] $p \leq 0.01$.
[d] $p \leq 0.001$.

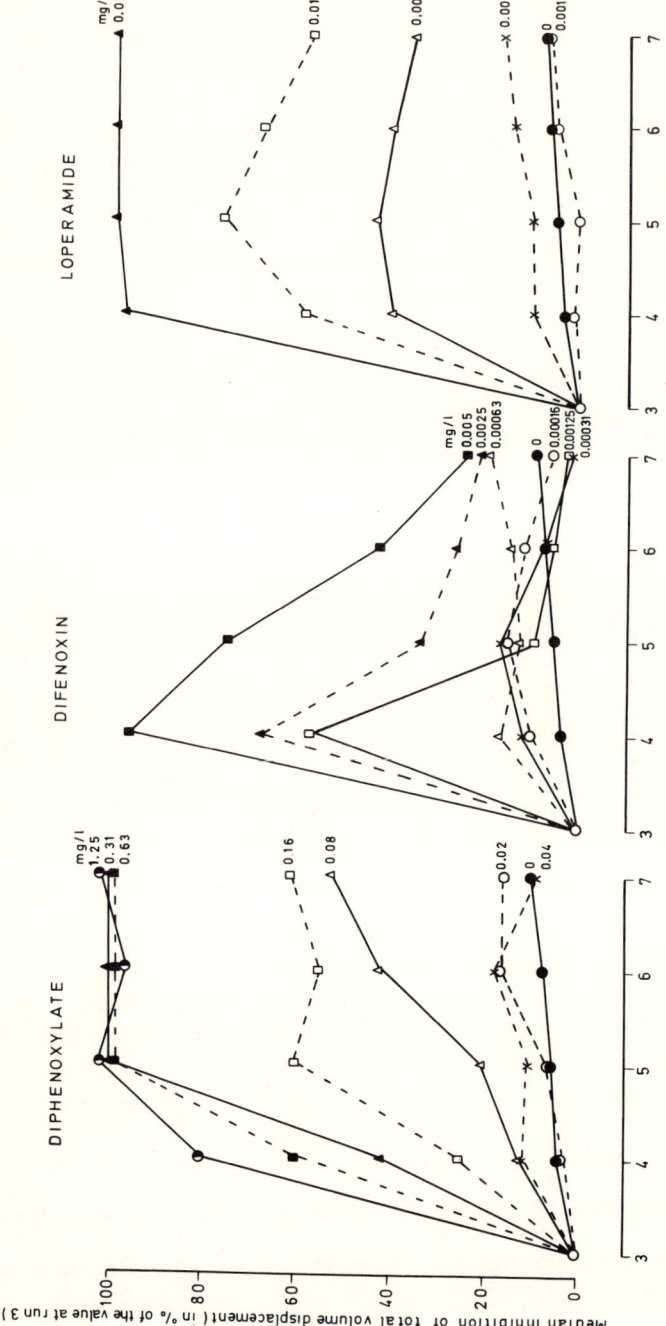

Fig. 25. Median inhibition of peristaltic reflex activity of guinea-pig ileum by diphenoxylate, difenoxin, and loperamide (six experiments per dose). Compounds were added 3 min before run 4 and washed out at the end of the same run. Further washing took place at the end of each subsequent run.

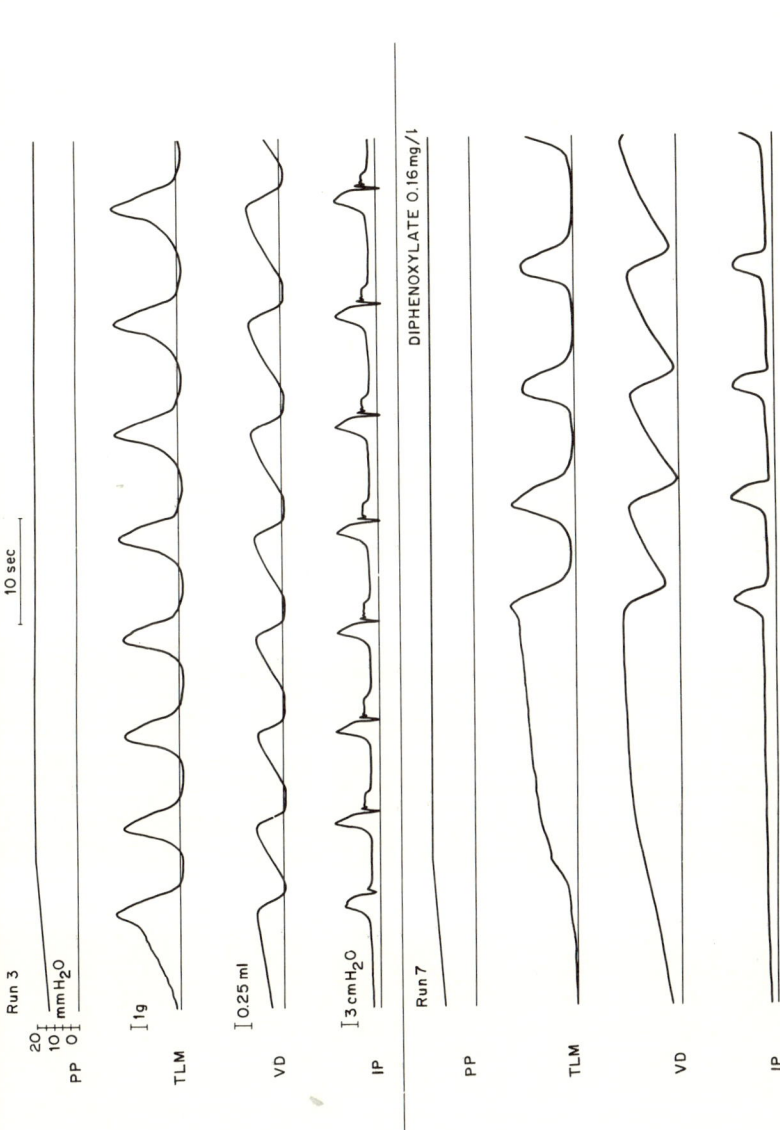

Fig. 26. Inhibition of peristaltic reflex activity of the guinea-pig ileum. Part of a typical experiment before (run 3) and after (run 7) diphenoxylate 0.16 mg/liter. The compound has been washed out at the end of runs 4, 5, and 6. Abbreviations: PP, passive pressure; TLM, tension of longitudinal muscle; VD, volume displacement; IP, intraluminal pressure.

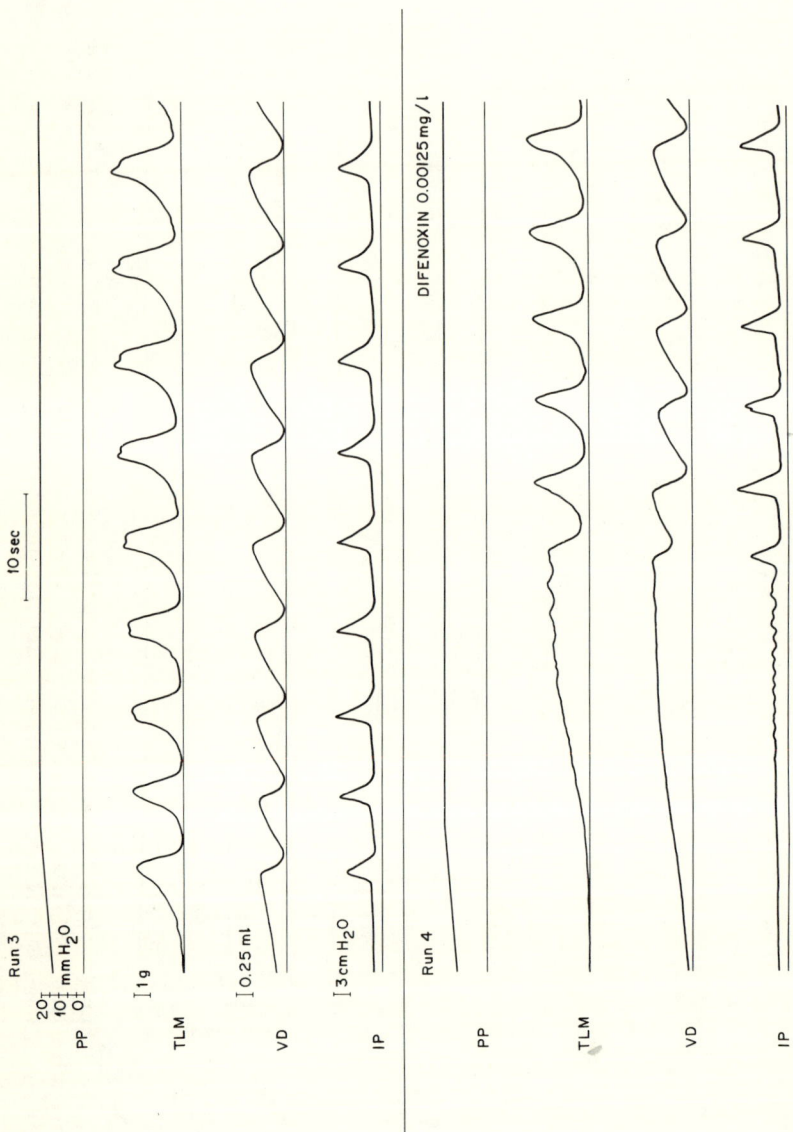

Fig. 27. Inhibition of peristaltic reflex activity of the guinea-pig ileum. Part of a typical experiment before (run 3) and in the presence (run 4) of difenoxin 0.00125 mg/liter. Abbreviations the same as in Fig. 26.

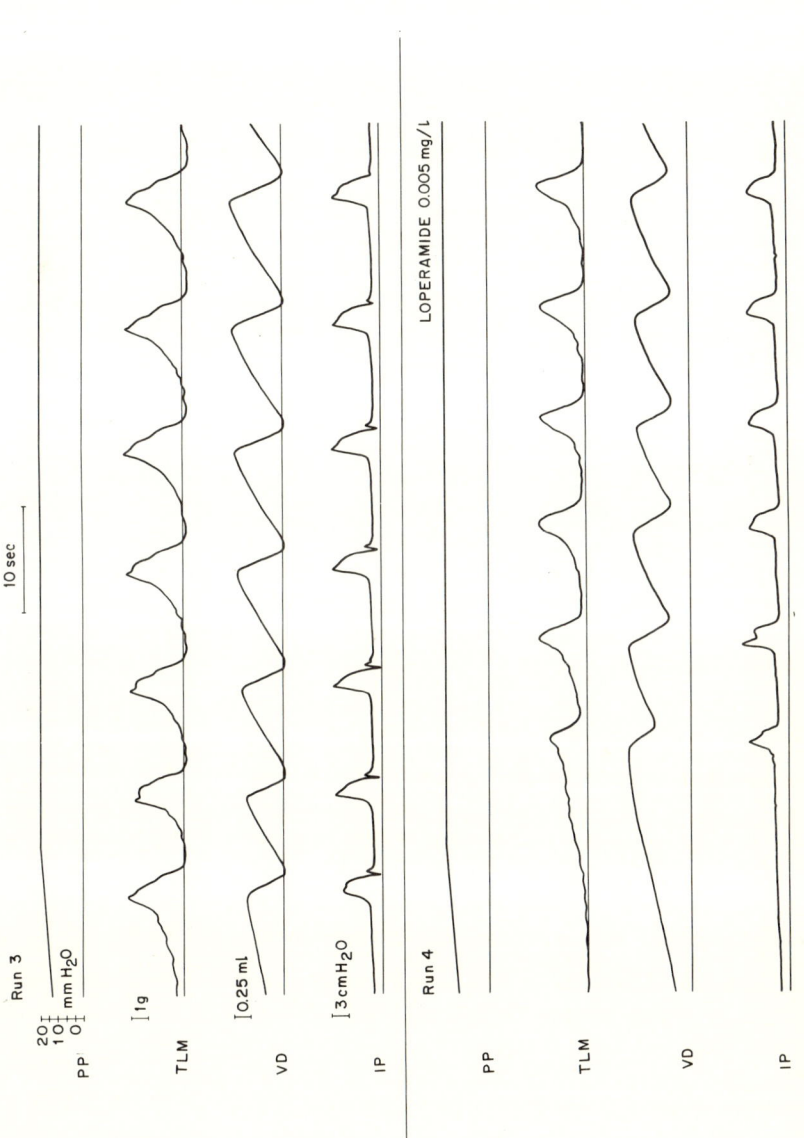

Fig. 28. Inhibition of peristaltic reflex activity of the guinea-pig ileum. Part of a typical experiment before (run 3) and in the presence (run 4) of loperamide 0.005 mg/liter. Abbreviations the same as in Fig. 26.

in contrast to the inhibitory effect of difenoxin, which was rapid in onset but readily reversible by washing. Loperamide effects were in-between, in the sense that its relatively fast onset of action is coupled to a long-lasting effect not reversible by washing.

Typical experiments are shown in Figs. 26-28, in which experimental runs are compared before and after addition of the compounds.

Phenomena observed include a later onset and advanced interruption of peristaltic cycles, together with an increased interval in-between these cycles. These changes from the normal pattern lead to a reduction of the number of cycles per experimental run. Furthermore, the activity of longitudinal and/or circular muscle layers decreased and the amount of fluid expelled per peristaltic cycle was reduced. Whether all or some of these phenomena occurred in a particular experiment was dependent on the dose and on the sensitivity of the intestine.

2.3.2. Interaction with Various Agonists and with the Response to Electrical Stimulation

The results obtained with diphenoxylate, difenoxin, and loperamide are shown in Tables 14 and 15.

The three compounds antagonized the contraction induced in the guinea-pig ileum by coaxial stimulation at doses which produced inhibition of the peristaltic reflex (Fig. 29).

Contractions produced in the same tissue by nicotine were inhibited at about the same low doses.

Diphenoxylate inhibited contractions induced in this tissue by 5-hydroxytryptamine (5-HT) at comparable doses. Antagonism of other agonists was observed at higher (e.g., angiotensin) or massive doses (e.g., histamine and bradykinin), or was absent ($BaCl_2$) in the guinea-pig ileum.

Difenoxin showed relatively little activity against 5-HT and angiotensin and almost none or absolutely none against histamine, bradykinin, and $BaCl_2$.

Loperamide's activity in inhibiting the response to all the agonists studied on guinea-pig ileum was very slight in view of its inhibiting action on the peristaltic reflex.

Cumulative dose-response curves for histamine showed that this unspecific antagonism, occurring at extremely high doses, was competitive for difenoxin, noncompetitive for loperamide, and both competitive and noncompetitive for diphenoxylate (Fig. 30). A 50% depression of the maximum was obtained at 1.25 mg/liter for loperamide (pA_h 5.60), and at 10 mg/liter for diphenoxylate (pA_h 4.69). A tenfold shift to the right of the dose-response curve was obtained for difenoxin at 10 mg/liter (pA_{10} 4.66).

TABLE 14

Inhibitory Activity[a] Against Muscular Response, Induced by Various Agonists In Vitro

Agonist	Test object	Contact time, min	ED_{50} with confidence limits, mg/liter		
			Diphenoxylate	Difenoxin	Loperamide
Coaxial stimulation	Guinea-pig ileum	0–15	0.1118 (0.03528–0.3547)	0.0008 (0.00043–0.00136)	0.0027 (0.00154–0.00487)
Nicotine	Guinea-pig ileum	3	0.3060[b] (0.1107–0.8461)	0.00126 (0.00068–0.00234)	0.0031 (0.00196–0.00517)
Angiotensin	Guinea-pig ileum	3	1.340 (0.415–4.38)	0.2056 (0.0228–1.853)	0.139 (0.0841–0.2306)
5-HT	Guinea-pig ileum	3	0.2718[b] (0.1045–0.7065)	0.0291 (0.0153–0.0554)	0.148 (0.0751–0.2919)
Bradykinin	Guinea-pig ileum	3	10	Inactive up to 10	0.293 (0.1275–0.6701)
$BaCl_2$	Guinea-pig ileum	3	Inactive up to 10	Inactive up to 10	0.580 (0.1251–2.687)
Histamine	Guinea-pig ileum	5	10[d]	10[c]	1.25[d]
5-HT	Rat fundus	3	Inactive up to 10	Inactive up to 10	Inactive up to 10
Epinephrine	Rabbit spleen	3	Inactive up to 10	Inactive up to 10	Inactive up to 10
Norepinephrine	Rabbit spleen	3	Inactive up to 10	Inactive up to 10	Inactive up to 10
Acetylcholine	Rabbit duodenum	3	Inactive up to 10	Inactive up to 10	Inactive up to 10
Isoprenaline	Guinea-pig trachea	30	Inactive up to 10	Inactive up to 10	Inactive up to 10
Isoprenaline	Hen rectal caecum	30	Inactive up to 10	Inactive up to 10	Inactive up to 10

[a] Expressed as ED_{50} values.
[b] Drug effects increased with time: the ED_{50} values given here were calculated after 9 min contact.
[c] Cumulative dose-response curves: 10-fold shift to the right.
[d] Cumulative dose-response curves: 50% depression.

TABLE 15

Ratio of ED_{50} Values for Inhibitory Effects on Guinea-pig Ileum Compared to the Antagonism of Peristaltic Reflex

Agonist	Diphenoxylate	Difenoxin	Loperamide
Peristaltic reflex	1	1	1
Coaxial stimulation	1.15	0.53	0.39
Nicotine	3.15	0.84	0.44
Angiotensin	13.81	137	19.86
5-HT	2.80	19.40	21.14
Bradykinin	103	>6000	41.86
$BaCl_2$	>103	>6000	82.86
Histamine	103	6000	179

The three compounds were inactive against 5-hydroxytryptamine on the rat-fundus preparation, and were devoid of α- or β-adrenergic blocking activity and of anticholinergic activity at concentrations as high as 10 mg/liter.

A pronounced decrease in tonus was observed on the hen rectal caecum with loperamide and difenoxin at 0.63 mg/liter and with diphenoxylate at 2.5 mg/liter. At doses four times higher, inhibition of both tonus and spontaneous movements was noted on the rabbit duodenum.

2.3.3. Study on Heart Tissues

The effects of the three compounds on the papillary muscle of the cat were studied in cumulative concentrations of 1, 3, and 10 mg/liter in comparison with solvent experiments over a total period of 90 min.

No changes in the contractile response to electrical stimulation were observed, except for a moderate negative inotropic effect with loperamide 3 mg/liter (35%) and 10 mg/liter (51%).

Negative chronotropic effects were observed on the guinea-pig right atria with diphenoxylate and difenoxin at 2.5 and 10 mg/liter and with loperamide at 0.16 and 0.63 mg/liter.

The main effect on dose-response curves for isoprenaline and histamine on this tissue was a depression of the maximal rise in heart rate without a parallel shift to the right. This was observed with diphenoxylate at 2.5 and 10 mg/liter, difenoxin at 10 mg/liter, and loperamide at 0.63 mg/liter. This inhibitory effect was purely noncompetitive and unspecific.

Preclinical Studies: In Vitro Pharmacology

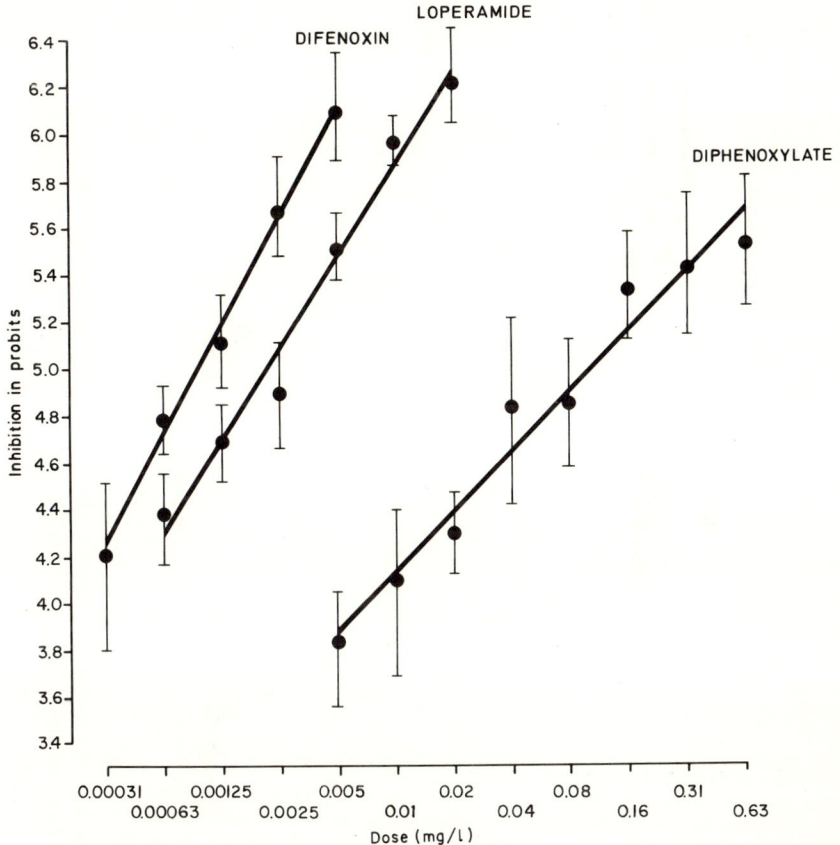

Fig. 29. Inhibition (in percent) of the response of the guinea-pig ileum to coaxial stimulation. Mean values and SEM (six experiments per dose) for diphenoxylate, difenoxin, and loperamide.

2.4. DISCUSSION AND CONCLUSIONS

Difenoxin, loperamide, and diphenoxylate inhibited the peristaltic reflex of guinea-pig ileum in vitro at doses as low as 0.16, 5 and 80 μg/liter respectively.

At these low doses the three compounds also inhibited the response of the same preparation to coaxial stimulation. This was not unexpected, since the contraction induced by electrical single pulses under the conditions described is due to acetylcholine release at the nerve endings (Paton and Zar,

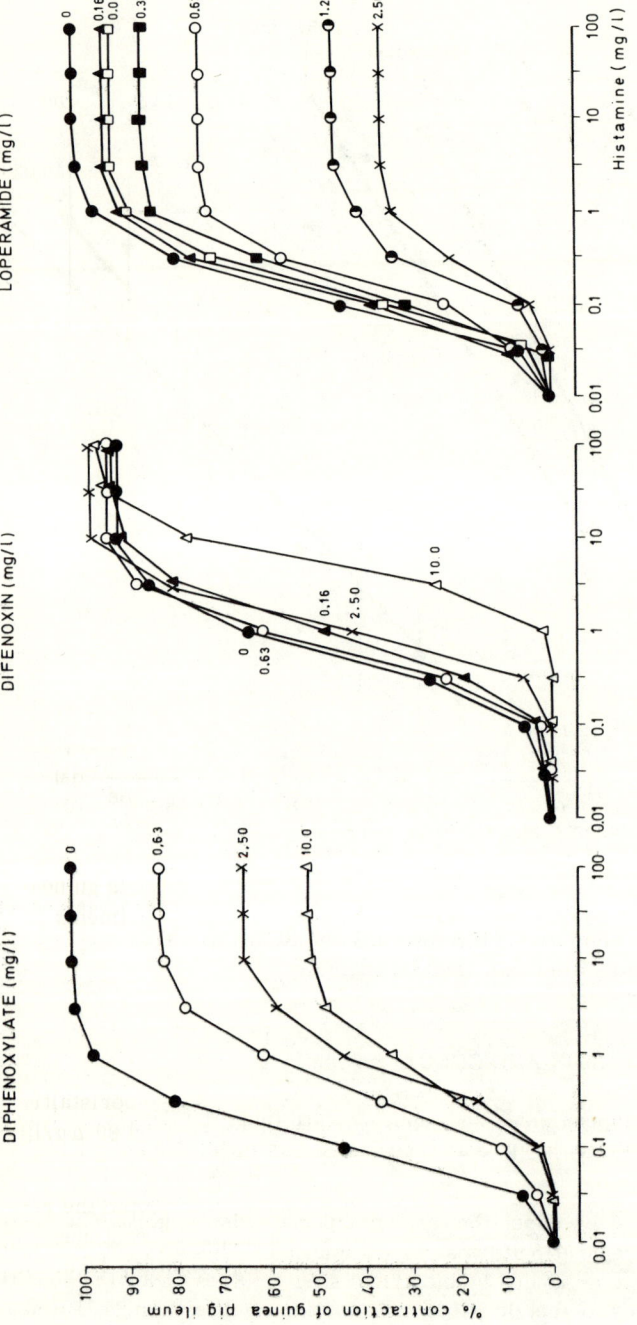

Fig. 30. Influence of diphenoxylate, difenoxin, and loperamide upon histamine-induced contraction of the guinea-pig ileum (cumulative dose-response curves).

1968), and since, on the other hand, there is convincing evidence for the cholinergic nature of part of the nervous pathway to the longitudinal muscle layer, activated during peristalsis (Kottegoda, 1969; Fontaine et al., 1973).

Contractions produced on the same tissue by the ganglionic stimulant nicotine were inhibited by the same low doses. This was also quite expected. Indeed, cholinergic receptors play a role in nicotine-responses on intestinal smooth muscle, whereas autonomic intramural ganglia are involved in the emptying phase (circular muscle activity) of peristalsis (Kosterlitz and Robinson, 1957).

Loperamide was four times less active than difenoxin in inhibiting the peristaltic reflex, and fourteen times more active than diphenoxylate. Administered orally in rats, loperamide is four times less active than difenoxin, and about two and a half times as active as diphenoxylate (Niemegeers et al., 1974c).

The real advantage of loperamide may well be that it combines the rapid onset of action of difenoxin with the long duration of action of diphenoxylate.

Inhibitory effects of both loperamide and diphenoxylate were not easily reversed by washing the compounds out of the bath fluid, which suggests that these compounds are more firmly bound to the intestinal tissues than difenoxin.

With diphenoxylate successive washing tend to increase the inhibitory activity which suggests that difenoxin might be formed in vitro from diphenoxylate by hydrolysis of the ester function.

All three substances inhibit increased propulsion of the intestinal content by a local effect on the intestinal wall. Inhibitory activity toward the contraction in response to coaxial stimulation and to nicotine are in favor of the hypothesis that they may interact with the release of acetylcholine at the postganglionic nerve endings, as well as with the intramural ganglia.

Loperamide inhibits the longitudinal muscle-reflex activity, affecting first the graded cholinergic part and also, some minutes later, the nongraded, noncholinergic part (Van Nueten et al., 1976).

On the other hand, we observed very recently a partial reversal of this inhibitory activity by adding prostaglandins E_1 and E_2 (unpublished results). Therefore additional interaction of loperamide with the noncholinergic longitudinal component cannot be excluded.

The antagonism of diphenoxylate towards 5-HT on the guinea-pig ileum, but not on the rat fundus, is unexpected, and is observed only at higher doses with difenoxin and loperamide. The nature of 5-HT induced contractions of the guinea-pig ileum is rather complex, so that an explanation of their inhibition by diphenoxylate requires further studies.

Apart from this effect, inhibition of peristaltic reflex was highly specific, since much higher or even massive doses are required to obtain antagonism of various spasmogenic drugs on the same smooth muscle preparation (Table 15).

At doses up to 10 mg/liter no inhibition was observed of $BaCl_2$ induced contractions by diphenoxylate and difenoxin, or of bradykinin-induced contractions by difenoxin.

The specificity of the inhibition of peristaltic reflex is intensified by the absence of specific antagonism towards 5-HT on the rat fundus and the lack of anticholinergic effect as well as of α- nor β-adrenergic blocking properties.

Studies on heart tissues showed no overt effects, except some unspecific activity at rather massive doses.

IV.3. METABOLISM OF SYNTHETIC ANTIDIARRHEAL DRUGS, DIPHENOXYLATE, DIFENOXIN, AND LOPERAMIDE

Aziz Karim and Jozef Heykants

3.1. INTRODUCTION

Diphenoxylate, a widely used antidiarrheal drug, may be considered a structural analogue of the analgesic drug meperidine (Fig. 31). Recently, two new compounds, difenoxin (Rubens et al., 1972) and loperamide (Demeulenaere et al., 1974), have been added to the clinically effective antidiarrheal agents. Difenoxin, the hydrolysis product of diphenoxylate is its major metabolite both in the rat (van Wijngaarden et al., 1972) and man (Karim et al., 1972; Heykants et al., 1972b). Loperamide (Fig. 31) may be considered a structural analogue of the neuroleptic drug haloperidol (Stokbroekx et al., 1973).

This section provides a summary of published as well as unpublished information on the absorption, distribution, metabolism, and excretion of diphenoxylate, difenoxin, and loperamide in both laboratory animal and man. It should be noted that in the clinic diphenoxylate is used in combination with atropine sulfate. Difenoxin also should be used in combination with this agent (De Coster et al., 1972). However, in all the studies described here no atropine sulfate was added.

Sensitive and specific bioanalytical methods for all three antidiarrheal drugs and/or their major metabolites are not yet available; therefore, drug determinations were carried out by measurement of radioactivity after administration of the radiolabeled compounds. Diphenoxylate and difenoxin, both as hydrochloride salts, were available either as the ^{3}H- or the

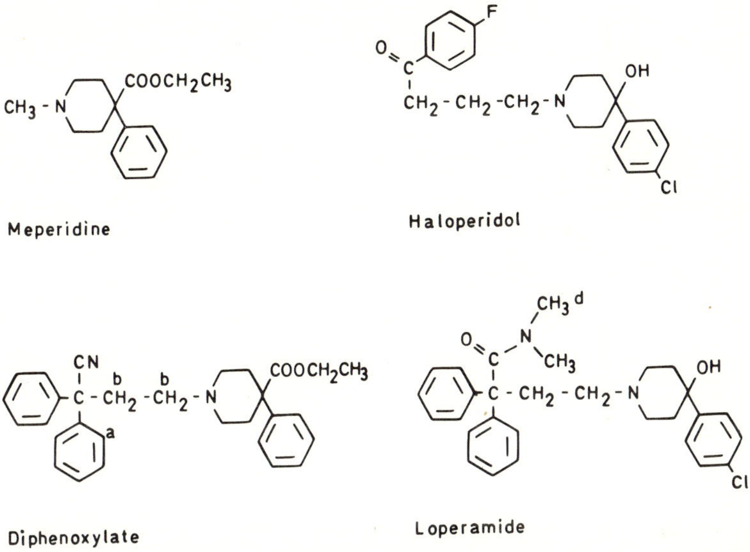

Preclinical Studies: Drug Metabolism

Fig. 31. Structural similarities between diphenoxylate and meperidine and between loperamide and haloperidol. The position of the ^{14}C label in [^{14}C]-diphenoxylate and [^{14}C]-difenoxin is indicated by b. The corresponding ^3H-labeled compounds are labeled at position a. [^3H]-Loperamide is labeled at position d. All three compounds were used as the hydrochloride salts.

^{14}C-labeled compounds; loperamide, also as a hydrochloride salt, was available only as the ^3H-labeled compound (Fig. 31).

3.2. ABSORPTION AND PLASMA LEVELS

3.2.1. Diphenoxylate and Difenoxin

3.2.1.1. Rat

The oral absorption of [^{14}C]-diphenoxylate in ethanolic solution was studied in rats by the measurement of plasma radioactivity after its oral or intravenous administration (Fig. 32). The peak ^{14}C level after an oral dose occurred at 3 hr, suggesting a relatively rapid absorption. The elimination half-life of the ^{14}C in the plasma was 9.9 hr. After intravenous administration an unusual plasma-level/time curve was obtained. Immediately after injection, the ^{14}C levels dropped rapidly with a half-life of 48 min; after 3 hr they increased to give a peak level at 4 hr and then dropped once again

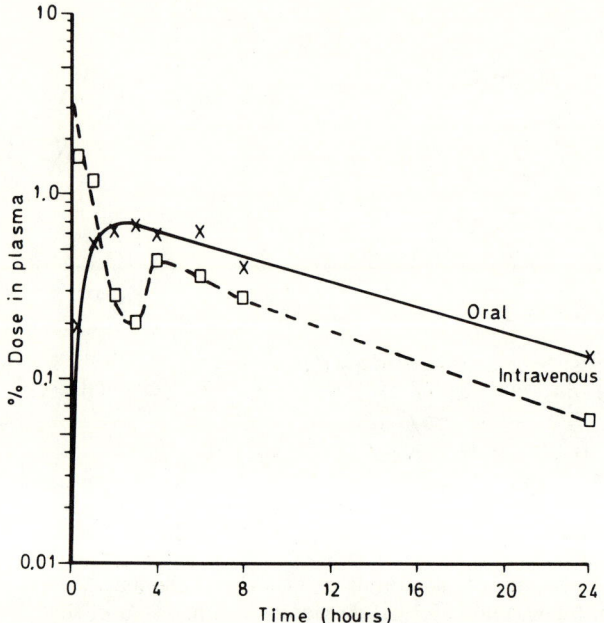

Fig. 32. Plasma ^{14}C levels in the rat after administration of [^{14}C]-diphenoxylate PO (1 mg/kg; x—x) and IV (5 mg/kg; □—□). Each point represents an average of three animals (male Charles River rats, 110-210 g). The drug was administered as the hydrochloride salt in 0.2 ml of ethanol. Y-axis: logarithmic scale, percentage of the administered radioactive dose in the plasma; x-axis: time in hours.

with a longer half-life of 7.1 hr. Comparison of the area under the plasma-level/time curves after the two different routes of administration indicated oral absorption of over 90%. It should be emphasized, however, that this estimate was based on the measurement of total ^{14}C levels; corresponding absorption of the pharmacologically active molecule cannot be assumed. Thin-layer chromatographic (TLC) analysis (Fig. 33) of the ^{14}C materials in the plasma at a peak period showed that the unchanged drug accounted for only 6% of the plasma radioactivity. The major compound (66%) was the de-esterified metabolite, difenoxin.

The ^{14}C levels in the plasma after identical oral doses of [^{14}C]-diphenoxylate or [^{14}C]-difenoxin, as shown in Fig. 34, indicate that the ^{14}C levels with the acid, relative to the ester, were lower; the absorption rate of the acid was also slower resulting in a peak ^{14}C level at 6 hr. Thin-layer chromatography showed that after the acid administration virtually all the

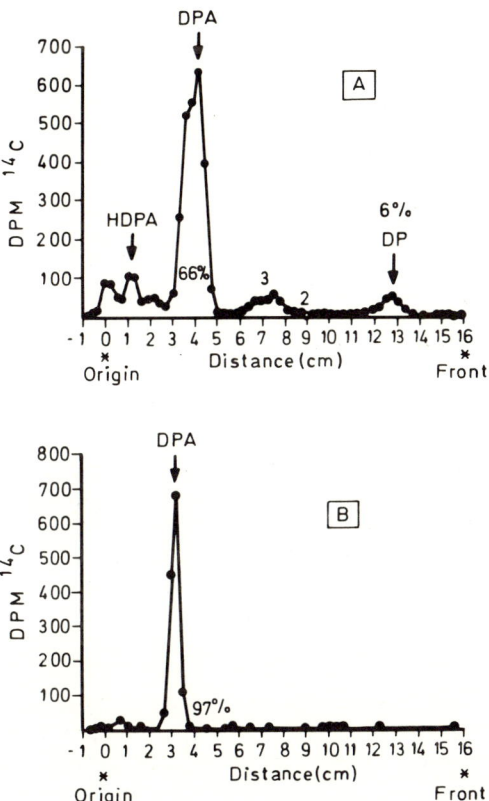

Fig. 33. Representative thin-layer chromatograms of the radioactive compounds in the plasma of the rat at a peak period following oral administration of [^{14}C]-diphenoxylate (curve A) and [^{14}C]-difenoxin (curve B). Percentage values refer to the amount of radioactivity applied to the plate which was associated with each peak. The chromatographic mobilities of the reference compounds diphenoxylate (DP), difenoxin (DPA), and hydroxydifenoxin (HDPA) are indicated by arrows. Chromatograms were developed on 250 μ silica-gel HF$_{254}$ plates using chloroform : methanol : acetic acid (94 : 5 : 1) as the solvent system. Radioactive compounds on the plate were detected by the zonal scraping method. Y-axis: DPM; x-axis: cm from origin.

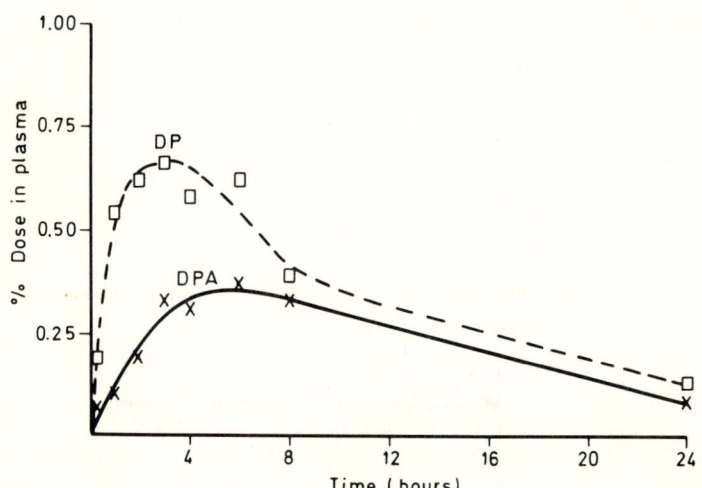

Fig. 34. Plasma ^{14}C levels in the rat after 1 mg/kg oral dose of [^{14}C]-diphenoxylate (DP) or [^{14}C]-difenoxin (DPA). Each point represents an average of three animals (male Charles River rats, 110-210 g). Both drugs were administered as the hydrochloride salt in 0.2 ml of ethanol. Y-axis: percentage of the administered radioactive dose in the plasma; x-axis: time in hours.

radioactivity at a peak period was associated with the unchanged drug (Fig. 33). Similar results were also obtained after the oral administration of the tritium-labeled drugs (Fig. 40): diphenoxylate plasma levels were low in comparison with the ^{3}H levels, while the difenoxin levels were almost identical to the total radioactivity levels.

3.2.1.2. Man

The plasma levels of the drug-related compounds in man following diphenoxylate administration (Karim et al., 1972) are shown in Fig. 35. In this study 5 mg oral doses of [^{14}C]-diphenoxylate hydrochloride in ethanolic solution were given to three healthy men. Radioactive compounds in the plasma at various intervals were analyzed by TLC. The levels of the total ^{14}C materials and of the separated diphenoxylate and difenoxin were converted to the concentration units (ng/ml) using the specific activity of the ingested dose. The average peak concentration of total ^{14}C was 102 ng/ml, while that of difenoxin, the major metabolite, was 40 ng/ml. The peak concentration of the unchanged drug was only 10 ng/ml. The plasma

Preclinical Studies: Drug Metabolism

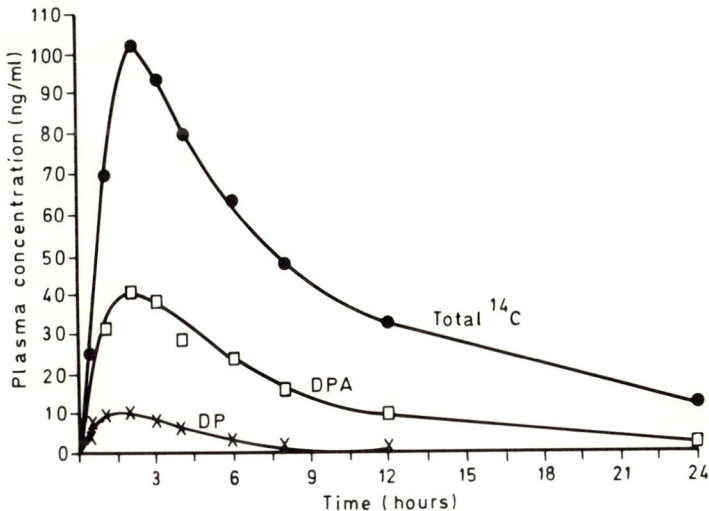

Fig. 35. Average (three subjects) plasma levels of total radioactive compounds (total ^{14}C), difenoxin (DPA) and unchanged diphenoxylate (DP) after oral administration (in ethanolic solution) of a single 5 mg dose of [^{14}C]-diphenoxylate hydrochloride. Y-axis: plasma radioactivity levels converted to the concentration units (ng/ml); x-axis: time in hours.

concentrations of these compounds declined with half-lives of 6.2 hr (total ^{14}C), 4.4 hr (difenoxin) and 2.5 hr (diphenoxylate).

In another unpublished study ^{14}C levels in the plasma of men after identical oral doses of [^{14}C]-diphenoxylate and [^{14}C]-difenoxin were compared. In this study, 2-mg capsules of these drugs were given to eight healthy men using the crossover technique. The results, presented in Fig. 36, indicate marked differences in the absorption characteristics of the two drugs. The essential pharmacokinetic parameters of the average ^{14}C levels, given in Table 16, show that, as compared with diphenoxylate, the peak level with difenoxin was about five times higher and the time taken to reach the peak levels with the acid was shorter. The area under the plasma-level/time curve following the acid intake was also higher than that after diphenoxylate; about four times higher from 0-4 hr and about three times higher from 0-72 hr. A biphasic decline in the plasma-^{14}C levels was seen both for diphenoxylate and difenoxin. With the former drug the half-life from 2 to 24 hr was 6.13 hr, and that from 24 to 72 hr was 23 hr. With difenoxin slightly shorter half-lives (3.48 hr from 2 to 24 hr and 12.6 hr from 24 to 72 hr) were obtained. The plasma-^{14}C levels for both drugs at 24 hr were less than 16% of the peak value. Thin-layer chromatography at each peak period showed that difenoxin was the major compound present after administration of either drug.

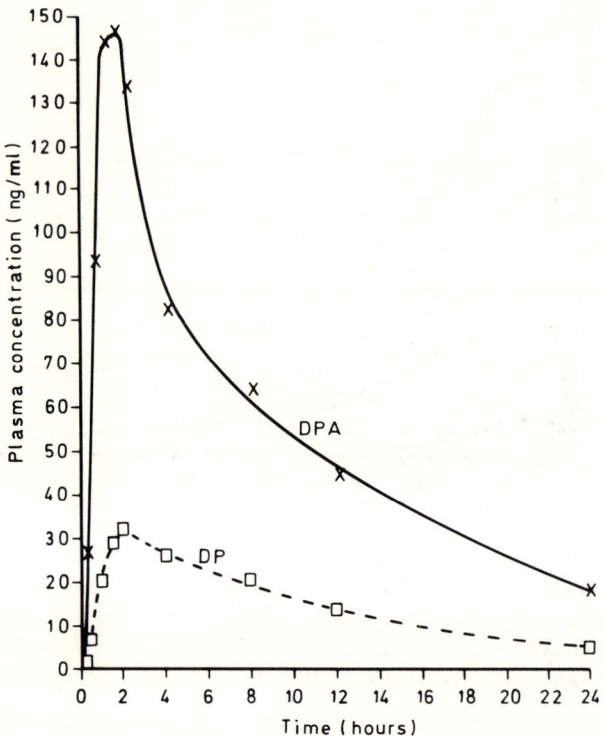

Fig. 36. Plasma ^{14}C levels in men following 2 mg oral doses of $[^{14}C]$-diphenoxylate (DP) or $[^{14}C]$-difenoxin (DPA). Each point is an average of eight subjects. See Table 16 for details of the study and the results of the pharmacokinetic analysis of the above curves. Y-axis: plasma radioactivity levels converted to the concentration units (ng/ml); x-axis: time in hours.

At 24 hr, however, more than 90% of the ^{14}C was present as compounds more polar than this acid. The long half-lives seen from 24 to 72 hr probably reflect the slow elimination of these very polar materials after the administration of either drug.

The comparative absorption in man of diphenoxylate and difenoxin has also been reported by Heykants and his co-workers (1972b). In their studies 0.5 mg and 1 mg tablets of ^{3}H-labeled compounds were given to three healthy subjects using the crossover technique. Here also the peak ^{3}H levels in the plasma following the acid intake were four to eight times higher than those after diphenoxylate administration.

TABLE 16

Summary of Pharmacokinetic Parameters[a]
of Total ^{14}C Materials in the Plasma after a 2 mg
Oral Dose of [^{14}C]-Diphenoxylate (DP) or [^{14}C]-Difenoxin (DPA)

Parameters	DP	DPA	Ratio DPA/DP
1. Average peak plasma concentration, ng/ml	32	146	4.6
2. Time at which the average peak concentration was attained, hr	2	1.5	0.75
3. Average plasma concentration at 24 hr (ng/ml)	5	18	3.6
4. Area under the average plasma concentration-time curve, (ng/ml) × hr			
0-4 hr	95	422	4.4
0-72 hr	492	1603	3.3
5. Half-life of total ^{14}C (hr)			
From 2-24 hr	6.13	3.48	
From 24-72 hr	23.0	12.6	

[a]The pharmacokinetic parameters obtained from average plasma concentration of total ^{14}C materials in eight healthy male subjects who received 2 mg of [^{14}C]-diphenoxylate hydrochloride followed, after a three-week interval, by 2 mg of [^{14}C]-difenoxin hydrochloride in a crossover design study. Both drugs were administered in a specially prepared capsule.

The above data show interesting species differences in the absorption properties of diphenoxylate and difenoxin. In the rat both the extent and the rate of diphenoxylate absorption were greater than for difenoxin. On the other hand, in man, these absorption parameters are much higher for the acid than for the ester. An interesting pharmacological correlation can also be seen in these data. In man the peak plasma-^{14}C levels after difenoxin treatment were about five times higher than those after the treatment with diphenoxylate, the antidiarrheal potency of difenoxin is also reported to be five times that of the ester (Rubens et al., 1972). Thus the higher potency of the acid may simply be due to its greater bioavailability (Table 16). These data also lead to speculation that the effect of antidiarrheal drugs may not be entirely local; absorption appears to play an important role.

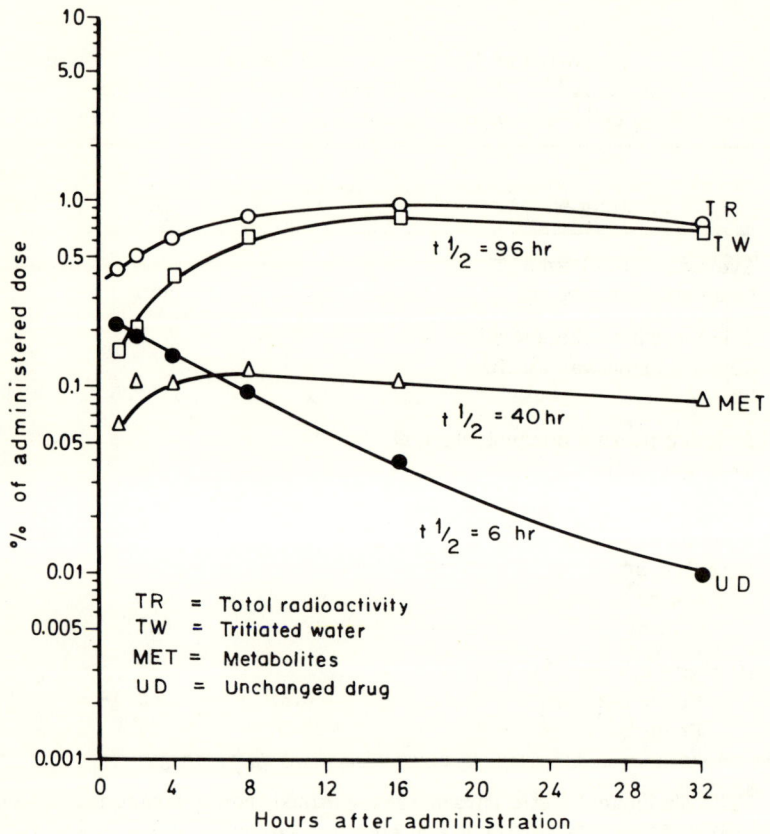

Fig. 37. Plasma levels of the drug-related compounds in the rat following oral administration of [^{3}H]-loperamide. Each point is an average of five animals (male Wistar rats, 240-260 g). [^{3}H]-Loperamide (1.25 mg/kg) was administered in aqueous solution (2.5 ml). Y-axis: logarithmic scale, percentage of the administered dose in the plasma; X-axis: time in hours. The in vitro data of Van Nueten et al. (1972), however, do not support this hypothesis since they found difenoxin also to be more potent than diphenoxylate in inhibiting peristaltic activity in the isolated guinea pig ileum.

3.2.2. Loperamide

The plasma levels of the drug-related compounds following a single oral administration of 1.25 mg/kg dose of [^{3}H]-loperamide to the rat and a 2 mg dose to men are shown in Figs. 37 and 38, respectively. In these studies the concentration of the unchanged drug was determined by inverse isotope dilution analysis. The peak concentration of loperamide (about 2 ng/ml) in man was attained at 2 hr suggesting a relatively rapid rate of drug absorption. The unchanged drug in the plasma of both species was only a small proportion of the total radioactivity. A substantial amount of the radioactivity was present either in tritiated water or in other volatile materials. This was confirmed by determining plasma radioactivity levels before and after lyophilization of the samples.

The half-life of ^{3}H in the plasma of the rat was about 96 hr and nearly 10 days in man. These long half-lifes were attributed to the presence of tritiated water. The half-life of the unchanged loperamide in the rat was 6 hr, and in man it was 40 hr, which is about ten times longer than that of difenoxin. If the plasma half-life is a measure of the duration of antidiarrheal activity for this series of compounds, then loperamide may be expected to be a much longer-acting drug in man than either diphenoxylate or difenoxin.

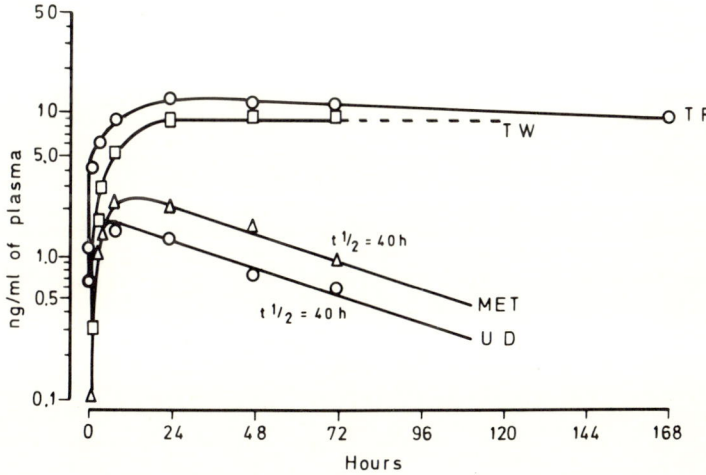

Fig. 38. Plasma levels of drug-related compounds in men following oral administration of [^{3}H]-loperamide. Each point is an average of three subjects. [^{3}H]-Loperamide (2 mg) was administered in gelatin capsules. TR = total radioactivity; TW = tritiated water; MET = metabolites; and UD = unchanged drug. Y-axis: logarithmic scale, plasma radioactivity levels converted to the concentration units (ng/ml); x-axis: time in hours.

3.3. DISTRIBUTION

A common distribution property in the rat of all three drugs was that, after oral administration of the radioactive compounds, more than 60% of the radioactive dose was present in the gastrointestinal tract at 4 hr (Heykants et al., 1972a). The extensive biliary excretion of the drug and/or its metabolites was the major contributing factor for the presence of large amounts of radioactivity in the gut. Table 17 shows that between 30 and 40% of the orally administered radioactivity of all three drugs was excreted in the bile. The enterohepatic recirculation of the drug and/or its metabolites appears to be a common property of these agents. This phenomenon results in the removal of the bulk of the drug-related materials from the general circulation and, at the same time, it supplies constant and large amounts of these materials to the intestine. This may be an important part of the mechanism of the antidiarrheal action of these compounds.

The percentages of the orally administered radioactivity present in the plasma, liver, and brain of the rat at various intervals are shown in Fig. 39. The percentage of the dose found in the brain for all three agents was about 10 to 20 times lower than that found in the plasma. In contrast, the liver contained 10 to 20 times as much radioactivity as the plasma in the case of the more lipid-soluble drugs, i.e., diphenoxylate and loperamide. The distribution properties of difenoxin differed from these two agents in that the percentage of the dose in the liver was only twice that in the plasma. The dissimilarity between the uptake of radioactivity in the liver after oral doses

TABLE 17

Percentage of the Radioactive Dose Excreted in the Bile of Bile-Cannulated Rats after Oral Administration of [^{14}C]-Diphenoxylate, [^{14}C]-Difenoxin, and [^{3}H]-Loperamide

Drug	Dose excreted, %
Diphenoxylate	29.7 ± 2.23[a]
Difenoxin	29.5 ± 8.08[b]
Loperamide	39.0[c]

[a] Mean ± SEM (from 0-48 hr) for three animals (male Charles River rats). Each animal received 1 mg/kg orally in 0.2 ml of propylene glycol.

[b] Mean ± SEM (from 0-24 hr) for three animals (male Charles River rats). Each animal received 1 mg/kg orally in 0.2 ml ethanol.

[c] Value (from 0-48 hr) in one animal (male Wistar rat) after receiving 1.25 mg/kg orally in aqueous solution.

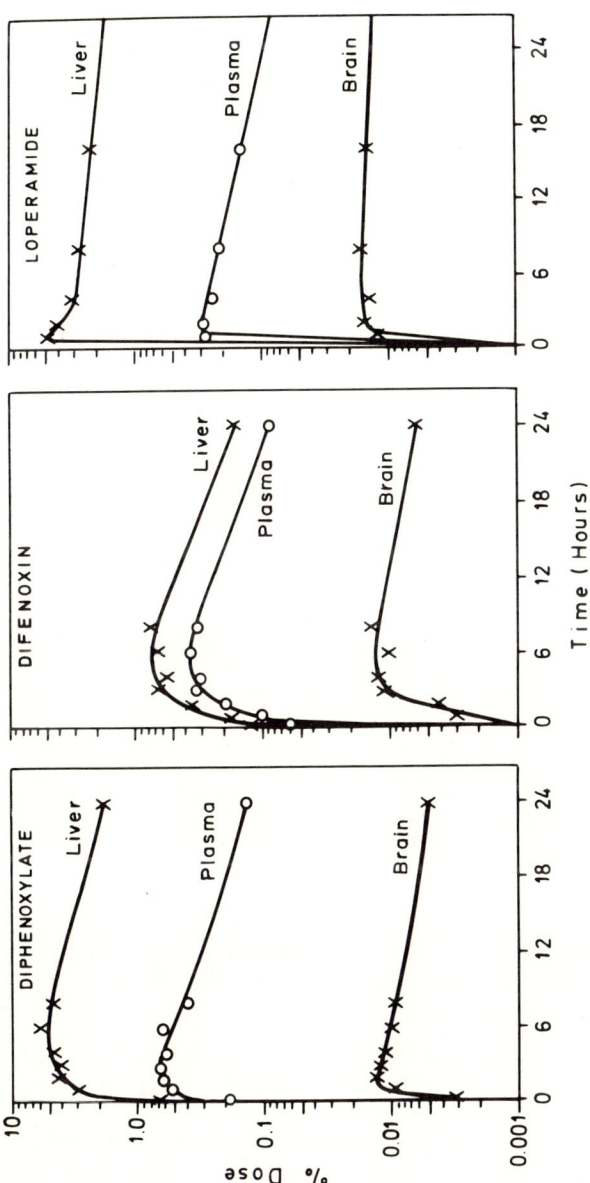

Fig. 39. Percentage of the administered radioactivity present in the plasma, liver, and brain of the rat following 1 mg/kg oral doses of $[^{14}C]$-diphenoxylate or $[^{14}C]$-difenoxin and 1.25 mg/kg oral dose of $[^{3}H]$-loperamide. For diphenoxylate and difenoxin each point is an average of three animals (male Charles River rats, 110–210 g). For loperamide each value is an average of five animals (male Wistar rats, 240–260 g). Radioactivity refers to that of the nonvolatile materials. Y-axis: logarithmic scale, percentage of the administered radioactive dose; x-axis: time in hours.

of diphenoxylate and of difenoxin suggests that the ester hydrolysis of the former probably does not occur in the gut. If diphenoxylate were hydrolyzed in the gut prior to its absorption, then one would expect close similarity in the liver plasma-distribution profiles. The radioactivity levels in the liver dropped with half-lives of 12.4 hr for diphenoxylate, 8.4 hr for difenoxin, and 33 hr for loperamide.

The percentages of total radioactivity and of unchanged drug, with respect to the administered dose, in the plasma, liver, and brain of the Wistar rat at various intervals, are shown in Fig. 40. Although the amounts

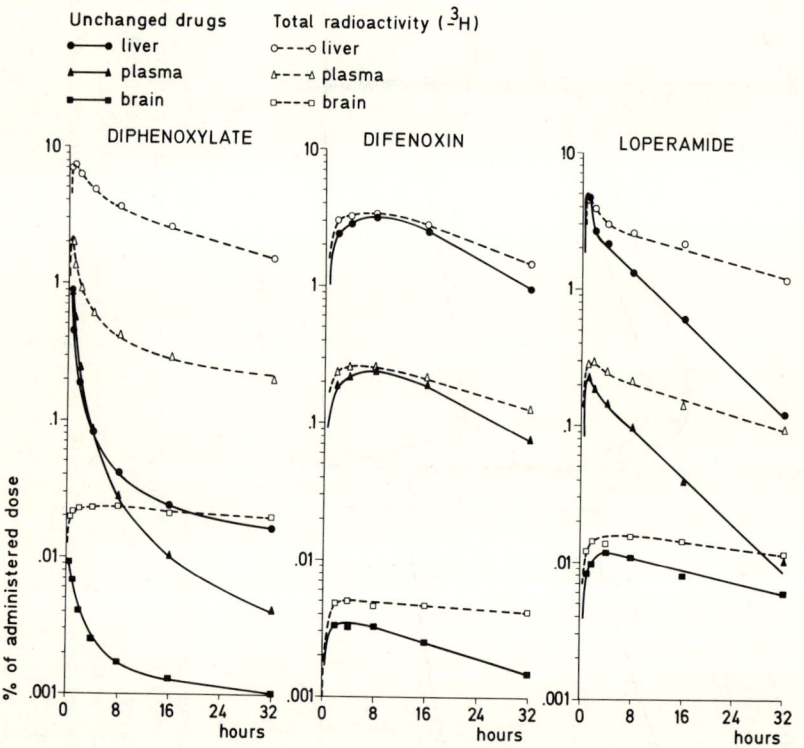

Fig. 40. Levels of total radioactivity and of unchanged drug in plasma, liver, and brain as a function of time for oral doses of [^{3}H]-diphenoxylate (1 mg/kg), [^{3}H]-difenoxin (1 mg/kg) and [^{3}H]-loperamide (1.25 mg/kg). The first two drugs were given in a Tween 80 suspension to male Wistar rats of 250 g, starved overnight. Loperamide was given in aqueous solution (as the hydrochloride salt).

of ^{3}H in the three organs were comparable, the levels of the unchanged drug were not. Even shortly after administration, the radioactive contents of the plasma, liver, and brain of rats treated with diphenoxylate were mainly metabolites, indicating a rapid metabolic breakdown of this drug. Difenoxin levels, however, did not differ greatly from those of total radioactivity.

In an interesting clinical study Heykants and his co-workers (1972b) investigated the distribution of the radioactive materials in the blood, plasma, and cerebrospinal fluids in seven subjects. Four of these subjects received 0.5-mg oral doses of [^{3}H]-diphenoxylate and three received [^{3}H]-difenoxin. This study showed that the radioactive materials in the blood were present exclusively in the plasma. At 4 hr, the average ^{3}H levels in the plasma were 8 ng/ml after diphenoxylate intake and 28 ng/ml after the acid. At this period the ^{3}H level in the cerebrospinal fluid was about 50 times less than that in the plasma in the case of diphenoxylate and about 100 times less in the case of difenoxin.

3.4. EXCRETION

The excretion of radioactivity in the urine and feces of the rat after the oral or intravenous administration of [^{14}C]-diphenoxylate or [^{14}C]-difenoxin and after the oral administration of [^{3}H]-loperamide is shown in Table 18. The major route of excretion of all three drugs was via the feces. The excretion of radioactivity in the urine in all cases accounted for less than 8% of the dose. The fecal recovery of a large quantity of radioactivity, at least in the case of diphenoxylate and difenoxin, cannot be attributed to the unabsorbed drug since Table 18 shows that about 70% of the dose was also recovered in the feces after the intravenous administration of these two drugs.

The excretion of the radioactivity in the urine and feces of man after oral administration of the three radiolabeled drugs is shown in Table 19. Here close similarities between excretion profiles of diphenoxylate and loperamide are seen. In both cases about 10% of the dose was excreted in the urine and about 40% in the feces. Difenoxin differs from these two drugs in that a much higher proportion (about 40%) of the dose was excreted in the urine. The total recovery (urine and feces) of the radioactivity following the acid treatment was also much higher than that of the other two drugs.

The graph plotting the percentages of the administered radioactive dose remaining to be excreted in the urine of men against time (sigma minus plot) for all three drugs is shown in Fig. 41. From this graph the half-lives of ^{14}C materials from diphenoxylate and difenoxin were calculated to be 19 hr and 16 hr, respectively. For loperamide the half-life of the total ^{3}H was 32 hr, and that of the nonvolatile ^{3}H was 26 hr.

TABLE 18

Comparative Recovery of Radioactivity in the Urine and Feces of the Rat Following Administration of [^{14}C]-Diphenoxylate, [^{14}C]-Difenoxin, and [^{3}H]-Loperamide

Time after which dose was recovered	Dose recovered, %					
	Diphenoxylate[a]		Difenoxin[b]		Loperamide[c]	
	Oral	Intravenous	Oral	Intravenous	Total ^{3}H	Nonvolatile ^{3}H
Urine						
Day 1	3.10	3.57	2.53	3.59	3.30	2.68
2	1.87	1.14	3.03	1.02	1.02	0.43
3	1.25	0.56	1.14	0.16	0.63	0.12
4	0.29	0.31	0.41	0.07	0.51	0.07
5	0.15	0.19	0.08	0.05		
Total in urine	6.66	5.77	7.19	4.89	5.46	3.30
Feces						
Day 1	22.0	32.8	45.0	36.7	56.3	
2	35.6	25.7	29.1	28.9	6.65	
3	19.8	9.64	11.3	2.64	0.97	
4	6.86	3.68	6.71	0.55	0.47	
5	4.91	2.26	1.45	0.22		
Total in feces	89.2	74.1	93.6	69.0	64.4	
Total dose recovered, %	95.9	79.8	101.0	73.9	69.9	

[a] Average values of three animals (male Charles River rats, 110–210 g). [^{14}C]-diphenoxylate hydrochloride (5 mg/kg PO and 1 mg/kg IV) was administered in 0.2 ml of ethanol.
[b] Average values of three animals (male Charles River rats, 120–180 g). [^{14}C]-difenoxin hydrochloride (5 mg/kg PO and 1 mg/kg IV) was administered in 0.2 ml of ethanol.
[c] Average values of five animals (male Wistar rats, 240–260 g). [^{3}H]-Loperamide (1.25 mg/kg PO) was administered in aqueous solution (1 ml). PO = orally; IV = intravenous.

TABLE 19

Comparative Recovery of Radioactivity in the Urine and Feces
of Men Following Oral Administration
of [^{14}C]-Diphenoxylate, [^{14}C]-Difenoxin, and [^{3}H]-Loperamide

Time after which dose was recovered	Dose recovered, %			
	Diphenoxylate[a]	Difenoxin[a]	Loperamide[b]	
			Total ^{3}H	Nonvolatile ^{3}H
Urine				
Day 1	10.7	34.3	3.10	2.63
2	1.90	5.78	2.28	1.59
3	0.64	1.51	1.47	1.05
4	0.31	0.43	1.20	0.75
5	0.21	0.34	0.92	0.50
6			0.60	0.24
7			0.50	0.18
Dose, %	13.8	42.4	10.1	6.94
Feces				
Day 1-5	39.8	56.2	41.7	
Total dose recovered, %	53.6	98.6	51.8	

[a] Average values of eight healthy male subjects who received in a crossover-design study 2 mg of [^{14}C]-diphenoxylate hydrochloride followed after a three-week interval by 2 mg of [^{14}C]-difenoxin hydrochloride. The drugs were administered in a specially prepared capsule.

[b] Average values of three healthy male subjects who received 2 mg of [^{3}H]-loperamide in a gelatin capsule.

3.5. BIOTRANSFORMATION

3.5.1. Diphenoxylate

The structures of the metabolites of diphenoxylate in the feces of the rat and the dog have been reported (Karim et al., 1971). A typical TLC profile of the methanol soluble radioactive materials in the feces of the rat is shown in Fig. 42. The unchanged drug accounted for less than 1% of the fecal radioactivity. Metabolite peaks 2 and 3 (curve A) each accounted for about 5% and difenoxin (DPA), the major metabolite, for about 50% of the radioactivity.

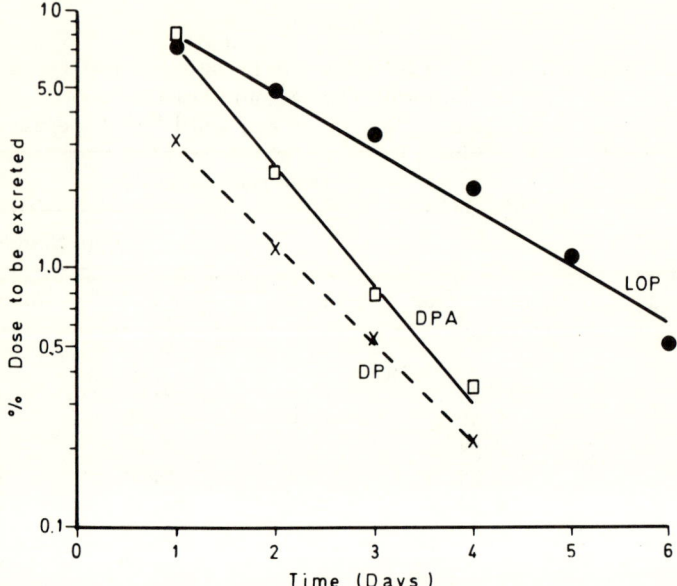

Fig. 41. The graph of percentage of the administered radioactivity remaining to be excreted in the urine with time (sigma minus plot) in men who received the oral dose of [^{14}C]-diphenoxylate (DP, x—x), [^{14}C]-difenoxin (DPA, □—□) and [^{3}H]-loperamide (LOP, ●—●). Y-axis: logarithmic scale, percentage of the administered radioactive dose remaining to be excreted in the urine; x-axis: time in days.

The remainder of the radioactivity was associated with compounds more polar than this acid. One of these polar metabolites was hydroxydifenoxin (HDPA). The Rf values and the mass spectral characteristics of these metabolites are given in Table 20. Besides these Heykants and co-workers (1972) using inverse isotope dilution analysis, also indentified 3-cyano-3,3-diphenylpropionic acid (CDPA) as a metabolite of diphenoxylate in the feces of men. The chemical structure of the above metabolites are shown in Fig. 43.

In the metabolism study by Karim and co-workers (1971) the identity of diphenoxylate and difenoxin in the feces of the rat was confirmed by comparing the IR and mass spectra and the thin-layer and gas-liquid chromatographic properties of the isolated materials with the authentic samples. The mass spectrum of diphenoxylate (Fig. 44) showed only a low-intensity molecular-ion peak was presented at m/e 452. The base peak at m/e 246 was very diagnostic in the structural assignment of the phenolic metabolites, peaks 2

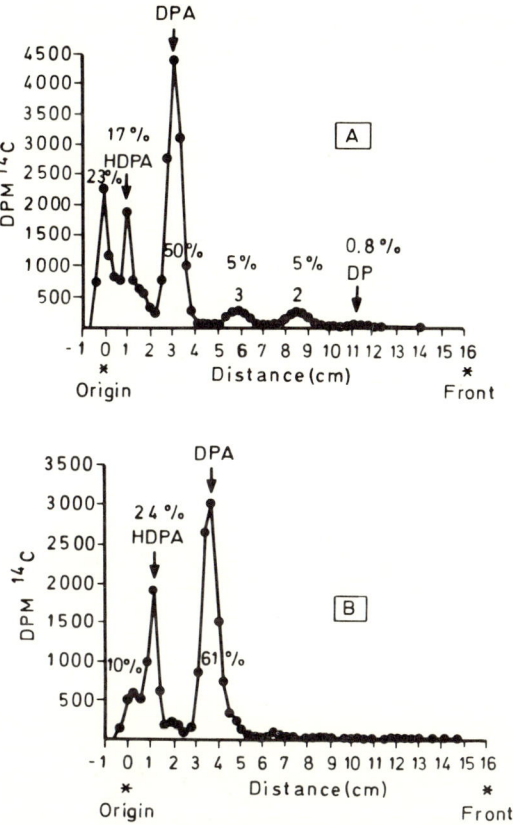

Fig. 42. Representative thin-layer chromatograms of the methanol extractable radioactive compounds in the 0-5 day freeze-dried feces of the rat after oral doses of [^{14}C]-diphenoxylate (curve A) and [^{14}C]-difenoxin (curve B). For details on chromatographic conditions, see legend of Fig. 33. The chromatographic mobilities of the reference compounds diphenoxylate (DP), difenoxin (DPA), and hydroxydifenoxin (HDPA) are indicated by arrows. Y-axis: DPM; x-axis: cm from origin.

and 3. The molecular ion of the metabolite peak 2 at m/e 498 indicated that it was diphenoxylate containing an additional -OH and -OMe group. Peak 3, on the other hand, gave a molecular ion peak at m/e 468 indicating that this metabolite contained only one additional -OH group. The base peaks in the mass spectra of both these metabolites were present at m/e 246 (Table 20) indicating that the oxidative transformation in both had occurred in the

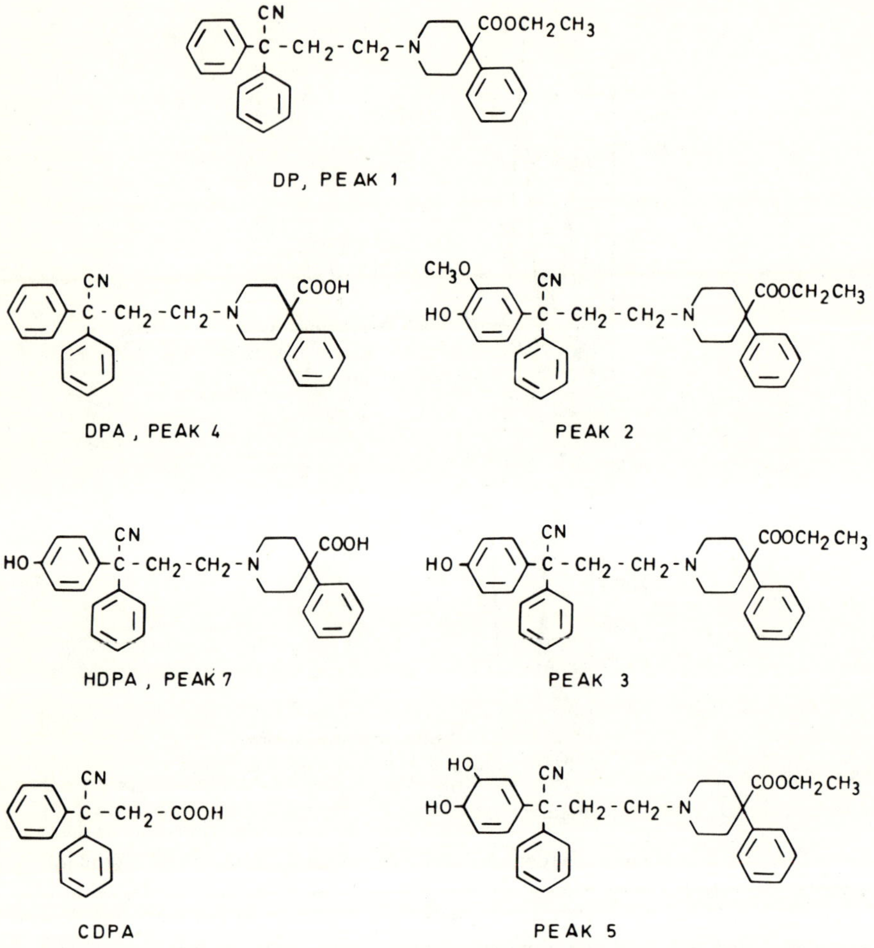

Fig. 43. Proposed structures of the metabolites of diphenoxylate.

3-cyano-3,3-diphenyl part of the diphenoxylate molecule. Besides being useful in structural elucidation, the high-intensity peak at m/e 246 may also be utilized in the mass fragmentographic assay of diphenoxylate and its metabolites in biological fluids.

Another interesting hydroxylated metabolite of diphenoxylate was peak 5 (Fig. 43). This metabolite was isolated from the feces of the dog only (Karim et al., 1971). In this species a much higher proportion of the fecal radioactivity was present as hydroxylated metabolites. The molecular-ion

TABLE 20

Thin-layer and Mass Spectral
Characteristics of Diphenoxylate and its Metabolites[a]

Compound	TLC, Rf[b]	Mass spectral data		
		M[+]	Molecular formula[c]	Base peak
Diphenoxylate (DP)	0.71	452	$C_{30}H_{32}N_2O_2$	246
Peak 2	0.53	498	$C_{31}H_{34}N_2O_4$	246
Peak 3	0.34	468	$C_{30}H_{32}N_2O_3$	246
Peak 4 (DPA)	0.18	424	$C_{28}H_{28}N_2O_2$	218
Peak 5	0.13	486	$C_{30}H_{34}N_2O_4$	246
Peak 7 (HDPA)	0.04			

[a] See Fig. 43 for proposed structures.

[b] Rf value in solvent system of chloroform-methanol-acetic acid (94 : 5 : 1) using silica gel HF_{254} (250 μ) plates.

[c] Molecular formula obtained by high resolution mass spectrometry.

peak at m/e 486 in peak 5 indicated that it was diphenoxylate containing two additional hydroxyl groups as well as a reduction of one double bond. Ultraviolet spectral analysis showed that this metabolite was not phenolic. On treatment with acid, however, it was converted to a mixture of products, one of which was phenolic metabolite peak 3. On the basis of these observations the dihydrodiol structure (Fig. 43) was assigned to peak 5.

In man the nature of the radioactive materials excreted in the feces following ingestion of radioactive diphenoxylate was dependent on the dosage form of the drug. In the studies in which the drug was administered in ethanolic solution (Karim et al., 1972) very little radioactivity was present as the unchanged drug and difenoxin, together with compounds more polar than this acid, were the major excretory products. However, in the studies in which diphenoxylate was given either as a tablet (Heykants et al., 1972b) or as a capsule (unpublished observations) more than 50% of the fecal radioactivity was associated with the unchanged drug. This finding suggests greater absorption of the drug when administered in ethanolic solution than when given as a solid formulation. This is not unreasonable since diphenoxylate has low solubility in water, and the dissolution of the drug from the solid dosage form may be expected to be a rate-limiting factor in its absorption. Comparison of the chromatograms of the methanol-soluble radioactive compounds in the feces of the rat and man indicated overall similarities in the biotransformation pathway in these two species (Karim et al., 1971,

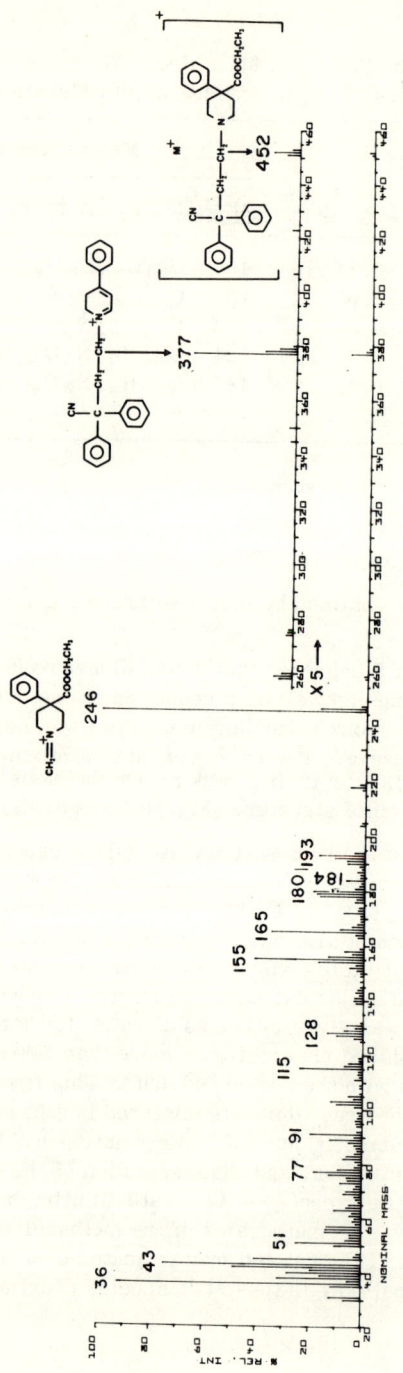

Fig. 44. Mass spectrum (electron impact) of diphenoxylate.

TABLE 21

Fractionation of Radioactivity[a] in the 0-24 hr
Urine of Men after Oral Dose of [^{14}C]-Diphenoxylate

Drug-related compounds	Urinary ^{14}C, %	Dose, %
Total ^{14}C	100.0	11.0
Chloroform extractable ^{14}C	26.0	2.85
Water-soluble ^{14}C	65.0	7.15
Unchanged diphenoxylate	0.41	0.04
Free DPA	5.0	0.55
Free plus conjugated DPA	26.0	2.85
Free HDPA	10.9	1.19
Free plus conjugated HDPA	20.0	2.20

[a] Average value of three subjects who received 5 mg oral dose of [^{14}C]-diphenoxylate hydrochloride in ethanolic solution.

1972). The proportion of the compounds more polar than difenoxin in the feces of man, however, was much higher than that in the feces of the rat.

The nature of the urinary excretory products in man following diphenoxylate ingestion is given in Table 21. The radioactivity in the 0-24 hr pooled urine was fractionated into chloroform extractable material and water-soluble conjugated material (Karim et al., 1972). The water-soluble fraction was subjected to both base and enzyme (β-glucuronidase) hydrolysis. The extracted compounds before and after hydrolyses were analyzed by TLC. As shown in Table 21, the unchanged drug and free, plus conjugated, difenoxin accounted for about 0.04 and 3% of the dose, respectively.

3.5.2. Difenoxin

The TLC of the methanol-soluble radioactive materials in the feces of the rat following oral administration of [^{14}C]-difenoxin is shown in Fig. 42 (curve B). Here, 61% of the fecal radioactivity (57% of the dose) was present as the unchanged drug and 24% as the hydroxydifenoxin. Using isotope dilution analysis, van Wijngaarden and Soudijn (1972) have also identified the primary amide metabolite A (Fig. 45) and the metabolite B without the nitrile group. These two compounds accounted for about 4 and 10%, respectively, of the fecal radioactivity. All three metabolites (HDPA, metabolite A, and metabolite B) were tested for their antidiarrheal activity in the rat and were found inactive.

In man, Heykants and his co-workers (1972b) showed that in one subject who received [^{3}H]-difenoxin about 33% of the dose was recovered in the urine

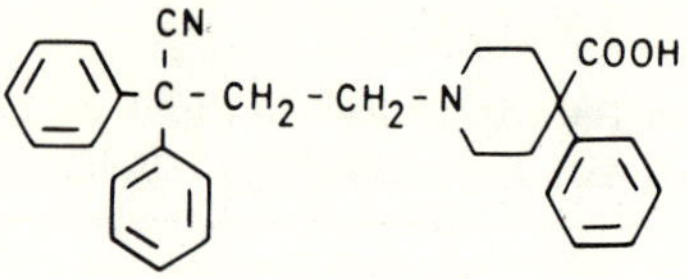

DPA

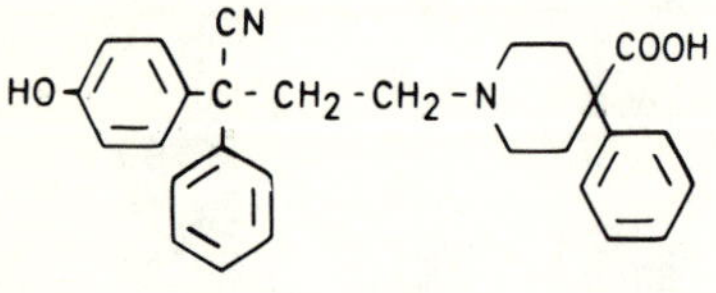

HDPA

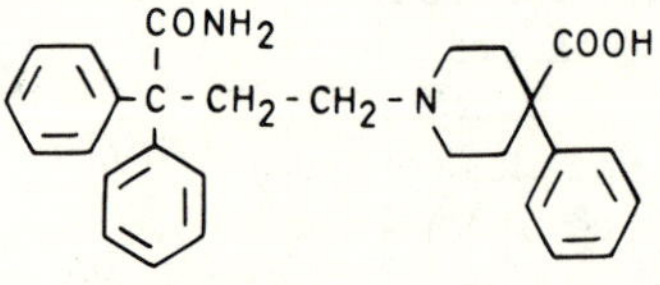

METABOLITE A

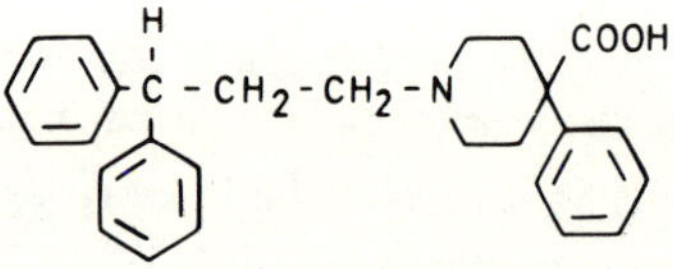

METABOLITE B

Fig. 45. Proposed structures of the metabolites of difenoxin.

in two days; about 60% of this radioactivity (20% of the dose) was present as the unchanged drug. These results indicate that in man there is considerably less metabolism of difenoxin than of diphenoxylate.

3.5.3. Loperamide

Detailed biotransformation pathways of loperamide have not been studied; only the proportions of the unchanged drug excreted in the urine and feces have been examined by inverse isotope-dilution analysis. In the rat about 20% of the urinary radioactivity (1% of the dose) and 80% of the fecal radioactivity (40% of the dose) were present as the unchanged loperamide. In man, the unchanged drug constituted 20% of the radioactivity in the urine (1.2% of the dose) and 40% of the radioactivity in the feces (10% of the dose). In both the rat and man about half the radioactivity excreted in the urine was present as the volatile materials (Tables 18 and 19). This may be due to the metabolic cleavage of the tritium-bearing methyl groups of the [^{3}H]-loperamide

Preclinical Studies: Safety Evaluation   155

(Fig. 31). This hypothesis has been confirmed very recently in a metabolic study in rats using [^{3}H]-loperamide with the label on the phenyl ring ortho to the chlorine atom. Preliminary unpublished results (Heykants et al., 1975) have shown that the main metabolic pathway of loperamide in the rat was oxidative N-demethylation, resulting in the corresponding N-desmethyl- (R 20 905) and N-bisdesmethylloperamide (R 21 345). Loperamide and these metabolites were excreted with the bile (about 50% in 24 hr), mainly as their glucuronides. In the urine of rats, 4-(4-chlorophenyl)-4-hydroxypiperidine was found as a major metabolite, indicating that oxidative N-dealkylation was another metabolic pathway. In addition to this compound, the N-desmethyl- analogs of loperamide were also excreted with the urine.

IV.4. SAFETY EVALUATION

Herman Blaton, Carlos Niemegeers, and Robert **Marsboom**

4.1. INTRODUCTION

The potential toxicity of the synthetic antidiarrheal agents diphenoxylate, fetoxylate, difenoxin, loperamide, and fluperamide, intended for use in man, has been determined by the measurement of acute oral toxicity in mice, rats, guinea-pigs, and dogs and by the measurement of subacute and chronic oral toxicity in rats and dogs. Fertility, teratogenesis and perinatal toxicity, as a phase of animal safety evaluation of these drugs, were studied in rats and rabbits with emphasis on the investigation on the effect of these compounds on the embryo during the period of organogenesis.

All toxicity studies described in this chapter were designed to meet the requirements of the initial pharmacological and therapeutic clinical evaluation, to support more extensive clinical trials, and ultimately to permit the acceptance of the new drug candidates. The experimental designs were governed by a realistic compromise with respect to regulatory demands and research interests. In view of the rapid advances made in recent years in improving the effectiveness and significance of the safety evaluation program, the work that has been carried out for the more recently developed compounds like loperamide was considerably more far-reaching.

4.2. METHODS

4.2.1. Acute Toxicity

The acute toxicity studies were performed in animals of closed laboratory-breeding colonies: adult male albino mice (Swiss) weighing 24 ± 4 g, adult male albino rats (Wistar) weighing 240 ± 40 g, young weaned albino rats

(Wistar) of both sexes weighing 50 ± 5 g, adult male albino guinea pigs weighing 350 ± 50 g, and adult Beagle dogs of both sexes.

The experimental animals were transferred from their rearing quarters to the air-conditioned laboratories 24 hr before the experiments (21 ± 1 °C; 65 ± 5% RH). After being starved overnight, tap water being available ad libitum, they were treated orally by gavage with either diphenoxylate, fetoxylate, difenoxin, loperamide, or fluperamide. All compounds were administered in freshly prepared aqueous solutions or, if insoluble, in aqueous suspensions containing 1% polysorbate 80, micronized with an ultrasonic sonifier. The dose levels were selected from the following geometrical series: 2560, 1280, 640 ... to 0.63, 0.31, 0.16 mg/kg and 10 animals per dose level were used. In mice, rats, and guinea-pigs 1 ml/100 g body weight, in dogs 0.5 ml/kg was administered. One, three, and seven days after treatment, gross behavioral symptoms and mortality were recorded and LD_{50} values with 95% fiducial limits were computed.

4.2.2. Subacute and Chronic Toxicity

The subacute and chronic toxicity studies were carried out in young male and female Wistar rats and in young male and female Beagle dogs, both from closed laboratory-breeding colonies. The subacute toxicity studies extended over a 12-to-15-week period, whereas the chronic toxicity studies covered a period of 18 months in rats and of 12 months in dogs.

The compounds were administered as a microcrystalline powder admixed in the rats' food, 7 days per week at different dosages. A control group received the basic laboratory diet. At the start of the experiment the rats were 6 to 8 weeks old, weighed between 150 and 200 g, and were divided into four to five comparable groups of 10 males and 10 females per dose (80 to 100 animals in the subacute studies) or into four comparable groups of 30 males and 30 females per dose (240 animals in the chronic studies). The animals were individually housed and acclimatized in the experimental rooms for 1 week before the first drug administration (12 hr light per day, temperature 21-23 °C, and relative humidity 55-60%).

The young purebred Beagle dogs, 24 to 32 divided into four groups, each containing three to four males and females, were individually housed and maintained on a commercial dog food and supplied with water ad libitum. When they were 12 weeks old, the animals were vaccinated against distemper and canine hepatitis. At the start of the experiments the dogs were about 7 to 8 months old. The compounds were administered orally as a microcrystalline powder in gelatin capsules at different dosages 6 days per week. Dosages were adjusted during the course of the experiment according to weekly recorded body weight. The control capsules contained 250 mg of lactose. Base-line preparation involved a 4-to-6-week acclimatization period and consisted of a

TABLE 16

Compounds Studied in Rats and Dogs

Compound	Species	Duration of study, weeks	Dosage, mg/kg				
Diphenoxylate	Rat	12	0	0.16	2.5	20	
	Rat	13	0	1.25	10	80	
	Rat	26	0	2	10	40	
	Dog	16	0	2	8	32	
Fetoxylate	Rat	15	0	0.16	2.5	20	
	Dog	52	0	5	20	80	
Difenoxin	Rat	13	0	1.25	10	20	80
	Rat	78	0	1.25	5	20	
	Dog	13	0	0.5	3	10	
	Dog	52	0	0.16	2.5	5	
Loperamide	Rat	15	0	2.5	10	40	
	Rat	78	0	2.5	10	40	
	Dog	52	0	0.31	1.25	5	
Fluperamide	Rat	13	0	2.5	10	40	
	Rat	78	0	1.25	5	20	
	Dog	12	0	0.31	1.25	2.5	
	Dog	52	0	0.16	0.31	0.63	

complete physical examination, including an ophthalmoscopic and slit-lamp examination of the eyes, electrocardiogram, blood pressure, hematology, serum analysis, and urinalysis.

Table 16 lists the subacute and chronic toxicity studies in rats and dogs discussed in this section.

During the subacute and chronic experiments all animals were examined daily for signs of waning health, abnormal behavior, or unusual appearance, and occurrence of untoward clinical effects and manifestations of toxic and pharmacologic responses. Body weight in dogs and rats, and food consumption in rats were recorded at weekly intervals. Electrocardiograms (Elema Mingograph 34) and blood pressure (physio-control mm Hg) were recorded in dogs at monthly intervals. At the same time in dogs and terminally in rats, hematology, serum analysis, and urinalysis were done. For hematology the following determinations were made: hematocrit, hemoglobin, red and white blood-cell count, differential count, thrombocytes count, and eventually coagulation and sedimentation time. For serum analysis the following determinations were made: sodium, potassium, chloride, carbon dioxide, total protein, albumin, calcium, alkaline phosphatase, bilirubin, blood-urea-nitrogen, glucose, SGOT, SGPT, LDH, inorganic phosphor, haptoglobin, cholesterol, and creatinine. In the urine the following measurements were made: pH, protein, glucose, acetone, bilirubin, urobilinogen, creatinine, UGOT, specific gravity, and sediment. Prior to sacrifice a complete physical and ophthalmoscopic examination was performed on all animals. At the end of the experiment all surviving animals were weighed. In the chronic study one third of the animals were sacrificed after 6, 12, or 18 months respectively. Rats were anesthetized with ether. Dogs received heparin (7 mg/kg IV) to prevent blood coagulation and were anesthetized with sodium pentobarbital (30 mg/kg IV). Autopsy was performed as soon as possible after sacrifice by exsanguination and all macroscopic pathologic changes were noted. The organs were then removed, weighed and preserved in 10% formalin or other fixatives as appropriate. The criteria chosen for statistical analysis included survival, body weight, food consumption, organ weight, urinalysis, and biochemical and hematological values. All statistical analyses were carried out by computer, using the Mann-Whitney U-test (Siegel, 1956) to compare the values obtained from the treated animals with those of the controls.

4.2.3. Reproduction Studies

The reproduction studies were divided into three sections, each of which pertained to a specific phase of the reproductive process.

4.2.3.1. Fertility and General Reproductive Performance

The effect on fertility and general reproductive performance was studied in male and female Wistar rats of a closed laboratory-breeding colony.

At the start of the studies the animals were sexually mature. Males were 60 days old before first administration of the compounds and they were treated for 60 days before mating and further till copulation. Females were 3 months old when they were treated for 14 days before being exposed to males and further till mating occurred and throughout gestation. Virgin females in the proestrus stage were coupled with breeding males: a treated animal was mated with a nontreated one. The occurrence of copulation was established by daily vaginal inspection for sperm and as soon as pregnancy was noted, the female was isolated until parturition. Groups of 20 males and 20 females each received the compound admixed in the diet, control animals received the basic laboratory diet. Difenoxin was tested at 0.16, 2.5, and 20 mg/kg, and loperamide at 2.5, 10, and 40 mg/kg. The females were sacrificed on day 22 of pregnancy and the fetuses were delivered by cesarean section. The dams were examined for number and distribution of embryos in each uterine horn,

Preclinical Studies: Safety Evaluation   159

presence of empty implantation sites and embryos undergoing resorption.
Any abnormal condition in the uterus that could have contributed to embryonic
death was also noted. All fetuses were carefully examined for any external
anomalies and radiographically examined. Rat fetuses of each litter were
further randomized for dissection (one third) and clearing and bone staining
with alizarin (two thirds).

4.2.3.2. Teratogenesis and Embryotoxicity

The teratogenic and embryotoxic effects were studied in sexually mature
virgin female Wistar rats and in New Zealand female rabbits, both from
closed laboratory-breeding colonies.

At mating the virgin female rats were 3 to 4 months old and weighed 200
to 220 g. Groups of 20 rats or more received the compound admixed in the
diet at various doses from day 6 through day 15 of pregnancy. A control
group received the basic laboratory diet. Diphenoxylate was tested at two
dose levels, 5 and 10 mg/kg, and difenoxin at 0.16, 2.5, 10, 20, and 80
mg/kg. For loperamide and fluperamide, the dosage groups received either
2.5, 10, or 40 mg/kg. The females were sacrificed the morning of the 22nd
day after insemination. The fetuses were delivered by cesarean section and
the dams were examined for number and distribution of dead and live embryos
in each uterine horn, presence of empty implantation sites, and embryos
undergoing resorption. Any abnormal condition in the uterus that could have
contributed to embryonic death was also noted. All fetuses were carefully
examined macroscopically and radiographically. Rat fetuses of each litter
were randomized for dissection (one third) and clearing and bone staining
with alizarin (two thirds).

Young virgin adult female rabbits were fertilized by artificial insemination.
Chorionic gonadotropin, 300 IU/kg rabbit, was given in the marginal
ear vein of the does, on the morning the experiment started. Within three
hours the does were inseminated; an artificial vagina was used to collect the
sperm of the buck. After removing the strings of mucus, the volume was
recorded. Semen was mixed and diluted with warm saline to obtain 3-4
million sperm/0.25 ml diluted sample. Sperm was checked for mobility
before insemination of 0.25 ml diluted sample per doe. From day 6 through
18 after insemination groups of 20 rabbits received the compounds orally by
gavage at different doses in a 0.2 ml/kg vol. The controls received identical
volumes of isotonic NaCl. The difenoxin dose levels were 2.5 and 10 mg/kg.
Loperamide was given at 5, 20, and 40 mg/kg and fluperamide at 1.25, 5,
and 20 mg/kg. All surviving animals were sacrificed the morning of the 28th
day after insemination. The does were necropsied and checked for pregnancy.
The fetuses were weighed individually and immediately examined for any
external anomalies. Radiographic examinations were carried out for all the

fetuses of every litter. One third of the fetuses were also examined for visceral anomalies, the others, being preserved in 95% ethanol. Within one month these two-thirds were used for clearing and bone staining with alizarin.

4.2.3.3. Perinatal and Postnatal Toxicity

The perinatal and postnatal studies were carried out in sexually mature virgin female Wistar rats of a closed laboratory-breeding colony. At mating, these rats were 3 to 4 months old and weighed 200 to 220 g. Groups of 20 rats received the compounds admixed in the diet at various doses from day 16 of pregnancy throughout a three-week lactation period. Control animals received the basic laboratory diet. Difenoxin was given at 0.16, 2.5, 20, and 80 mg/kg and loperamide was given at 2.5, 10, and 40 mg/kg. The young rats of each litter were counted and weighed 8 to 12 hr after birth. Live and dead animals were examined macroscopically and radiographically. When birth had not occurred at the expected date, the females were sacrificed the morning of the 24th day after insemination. After opening the uterus, the distribution of placental sites, resorptions, and dead and live fetuses were noted. Abnormalities were also recorded. Young animals were further individually weighed at 4, 14, and 21 days of age and survival rate at weaning was calculated. Table 17 lists the reproduction studies in rats and rabbits discussed in this section.

TABLE 17

Reproduction Studies in Rats and Rabbits

Compound	Species	Type of study [a]	Dosage, mg/kg					
Difenoxin	Rat	1	0	0.16	2.5	20		
Loperamide	Rat	1	0	2.5	10	40		
Diphenoxylate	Rat	2	0	5	10			
Difenoxin	Rat	2	0	0.16	2.5	10	20	80
	Rabbit	2	0	2.5	10			
Loperamide	Rat	2	0	2.5	10	40		
	Rabbit	2	0	5	20	40		
Fluperamide	Rat	2	0	2.5	10	40		
	Rabbit	2	0	1.25	5	20		
Difenoxin	Rat	3	0	0.16	2.5	20	80	
Loperamide	Rat	3	0	2.5	10	40		

[a] 1: Fertility and reproductive performance; 2: Teratogenesis and embryotoxicity; 3: Perinatal and postnatal toxicity.

TABLE 18

Acute Oral Toxicity of Diphenoxylate, Mortality after Indicated Number of Days

Dose, mg/kg	Mice			Adult rats			Young ♂ rats			Young ♀ rats			Guinea pigs		
	1	3	7	1	3	7	1	3	7	1	3	7	1	3	7
2.5													0	0	0
5.0													0	0	0
10.0													0	0	2
20.0				0	0	0							1	2	2
40.0	0	0	0	0	0	0	0	1	1	0	0	0	0	0	7
80.0	0	0	0	0	0	0	0	7	8	0	3	5	0	4	9
160.0	0	0	0	1	1	2	0	5	6	0	0	4	0	4	10
320.0	0	0	0	0	1	4	0	6	7	0	5	8	1	5	9
640.0	0	0	0	1	1	7		10	10	0	6	8	0	5	10
1280.0	0	1	2		3	8									
2560.0	0	1	2												
LD_{50}	>2560	>2560	>2560	>640	≥640	221	>320	58.0	40.0	>320	137	84.0	>640	231	31.1
LL	–	–	–	–	–	133	–	36.3	25.5	–	85.5	49.2	–	132	21.3
UL	–	–	–	–	–	367	–	92.7	62.7	–	219	143	–	404	45.3

TABLE 19

Acute Oral Toxicity of Fetoxylate, Mortality after Indicated Number of Days

Dose, mg/kg	Mice			Adult rats			Young ♂ rats			Young ♀ rats			Guinea pigs		
	1	3	7	1	3	7	1	3	7	1	3	7	1	3	7
20.0	0	0	0	0	0	0	0	0	0	0	0	0	0	0	0
40.0	0	0	0	0	0	0	0	0	0	0	0	0	1	1	3
80.0	0	0	0	0	0	0	0	1	2	0	4	1	0	0	2
160.0	0	0	1	0	0	0	0	7	9	0	4	4	0	0	1
320.0	0	0	0	1	1	2	0	7	9	2	5	6	2	3	7
640.0	0	1	1	0	1	2	0	7	7	0	3	7	0	2	4
1280.0	0	0	1	1	1	3				2			2	8	8
2560.0				0	1	6									
LD$_{50}$	>2560	>2560	>2560	>2560	>2560	1535	>640	172	129	>640	>640	258	>2560	743	399
LL						849	—	110	89.5	—	—	164	—	500	151
UL						2776	—	269	186	—	—	407	—	1104	1054

TABLE 20
Acute Oral Toxicity of Difenoxin, Mortality after Indicated Number of Days

Dose, mg/kg	Mice			Adult rats			Young ♂ rats			Young ♀ rats			Guinea pigs		
	1	3	7	1	3	7	1	3	7	1	3	7	1	3	7
2.5	0	0	0	0	0	0	0	0	0	0	0	0	0	0	0
5.0	0	0	0	0	0	0	0	0	0	0	0	0	0	0	3
10.0	0	0	0	0	0	0	0	3	3	0	2	2	0	3	4
20.0	0	0	0	0	0	1	3	8	8	0	2	2	1	4	7
40.0	0	0	0	0	0	1	1	7	7	0	3	3	0/5	4/5	5/5
80.0	0	1	1	0	0	0	1	7	7	1	7	7	1/5	4/5	5/5
160.0	1	1	1	0	0	4	1	10	10	0	6	6	1/5	5/5	5/5
320.0	0	0	2	2	3	10				1	10	10			
LD₅₀	>320	>320	>320	>320	>320	149	>160	30.0	30.0	>320	57.0	57.0	>160	23.2	11.0
LL	—	—	—	—	—	89.4	—	20.1	20.1	—	31.2	31.2	—	14.0	7.49
UL	—	—	—	—	—	24.9	—	44.8	44.8	—	104	104	—	38.4	16.3

TABLE 21

Acute Oral Toxicity of Loperamide, Mortality after Indicated Number of Days

Dose, mg/kg	Mice			Adult rats			Young ♀ rats			Young ♂ rats			Guinea pigs			Dogs		
	1	3	7	1	3	7	1	3	7	1	3	7	1	3	7	1	3	7
0.31																0	0	0
0.63																0	0	0
1.25													0	0	0	0	0	0
2.5													0	0	0	0	0	0
5.0													0	0	0	0	0	0
10.0	0	0	0	0	0	0	0	0	0	0	0	0	0	0	1	0	0	0
20.0	0	0	0	0	0	0	0	0	0	0	0	0	2	0	0	0	0	0
40.0	0	0	0	0	0	0	0	0	0	0	0	0	4	3	3			
80.0	0	2	2	1	2	4	1	4	4	0	2	2		8	10			
160.0	4	6	9	6	8	9	0	6	6	1	3	6						
320.0	9	10	10	10	10	10		8	8	2	9	10						
640.0																		
LD$_{50}$	186	129.0	105.0	276	226	185	>320	135.0	135.0	>640	360	261	≈100	53.3	41.5	>40	>40	>40
LL	135	91.5	79.3	202	166	135	—	74.4	74.4	—	244	158	—	37.8	26.6	—	—	—
UL	254	181.0	140.0	378	309	254	—	245.0	245.0	—	532	430	—	75.3	64.6	—	—	—

TABLE 22
Acute Oral Toxicity of Fluperamide, Mortality after Indicated Number of Days

Dose, mg/kg	Mice			Adult rats			Young ♂ rats			Young ♀ rats			Guinea pigs		
	1	3	7	1	3	7	1	3	7	1	3	7	1	3	7
5.0	0	0	0												
10.0	0	0	0												
20.0	0	1	1	0	0	0	0	0	0	0	0	0	0	0	0
40.0	5	8	8	1	1	3	0	1	1	0	0	0	0	0	0
80.0				5	6	7	0	1	1	0	1	2	1	1	1
160.0				8	9	9	0	6	6	0	6	8	1	2	4
320.0				10	10	10	4	10	10	3	9	10	8	10	10
640.0															
LD$_{50}$	160.0	122.0	122.0	160	147	120.0	≥320	132.0	132.0	>320	147	114.0	57.2	45.5	41.7
LL	126.0	91.4	91.4	118	105	86.7	—	90.2	90.2	—	101	88.6	41.4	31.8	25.8
UL	203.0	163.0	163.0	217	207	166.0	—	193.0	193.0	—	214	147.0	79.0	65.1	67.5

4.3. RESULTS

4.3.1. Acute Toxicity Studies

Aqueous solutions or suspensions of the various microcrystalline compounds, prepared with a sonifier, were well tolerated by mice, rats, guinea-pigs, and dogs. The detailed results of the acute toxicity tests are given in Tables 18-22.

From Tables 23 and 24 it is clear that the safety of all tested compounds is extremely high. The safety margin, i.e., the ratio of the toxic dose to the antidiarrheal dose, exceeds 800 for all compounds. Young animals seemed to be more sensitive than adults to diphenoxylate and difenoxin, but this was not the case for loperamide and fluperamide.

The behavioral phenomena at the very high doses tested were as follows:

a. In mice with diphenoxylate, fetoxylate and difenoxin: compulsive circling behavior, arched back and Straub tail; with loperamide and fluperamide: palpebral ptosis, hypertonia, and sedation.

b. In rats with diphenoxylate, fetoxylate and difenoxin: hypertonia, catatonia, and hypothermia; with loperamide and fluperamide: hyper- and hypotonia, and ataxia and palpebral ptosis.

c. In guinea-pigs with diphenoxylate, fetoxylate, difenoxin, loperamide, and fluperamide: behavioral phenomena were less pronounced and more difficult to evaluate. Generally they consisted of hyper- and hypotonia and occasionally of prelethal tremors and dyspnea.

d. In dogs: only loperamide was tested and emesis and paresia of the hind legs were observed.

TABLE 23

Oral LD_{50} Values (mg/kg) of Various Synthetic Antidiarrheal Agents[a]

Compound	Mice	Rat			Guinea pig	Dog
		Adult	Young ♂	Young ♀		
Diphenoxylate	>2560	221	40	84	31.1	
Fetoxylate	>2560	1535			399	
Difenoxin	>320	149	30	57	11.0	
Loperamide	105	185	135	261	41.5	>40
Fluperamide	122	120	132	114	41.7	

[a] After a 7-day observation period.

TABLE 24
Safety Martin in Rats[a]

Compound	Lowest ED_{50}, mg/kg	LD_{50} mg/kg	Safety ratio
Diphenoxylate	0.15	221	1473
Fetoxylate	0.43	1535	3570
Difenoxin	0.04	149	3725
Loperamide	0.15	185	1233
Fluperamide	0.15	120	800

[a] Defined as the ratio of the LD_{50} dose over the lowest ED_{50} dose protecting against diarrhea.

4.3.2. Subacute and Chronic Study

The results of the different subacute and chronic toxicity tests are discussed separately for each compound.

4.3.2.1. Diphenoxylate

<u>Subacute Toxicity in rats (12-13 weeks)</u>: In the subacute toxicity studies in rats no dose or drug-related mortality was observed. In the 12-week study, all animals survived, except one control and one 20 mg/kg dosed female. Control and treated animals were indistinguishable from each other with regard to health, behavior, and appearance. Food consumption decreased slightly in the 20 mg/kg dosed females of the 12-week study and also in the 80 mg/kg dosed males of the 13-week study. Although a slight decrease in body weight gain was observed in the high-dosed 20 and 80 mg/kg groups during the initial weeks of drug administration, no dose-related effect on terminal body weight was observed (see Table 25).

Terminal slit-lamp examinations, hemograms, serum analyses, and urinalyses gave normal results. At autopsy the recorded values of the organ weights fell within the range of normal laboratory values of a compounded laboratory series. The microscopic examinations failed to detect any drug-induced modifications.

<u>Subacute toxicity in dogs (16 weeks)</u>: All controls and all 2, 8, and 32 mg/kg dosed animals survived. No influence on body weight could be detected. Hematological examinations and blood chemistry tests in these dogs gave

TABLE 25

Mean Terminal Body Weight and Food
Consumption of Rats Treated with Diphenoxylate[a]

Diphenoxylate, mg/kg	Body weight, g		Food consumption, g	
	Male	Female	Male	Female
12 Weeks				
0	446	289	2384	1869
0.16	455	294	2441	1826
2.5	469	287	2484	1782
20	445	279	2372	1704[b]
13 Weeks				
0	431	308	2573	1939
1.25	469	289[b]	2704	1908
10	471	315	2605	2055
80	423	304	2402[b]	1959

[a] Admixed in the diet for a 12-to-13-week period.
[b] $p < 0.05$.

essentially normal values. No gross pathological changes attributable to the compound were seen in the dogs at sacrifice. The adrenal to body-weight ratios slightly increased in two 32 mg/kg dosed males but no dose or drug-related histopathology was seen in any organs or tissues.

Chronic toxicity in rats (26 weeks): In this study three 40 mg/kg and one 10 mg/kg dosed males died during the experiment, whereas all females survived. No significant differences in body weight were noted. No changes were seen in the hemograms of the rats and no gross pathology was detected at autopsy. The adrenal to body-weight ratios increased in the treated male rats but not in the females. Histologically the tissues examined were within normal limits (see Table 26).

4.3.2.2. Fetoxylate

Subacute toxicity in rats (15 weeks): All controls and all experimental animals survived, except one 0.16 mg/kg dosed male. Controls and dosed animals were indistinguishable with regard to health and behavior. Final body weight in 0.16 and 2.5 mg/kg dosed males and females and in 20 mg/kg

TABLE 26

Adrenal-to-body-weight Ratio in Rats Orally Treated with Diphenoxylate[a]

Diphenoxylate, mg/kg	Adrenal-to-body-weight ratio, mg/100 g	
	Male	Female
0	9.6	22.2
2	12.6	22.2
10	14.6	21.4
40	14.2	20.4

[a] For a period of 26 weeks.

dosed females was not adversely affected. At 20 mg/kg body-weight gain of males was significantly reduced. A significant decrease in food consumption occurred in the same males, weight gain being correlated with food consumption (see Table 27).

Terminal hemograms and serum analyses gave normal values at all dose-levels. Terminal urinalyses also gave normal results except that specific gravity decreased in the 2.5 mg/kg dosed females and in the 20

TABLE 27

Terminal Mean-Body Weight and Food Consumption of Rats Treated with Fetoxylate[a]

Fetoxylate, mg/kg	Body weight, g		Food consumption, g	
	Male	Female	Male	Female
0	467	334	2958	2414
0.16	469	317	3086	2377
2.5	451	324	2910	2350[b]
20	416[b]	318	2716[c]	2330

[a] Admixed in the diet for a 15-week period.
[b] $p < 0.05$.
[c] $p < 0.01$.

mg/kg dosed males and females. No dose or drug-related pathology was observed at autopsy. Organ weights gave normal values at all dose levels and the histological examination failed to reveal any drug-related pathological changes.

<u>Chronic toxicity in dogs (52 weeks)</u>: All animals (12 males and 12 females) survived the experiment. The body weight of all dosed groups (5, 20, and 80 mg/kg) decreased during the first and the second week of dosing. After this adaptation period the body weight of all dosed groups increased again and was normalized first for the low-dosage group and later also for the higher-dosed groups. Lacrimation, salivation, and vomiting were observed occasionally and irregularly in the 80 mg/kg dosed dogs and rarely in the lower-dosed animals till 6 hr after dosing. Electrocardiogram and indirect blood pressure values were normal. Hematology, serum analyses, and urinalyses failed to reveal significant changes. Histopathological examination of the organs and tissues showed no changes attributable to the drug administration.

4.3.2.3. Difenoxin

<u>Subacute toxicity in rats (13 weeks)</u>: All controls and all 1.25 and 10 mg/kg dosed animals survived. At 20 mg/kg two males out of ten and two females out of ten died. At 80 mg/kg five males out of ten and seven females out of ten died, apparently from constipation. At 1.25 and 10 mg/kg the dosed rats were indistinguishable from the controls regarding health and behavior. At higher doses constipation, roughness of the fur, stiff legs, and decreased general activity was noted. At 20 and 80 mg/kg, body-weight gain was significantly reduced when compared with the controls. This decrease in weight gain was correlated with a decrease in food consumption (see Table 28).

Terminal hemograms, serum analyses and urinalyses gave normal results at all dose levels. With the exception of constipation and haemorrhagic cystitis in animals dosed at 20 and 80 mg/kg, and sacrificed during the test period, no dose- or drug-related pathology could be observed at autopsy. The absolute weight of the liver and the heart decreased in the 20 and 80 mg/kg dosed males (see Table 29), but histological examination failed to reveal any significant changes.

<u>Subacute toxicity in dogs (13 weeks)</u>: During this 13-week study dogs were treated with 0.5, 3, or 10 mg/kg and no mortality occurred. Decreased activity was noted in the 10 mg/kg dosed dogs for about two weeks. In this

TABLE 28

Terminal Body Weight and Food
Consumption of Rats Treated with Difenoxin[a]

Difenoxin, mg/kg	Body weight, g		Food consumption, g	
	Male	Female	Male	Female
0	448	300	2859	2273
1.25	466	302	2869	2218
10	440	288	2769	2195
20	390[b]	278	2521[b]	2185
80	368[b]	294	2394[b]	2355

[a] Admixed in the diet for a 13-week period.
[b] $p < 0.01$.

group, a slight decrease in body weight was noted. Although a slight decrease of hemoglobin and hematocrit was noted in the 10 mg/kg dosed dogs, hematological values remained in the range of the accepted control values. Serum analyses and urinalyses gave normal results. Ophthalmoscopic examinations and electrocardiograms failed to reveal any effects. No distinctive histopathological alterations were found.

TABLE 29

Mean Liver and Heart Weight in Rats Treated with Difenoxin[a]

Difenoxin, mg/kg	Liver weight, mg		Heart weight, mg	
	Male	Female	Male	Female
0	16210	11890	1464	1090
1.25	15490	12330	1393	1139
10	14680	11490	1410	1048
20	12710[b]	11230	1254[b]	1078
80	12680[b]	11320	1183[b]	1085

[a] Admixed in the diet for a 13-week period.
[b] $p < 0.01$.

Chronic toxicity in rats (78 weeks): Difenoxin was admixed in the diet of male and female Wistar rats at dosages of 0, 1.25, 5, and 20 mg/kg. After 12 months of drug administration one half of the males and females was sacrificed, the other half was treated further and sacrificed after 18 months of drug administration. A total of 29 animals out of 160 died during the experiment and eight other animals had to be sacrificed in a moribund state. They were equally distributed among the various dosage groups and the control group. Controls and dosed animals were indistinguishable with regard to health, behavior, and physical appearance. However, at 20 mg/kg stiff legs and a swollen abdomen were noted during the first three weeks of drug administration. These phenomena gradually disappeared and after 3 to 4 weeks the behavior and appearance of these high-dosed rats were normal again. A slight decrease in food intake was noted at 5 and 20 mg/kg during the first month of the experiment; however, after 12 months, as well as after 18 months, there was no significant difference in total food intake between control and treated groups. Although food consumption did not significantly decrease, there was some negative effect on body weight gain at 5 and 20 mg/kg in the males of the 12-month trial. No effect on body weight could be seen in dosed females involved in the 12-month trial and in dosed males and females involved in the 18-month experiment. The results obtained in hematology, clinical chemistry, and urinalysis, fell within the range of our normal values. The gross pathology observations failed to reveal any dose or drug-related effects. Findings such as pneumonia, pleuritis, and local alopecia, were related to ageing processes, for they were encountered in dosed as well as in control rats. Organ weights fell within the normal range and no drug-related histopathological modifications could be observed.

Chronic toxicity in dogs (52 weeks): The dosage schedule for this study is given in Table 30.

The initial doses were reduced after one week as an abnormally high rate of emesis, salivation, and depression was noted during the first week of

TABLE 30

Schedule of Dosage

Group	Dosage, mg/kg/day		
	Week 1	Week 2-21	Week 22-52
Control	0	0	—
Low	0.63	0.16	0.16
Medium	2.5	0.63	2.5
High	10	2.5	5

Preclinical Studies: Safety Evaluation

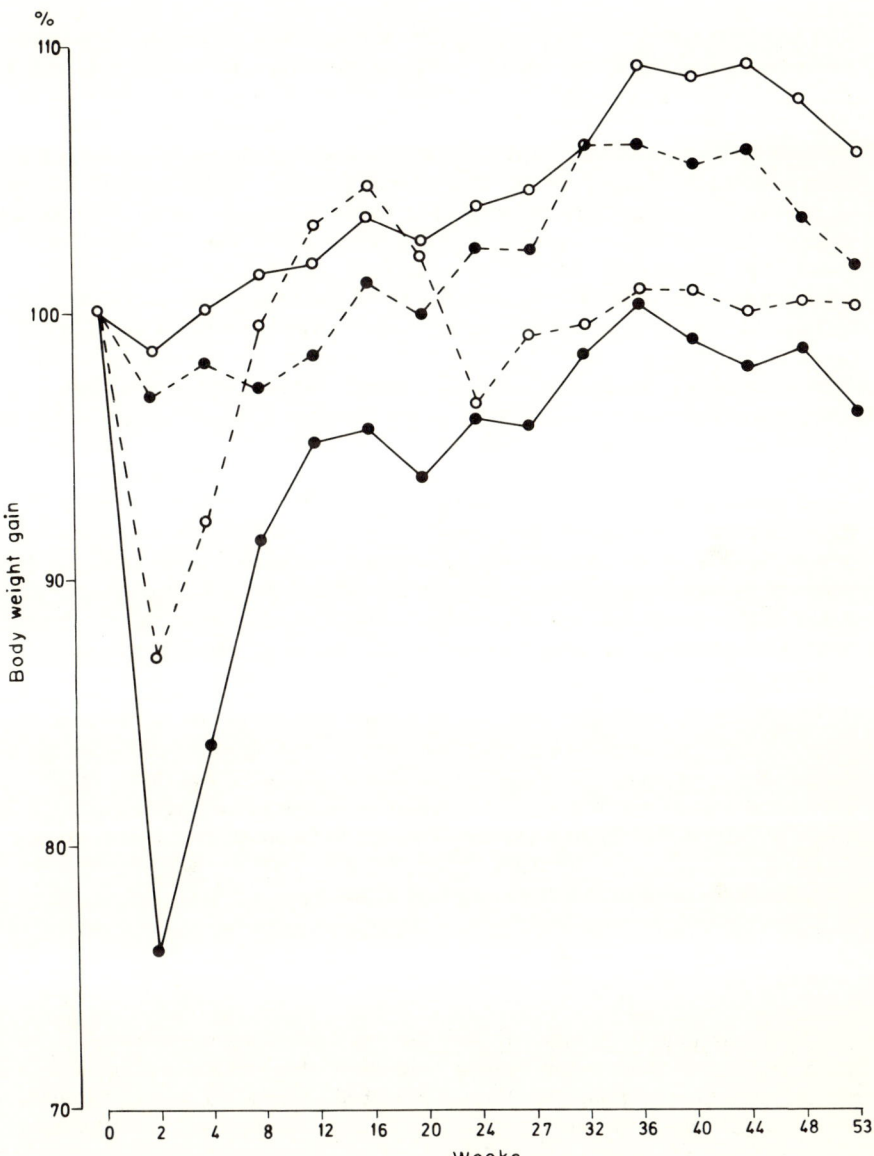

Fig. 46. Average body-weight gain (expressed in percentages) of dogs receiving difenoxin for a period of 53 weeks. Dose of drug: Control = 0 (o—o); low (●---●), 0.63 mg/kg (week 0-1), 0.16 mg/kg (week 2-53); medium (o---o), 2.5 mg/kg (week 0-1), 0.63 mg/kg (week 2-21), 2.5 mg/kg (week 22-53); high (●—●), 10 mg/kg (week 0-1), 2.5 mg/kg (week 2-21), 5 mg/kg (week 22-53).

drug administration. At 0.16 mg/kg the animals were indistinguishable from the controls with regard to health, behavior, and appearance. At 2.5 mg/kg one female died of enteritis (week 29) and at 5 mg/kg two males were sacrificed in a moribund state (week 4 and 25) with petechial bleeding in the stomach and with enteritis. All other animals survived. At 2.5 and 5 mg/kg, dosage had to be stopped once or twice for a few days in about half the animals as severe hemorrhagic stools were observed from time to time. This feature occurred for the various animals at various periods of the test: from a few weeks after the start of the trial up to several months later. Body-weight gain decreased with increasing dosages and the average terminal weight increase or decrease was +5.9% in the control group, +1.7% at 0.16 mg/kg, +0.2% at 2.5 mg/kg, and -3.8% at 5 mg/kg (see Fig. 46). Terminal electrocardiograms were satisfactory. Heart rates, however, increased when dosages were raised from 0.63 to 2.5 and from 2.5 to 5 mg/kg during week 22, and also during the period when the animals were affected by hemorrhagic stools. Blood pressure was not affected. The hematological values and the values obtained by serum analyses were within the normal limits, except a slight terminal decrease of total protein, albumin, and calcium at 5 mg/kg and of cholesterol at 2.5 and 5 mg/kg. Urinalyses gave normal results. No dose- or drug-related changes were found at necropsy, except the cases of enteritis observed in the three animals, dead or sacrificed during the experiment. Organ weights were within normal limits with a possible marginal increase of the liver weight in the 5 mg/kg dosed group.

Histological examination of the organs and tissues failed to reveal any dose- or drug-related effects. The testes of a few animals, especially those that had to be sacrificed during the experiment showed some giant cell formation, slight desquamation, and sometimes poor spermatogenic activity. However, as no obvious degenerative tubules were observed but only some arrest of the seminal maturation, it was believed that this effect occurred through impairment of the general status of health.

4.3.2.4. Loperamide

Subacute toxicity in rats (15 weeks): The dietary administration of loperamide provided an approximate dose of 40, 10, and 2.5 mg/kg. All controls and all experimental animals survived, except one 40 mg/kg dosed female which had to be sacrificed on the 56th day of the experiment because of an abscess under the bulbus olfactorius.

Controls and 2.5 mg/kg dosed animals were indistinguishable with regard to health and behavior. The 10 mg/kg dosed animals had unusually rough fur during the first two weeks of the experiment, and the 40 mg/kg dosed animals during the first four weeks. In the last group nasal discharge and swollen abdomen were also observed during the first three to four weeks but later disappeared. From the first week of treatment, weight gain and food

Preclinical Studies: Safety Evaluation

TABLE 31

Terminal Mean Body Weight and Food Consumption of Rats Treated with Loperamide[a]

Loperamide, mg/kg	Body weight, g		Food consumption, g	
	Male	Female	Male	Female
0	439	284	3089	2338
2.5	437	292	2974	2309
10	421	293	2844[b]	2345
40	319[c]	241[c]	2296[c]	1920[c]

[a] Admixed in the diet for a 15-week period.
[b] $p < 0.05$.
[c] $p < 0.001$.

consumption were significantly lower ($p < 0.001$) in the 40 mg/kg dosed males and females (see Table 31). Terminal slit-lamp examinations, hemograms, serum analyses and urinalyses were satisfactory, except for a decrease of creatinine in dosed males and females (see Table 32).

No gross pathology was observed, except a small prostate and a thin oblong-shaped uterus in some 40 mg/kg dosed animals. At this dose the weight of the brain, expressed as a percentage of body weight, increased

TABLE 32

Terminal Mean Creatinine Values in the Urine of Rats Treated with Loperamide[a]

Loperamide, mg/kg	Creatinine, mg %	
	Male	Female
0	150	131
2.5	113[c]	110
10	114[b]	104[b]
40	54[d]	58[d]

[a] Admixed in the diet for a 15-week period.
[b] $p < 0.05$.
[c] $p < 0.01$.
[d] $p < 0.001$.

TABLE 33

Mean Brain Weight of Rats Treated with Loperamide[a]

Loperamide, mg/kg	Mean brain weight			
	Males		Females	
	Absolute, mg	Relative[b]	Absolute, mg	Relative[b]
0	1898	0.44	1751	0.60
2.5	1880	0.44	1755	0.59
10	1906	0.46	1753	0.58
40	1795[c]	0.56[d]	1694	0.70[e]

[a] Admixed in the diet for a 15-week period.
[b] Percent body weight.
[c] $p < 0.05$.
[d] $p < 0.001$.
[e] $p < 0.01$.

TABLE 34

Mortality Rate in Rats Treated with Loperamide[a]

Loperamide, mg/kg	Number of deaths in indicated period					
	6 months		12 months		18 months	
	Male	Female	Male	Female	Male	Female
0	2	0	0	0	6	2
2.5	0	0	0	0	4	2
10	0	0	1	1	7	2
40	0	0	1	1	6	7

[a] Admixed in the diet for a 6-, 12-, or 18-month period (10 animals per group).

(see Table 33). All other recorded organ weights were satisfactory. The histological study failed to reveal dose- or drug-related changes, except less thyroid activity and less thyrotropin in the pituitary glands in the 40 mg/kg dosed males. Because of the creatinine findings, various muscles were examined histologically; they did not reveal any atrophy or dystrophy. At 40 mg/kg a slightly reduced secretory activity of the prostate was observed in a few males. The 40 mg/kg dosed females had a tendency to diestrus. Since no degenerative modifications were seen and since, in rats, similar changes are easily produced by partial starvation, the observed macroscopic and histological changes are probably related to the reduction of food consumption and not to the experimental compound.

Chronic toxicity in rats (78 weeks): The dietary administration of loperamide provided an approximate dose of 40, 10, and 2.5 mg/kg. A total of 24 animals out of 240 died and 18 other animals had to be sacrificed before the end of the 6-, 12-, or 18-month experiments (see Table 34). No dose- or drug-related effect could be observed.

Throughout the experiment, health and behavior were normal in all experimental groups. Weight gain and food consumption were lower (see Tables 35 and 36) in the 40 mg/kg dosed males and females throughout the entire experimental period, but especially during the first three months of drug administration.

TABLE 35

Terminal Mean Body Weight, g, of Rats Treated with Loperamide[a]

Loperamide, mg/kg	Body weight, g, after stated period					
	6 months		12 months		18 months	
	Male	Female	Male	Female	Male	Female
0	500	328	537	361	529	400
2.5	496	322	540	336[b]	597	379
10	481	321	524	360	492	403
40	421[c]	274[d]	410[d]	294[c]	441	302[c]

[a] Admixed in the diet for a 6-, 12-, or 18-month period.
[b] $p < 0.05$.
[c] $p < 0.01$.
[d] $p < 0.001$.

TABLE 36

Terminal Mean Food Consumption, g, in Rats Treated with Loperamide[a]

Loperamide, mg/kg	Food consumption, g, after stated period					
	6 months		12 months		18 months	
	Male	Female	Male	Female	Male	Female
0	5641	4435	10512	8444	16406	13607
2.5	5436	4322	10263	7874[b]	17579	12783
10	5478	4403	10319	8344	16063	14441
40	4815[b]	3806[c]	9019[d]	7433[c]	14134[b]	11787[b]

[a] Admixed in the diet for a 6-, 12-, or 18-month period.
[b] $p < 0.05$.
[c] $p < 0.01$.
[d] $p < 0.001$.

TABLE 37

Terminal Mean Creatinine, mg %, in the Urine of Rats Treated with Loperamide[a]

Loperamide, mg/kg	Creatinine, mg %, in stated period					
	6 months		12 months		18 months	
	Male	Female	Male	Female	Male	Female
0	125	106	143	93	161	114
2.5	111	147[b]	120	89	140	106
10	108[b]	137	95[d]	72[b]	137	135
40	63[c]	112	85[d]	71[b]	136	103

[a] Admixed in the diet for a 6-, 12-, or 18-month period.
[b] $p < 0.05$.
[c] $p < 0.001$.
[d] $p < 0.01$.

Terminal slit-lamp examinations, hemograms, serum analyses, and urinalyses were satisfactory, except, as in the subacute study, for a decrease of creatinine at 10 and 40 mg/kg in the males of the 6- and 12-month studies and the females of the 12-month study, but not in the 18-month study (see Table 37).

Gross pathology revealed a dose-related incidence of hyperemia of the vascular system of the intestines and mesenterium in the 6- and 12-month studies. The other observed necropsy findings were mainly related to ageing processes. No carcinogenic effect could be detected. Organ weights were also within normal limits, except for an increase of the relative weight of the brain in the 40 mg/kg dosed males and females of the 6- and 12-month studies (see Table 38). Histologically all organs and tissues were considered to be

TABLE 38

Mean Brain Weight in Rats Treated with Loperamide[a]

Duration of study, months	Loperamide, mg/kg	Mean brain weight			
		Males		Females	
		Absolute, mg	Relative	Absolute, mg	Relative[b]
6	0	1915	0.38	1786	0.54
	2.5	1973	0.40	1785	0.56
	10	1928	0.40	1866[c]	0.58[c]
	40	1918	0.46[d]	1823	0.66[e]
12	0	2036	0.38	1911	0.54
	2.5	2047	0.38	1898	0.57
	10	1985	0.38	1920	0.54
	40	1979	0.49[e]	1902	0.65[e]
18	0	2047	0.39	1863	0.47
	2.5	2180[c]	0.37	1953[c]	0.52
	10	2079	0.44	1927	0.48
	40	2046	0.47	1827	0.61[c]

[a] Admixed in the diet for a 6-, 12-, or 18-month period.
[b] Percent body weight.
[c] $p < 0.05$.
[d] $p < 0.01$.
[e] $p < 0.001$.

normal, except that the 40 mg/kg dosed animals of the 12- and 18-month studies frequently showed septal cell proliferation in the lungs, which is considered to occur normally in aged rats.

Chronic toxicity in dogs (52 weeks): All controls and all 0.31 and 1.25 mg/kg dosed animals survived. At 5 mg/kg one animal died of hemorrhagic enteritis during the 17th week of the experiment. From time to time five

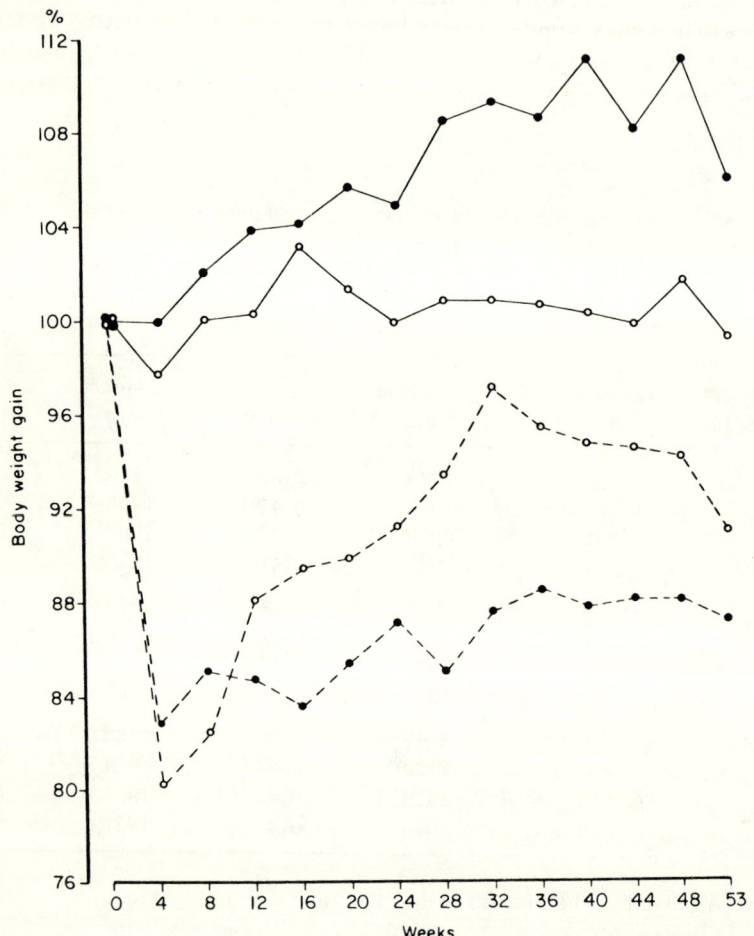

Fig. 47. Average body-weight gain (expressed in percentages) of dogs receiving loperamide orally for a period of 12 months. Dose of drug: Control = 0 (●—●); low = 0.31 mg/kg (o—o); medium = 1.25 mg/kg (●---●); high = 5 mg/kg (o---o).

other animals of this group had hemorrhagic stools; the 0.31 and 1.25 mg/kg dosed animals had soft stools. During the first week of the experiment, the 1.25 and 5 mg/kg dosed animals were depressed and vomited and salivated regularly after drug administration. From the second week onwards, behavior and appearance were normal in all experimental groups. During the first two weeks of dosing, body weight decreased in all dosed groups. At 1.25 and 5 mg/kg body weight fell to ±80% of the initial body weight and remained depressed till week 6. From that time onward, body weight increased without reaching its initial value (see Fig. 47).

Blood pressure, heart rate, electrocardiograms, hemograms, serum analyses, urinalyses, ophthalmoscopic, and slit-lamp examinations were satisfactory. Gross pathologic and histologic examination did not reveal any dose- or drug-related changes.

4.3.2.5. Fluperamide

Subacute toxicity in rats (13 weeks): The dietary administration of fluperamide provided an approximate dose of 2.5, 10, and 40 mg/kg. All control animals survived. At 2.5 mg/kg one male out of 20 animals died. At 10 mg/kg no mortality occurred, whereas at 40 mg/kg two males out of 10 and one female out of 10 died. Urinary retention and/or enteritis were probably the cause of death. Controls and 2.5 mg/kg dosed animals were indistinguishable with regard to health, behavior, and appearance. At 10 and 40 mg/kg slight to pronounced depression was observed during the entire experimental period. Terminal food consumption and weight gain decreased significantly in 40 mg/kg dosed males and females (see Table 39). These

TABLE 39

Terminal Mean Body Weight and Food Consumption in Rats Treated with Fluperamide[a]

Fluperamide, mg/kg	Body weight, g		Food consumption, g	
	Male	Female	Male	Female
0	413	285	2521	2033
2.5	424	282	2495	2013
10	410	291	2429	2062[b]
40	260[b]	220[b]	1571[b]	1528[b]

[a] Admixed in the diet for a 13-week period.
[b] $p < 0.001$.

effects were observed during the entire experimental period. At lower doses a transitional effect on food consumption was noted during the first week of dosing.

Hemograms were considered to be normal in all groups. Serum analyses gave normal results, except a marginal decrease of potassium in the 2.5 and 40 mg/kg dosed females, a marginal increase of total protein in 10 mg/kg dosed females, an increase of alkaline phosphatase and a decrease of glucose in both males and females dosed at 40 mg/kg, and a decrease of phosphorus in 40 mg/kg dosed males. Urinalyses gave normal results, except for a decrease of creatinine in 40 mg/kg dosed males and in 10 and 40 mg/kg dosed females (see Table 40).

No gross pathology was observed, except that the prostates of some 40 mg/kg dosed males were atrophic and that some constipation was seen in both males and females dosed at 40 mg/kg. The histological studies revealed changes in the following organs of the 40 mg/kg dosed animals. A slight chronic stimulation of the liver parenchyma with somewhat more densely nucleated tissue was noted. A tendency to more fatty cortex in the adrenals was noted. The male genital organs showed more changes than usually seen, namely, two out of eight (one of which was evidently atrophic) had no or very poor spermatogenic activity. The prostate showed an atrophic aspect more regularly with a reduced amount of secretion. The mammary gland had a tendency to some atrophy. The female genital organs were characterized by a tendency to more numerous atretic follicles, more abundant interstitial

TABLE 40

Terminal Mean Alkaline Phosphatase Values in Serum and Terminal Mean Creatinine Values in Urine of Rats Treated with Fluperamide[a]

Fluperamide, mg/kg	Alkaline phosphatase, KA units		Creatinine, mg %	
	Male	Female	Male	Female
0	32	21	135	143
2.5	30	20	169	146[b]
10	35	19[b]	95[c]	104[c]
40	46[c]	26[b]	77[c]	89[c]

[a] Admixed in the diet for a 13-week period.
[b] $p < 0.05$.
[c] $p < 0.01$.

glandular tissue, and a somewhat atrophic aspect of the uterus. The chromophobe tissue of the hypophysis was more extended in the 40 mg/kg dosed rats. The 40 mg/kg dosed males showed fewer or no cytoplasmic vacuoles in the gonadotrophs.

On the whole it was believed that most of these changes were the secondary consequences of an altered general health, as observed in the 40 mg/kg dosed group, and evidenced by very low weight gains.

Subacute toxicity in dogs (12 weeks): All six controls and all six 0.31 mg/kg dosed animals survived the experiment. At 1.25 mg/kg, one animal out of six died and at 2.5 to 5 mg/kg five animals out of nine died during the experiment. Health, behavior, and appearance were normal and comparable in controls and in the 0.31, 1.25, and 2.5 mg/kg dosed dogs, with the exception that sporadic soft and even bloody stools were seen in all dosed groups. At 5 mg/kg apathy, blood mucous feces, prostration, and decubitus were seen. After reduction of the 5 mg/kg dose to 2.5 mg/kg all surviving animals of this group recovered within a few weeks, and no clinical observations could be made, except for the above mentioned sporadic appearance of soft stools. At 0.31, 1.25, and 2.5 mg/kg an important decrease in body weight was observed after 2 to 3 weeks of dosing, whereafter a slight trend to increase was noted but the initial body weight was not reached again after 3 months of dosing. At 5 mg/kg the decrease in body weight was fatal. At 0.31, 1.25, and 2.5 mg/kg heart rates, electrocardiograms, blood pressure, hemograms, serum analyses, and urinalyses were considered to be normal. Gross pathology findings at 0.31, 1.25, and 2.5 mg/kg were considered to be normal, except that one 1.25 mg/kg dosed animal, which died during the 3rd week of the experiment, showed the same features as the animals which died after the 5 mg/kg dose, i.e., gastritis, duodenitis, enteritis with intestinal bleedings, and icterus. Organ weights at the 0.31, 1.25, and 2.5 mg/kg doses were considered to be normal. The histological examinations of the 0.31, 1.25, and 2.5 mg/kg dosed dogs failed to reveal any dose- or drug-related effects, except that impairment of general health could have resulted in some lowered spermatogenesis and germinal cell desquamation at 2.5 mg/kg. At 5 mg/kg, in the dogs which died or were sacrificed in extremis, general hyperemia of the tissues and/or more or less defined post-mortem changes were seen.

Chronic toxicity in rats (78 weeks): No dose- or drug-related mortality was noticed in the 6-, 12-, and 18-month studies. Mortalities observed in the 12- and 18-month studies were due to normally occurring diseases in aged rats. During the first weeks of drug administration, apathy and sedation with ptosis were seen in the medium (5 mg/kg) and high-dosage (20 mg/kg) animals. After these initial weeks the animals became excited and aggressive for the entire experimental period. At 1.25 mg/kg no drug-related effect could be

TABLE 41

Terminal Mean Body Weight, g, of Rats Treated with Fluperamide[a]

Fluperamide, mg/kg	6 months		12 months		18 months	
	Male	Female	Male	Female	Male	Female
0	522	348	567	375[b]	522	393
1.25	518	325	564	336[b]	495	382[b]
5	523	329[c]	535[c]	369[c]	545	360[b]
20	435[c]	295[c]	439[c]	294[c]	462	319[c]

[a] Admixed in the diet for a 6-, 12-, or 18-month period.
[b] $p < 0.05$.
[c] $p < 0.001$.

noted. The recorded observations are of no clinical importance since the ED_{50} in the castor-oil test (inhibition of diarrhea produced by castor oil in rats) equals 0.15 mg/kg (1 hr protection) to 0.89 mg/kg (8 hr protection). A decrease of food consumption was noted in males and females when dosed at 20 mg/kg for 6, 12, and 18 months. This effect was most pronounced during the first three months of dosing. At 1.25 and 5 mg/kg, food consumption slightly and temporarily decreased during the first weeks of dosing. A decrease of body weight gain was noted in males and females when dosed at 20 mg/kg for 6, 12, and 18 months. This effect was persistent during the entire experimental period and correlated with decreased food consumption. At 1.25 and 5 mg/kg no conspicuous effect on body weight could be detected. The differences in hematology between control and treated groups were devoid of any clinical importance, for most of the recorded values in the treated groups were within normal limits, and/or the recorded differences in these treated groups were not dose-related. The differences in biochemistry between control and treated animals were devoid of any clinical importance. Most of the changes occurred simultaneously in dosed and undosed animals. Changes occurring only in dosed animals were considered to be of no importance for they were either not dose-related, or remained within or were marginal to normal values. All values recorded were considered to be normal except that after 6 months a decrease in creatinine in the 5 and 20 mg/kg dosed males and in the 20 mg/kg dosed females was noted. There was also a decrease in the 20 mg/kg dosed males and females after 12 months.

No dose- or drug-related effects could be observed at autopsy. No dose- or drug-related effects on organ weights could be observed for the changes in

TABLE 42

Terminal Mean Food Consumption, g,
of Rats Treated with Fluperamide[a]

Fluperamide, mg/kg	6 months		12 months		18 months	
	Male	Female	Male	Female	Male	Female
0	5657	4537	11048	8513	17437[b]	14037
1.25	5481	4220[b]	10584	7961	16246[b]	13592
5	5778	4237[d]	10545[b]	8866[d]	17878	13177[c]
20	4819[c]	3956[d]	9611[b]	7348[d]	15842	12596[c]

[a] Admixed in the diet for a 6-, 12-, or 18-month period.
[b] $p < 0.05$.
[c] $p < 0.01$.
[d] $p < 0.001$.

treated animals were either within or marginal to normal values. No dose- or drug-related histopathology could be observed in the various organs and tissues of rats from the 6-, 12-, and 18-month studies.

Chronic toxicity in dogs (52 weeks): All controls and all 0.16, 0.31, and 0.63 mg/kg dosed animals survived the 12-month experiment. With the exception of some emesis and soft stools during the first week of dosing, especially at the 0.63 mg/kg level, behavior and appearance were normal in all groups during the entire experiment. A temporary body-weight decrease was noted in all dosed groups during the first 2 months at 0.16 mg/kg, the first 4 months at 0.31 mg/kg, and the first 6 months at 0.63 mg/kg. Thereafter a normal increase in body weight was noted in all groups. However, terminally, body-weight gain was lower with increasing dosages (see Fig. 48). Heart rate, electrocardiograms, and blood pressure were satisfactory during the entire experimental period. Hematology, serum analysis, and urinalysis gave normal results. Gross pathology failed to produce any abnormalities at 0.16 mg/kg, whereas at 0.31 and 0.63 mg/kg a thickened wall of the gastrointestinal tract was observed with bile-pigment coloration of the duodenal mucosa. Organ weights were considered to be normal. The histological examination of the various organs and tissues did not reveal any modifications which could be ascribed to the administration of fluperamide.

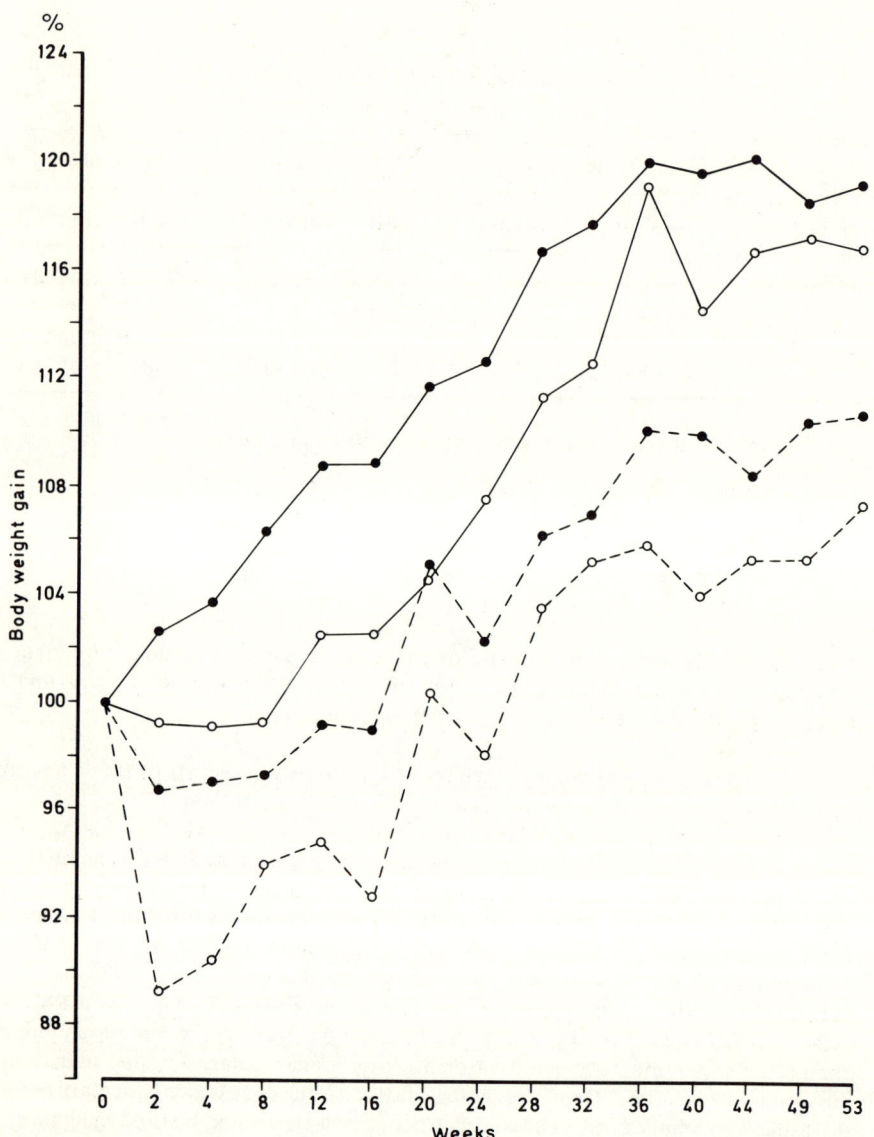

Fig. 48. Average body-weight gain (expressed in percentages) of dogs receiving fluperamide orally for a period of 53 weeks. Dose of drug: Control = 0 (●——●); low = 0.16 mg/kg (o——o); medium = 0.31 mg/kg (●---●); high = 0.63 mg/kg (o---o).

Preclinical Studies: Safety Evaluation   187

4.3.3. Reproduction Studies

   4.3.3.1. Fertility and General Reproductive Performance

   The results of these studies are listed in Tables 43 and 44. Difenoxin and loperamide, administered at the doses mentioned, did not affect the mating performance of the dosed rats. Neither did difenoxin and loperamide influence the fertility of treated female rats; except in the 40 mg/kg loperamide dosed group of females in which no pregnancies occurred. In the lower-dosed loperamide groups and in all difenoxin groups, there were no differences in the number of implantations per dam, litter size, percentage of live, dead, and resorbed fetuses; distribution of live, dead, and resorbed fetuses in the left and right uterine horns; and body weight of live pups. There was also no evidence of teratogenicity.

   4.3.3.2. Teratogenesis and Embryotoxicity

   The results of the rat studies are presented in Table 45. No dose-related mortalities were noted among the various experimental groups receiving diphenoxylate, difenoxin, loperamide, and fluperamide at the doses mentioned. With difenoxin one animal out of 20 died at 10, 20, and 80 mg/kg and with fluperamide one animal out of 20 died at 2.5 and 40 mg/kg. The pregnancy rate among the various experimental groups was considered to be normal, except at high doses where the number of pregnant animals decreased. Diphenoxylate at 5 and 10 mg/kg, difenoxin at 0.16, 2.5, and 10 mg/kg, loperamide and fluperamide at 2.5 and 10 mg/kg did not significantly influence the number of implantations per dam; litter size, percentage of live, dead, and resorbed fetuses; distribution of live, dead, and resorbed fetuses in the left and right uterine horns and body weight of live pups. No dose- or drug-related macroscopic, visceral or skeletal malformations were seen. A few cases of waved ribs were seen, but this is a commonly encountered feature in control animals of the particular Wistar substrain used.

   The results of the rabbit studies are presented in Table 46. No differences in pregnancy rate could be noted in the various dosed groups as compared with the control groups. The mortality rate of treated rabbits only increased in the high-dosed loperamide group (40 mg/kg) and the high-dosed fluperamide group (20 mg/kg) and was mainly due to enteritis. For difenoxin an increase in the percentage of resorptions was noted at the high-dose level of 10 mg/kg. In the high-dosed loperamide group (40 mg/kg) there was an increase in the percentage of dead fetuses; at this dosage there was also a decrease in the average weight of pups at delivery. In the high-dosed fluperamide group (20 mg/kg) there was a decrease in the average weight of pups at delivery and in the percentage of live fetuses, whereas the percentage of resorptions increased. In the treated animals no dose- or drug-related skeletal or visceral

TABLE 43

Pregnancy and Litter Data in Rats and Their Offspring After Oral Administration of Difenoxin to Males[a] or to Females[b]

Experimental conditions	Dosage, mg/kg							
	0		0.16		2.5		20	
	Control males + treated females	Treated males + control females	Control males + treated females	Treated males + control females	Control males + treated females	Treated males + control females	Control males + treated females	Treated males + control females
Adult rat								
Pregnancy rate, %	100	100	80	100	90	100	78.9	94
Mortality rate of females, %	0	0	0	0	0	0	0	0
Litter[c]								
Mean litter size	11.8	10.9	13.3	9.4	12.8	10.8	10.5	10.1
Average weight at birth, g	5.5	5.3	5.2	5.5	5.3	5.3	5.3	5.4
Alive fetuses, %	99.2	96.9	97.2	95.9	98.3	99.5	98.1	96.2
Dead fetuses, %	0	0	0	0	0	0	0	0
Resorbed fetuses, %	0.8	3.1	2.8	4.1	1.7	0.5	1.9	3.8

[a]Minimum 60 days before mating.
[b]Fourteen days before mating and further during pregnancy.
[c]No abnormalities.

TABLE 44

Pregnancy and Litter Data in Rats and Their Offspring After Oral Administration of Loperamide to Males[a] or to Females[b]

Experimental conditions	Dosage, mg/kg							
	0		2.5		10		40	
	Control males + treated females	Treated males + control females	Control males + treated females	Treated males + control females	Control males + treated females	Treated males + control females	Control males + treated females	Treated males + control females
Adult rat								
Pregnancy rate, %	100	100	100	100	95	85	0	80
Mortality rate of females, %	0	0	0	0	0	0	0	0
Litter[c]								
Mean litter size	11.3	10.6	10.3	11.1	11.0	11.5	—	11.0
Average weight at birth, g	5.3	5.4	5.4	5.3	5.5	5.3	—	5.4
Alive fetuses, %	96.6	95.5	92.4	98.7	98.1	99.0	—	98.3
Dead fetuses, %	0	0	5.2	0	0	0	—	0
Resorbed fetuses, %	3.4	4.5	2.4	1.3	1.9	1.0	—	1.7

[a] Minimum 60 days before mating.
[b] Fourteen days before mating and further during pregnancy.
[c] No abnormalities.

TABLE 45

Teratogenic Potential of Various Antidiarrheal Agents in Wistar Rats[a]

Diphenoxylate	Dosage, mg/kg		
	0	5	10
Adult rat			
Pregnancy, %	92	80	53
Mortality, %	0.85	0	0
Litter			
Mean litter size	11.1	11.2	10.4
Average weight at birth, g	5.0	4.7	4.7
Live fetuses, %	96.0	95.0	93.0
Dead fetuses, %	0.6	3.0	0
Resorbed fetuses, %	3.4	2.0	7.0
Abnormalities	0	0	0

Difenoxin	Dosage, mg/kg					
	0	0.16	2.5	10	20	80
Adult rat						
Pregnancy, %	90	100	100	16	0	0
Mortality, %	0	0	0	5	5	5
Litter						
Mean litter size	10.6	11.7	11.5	10.7		
Average weight at birth, g	5.4	5.2	5.1	4.6		
Live fetuses, %	97.4	96.7	96.2	94.1		
Dead fetuses, %	0	0.5	0	0		
Resorbed fetuses, %	2.6	2.8	3.8	5.9		
Abnormalities	0	+[b]	0	0		

Loperamide	Dosage, mg/kg			
	0	2.5	10	40
Adult rat				
Pregnancy, %	100	100	95	5
Mortality, %	0	0	0	0

Preclinical Studies: Safety Evaluation

Table 45 (Continued)

Loperamide	Dosage, mg/kg			
	0	2.5	10	40
Litter				
Mean litter size	10.6	9.3	9.9	8.0
Average weight at birth, g	5.3	5.5	5.2	4.5
Live fetuses, %	93.5	92.5	91.7	88.9
Dead fetuses, %	4.2	0.0	0.5	0.0
Resorbed fetuses, %	2.3	7.5	7.8	11.1
Abnormalities	0	0	0	0

Fluperamide	Dosage, mg/kg			
	0	2.5	10	40
Adult rat				
Pregnancy, %	100	65	65	0
Mortality, %	0	5	0	5
Litter				
Mean litter size	10.5	10.9	10.2	
Average weight at birth, g	5.5	5.3	5.5	
Live fetuses, %	99.1	95.3	95.7	
Dead fetuses, %	0.0	0.0	0.0	
Resorbed fetuses, %	0.9	4.7	4.3	
Abnormalities	0	0	+[b]	

[a] Treatment period: day 6 through day 15 of pregnancy.

[b] Abnormalities of the type commonly encountered in control fetuses of the same Wistar substrain.

anomalies were noted. In the difenoxin study one control fetus had one deformed thoracic bone. The same abnormality was observed in one fetus born to a mother treated at 2.5 and at 10 mg/kg. One case of deformed ribs (2.5 mg/kg) and one case of coelosomy (10 mg/kg) were also noted. In the loperamide study one control fetus had bifurcated ribs and one fetus of the 40 mg/kg group showed cyclotia. In the fluperamide study no abnormalities were seen at 20 mg/kg but two fetuses of the 1.25 mg/kg group and one fetus of the 5 mg/kg group showed minor skeletal variations. It was not believed that the above described abnormalities were dose- or drug-related effects, as analogous abnormalities have been encountered in control fetuses of many other studies using the same New Zealand rabbit strain under comparable laboratory conditions.

TABLE 46

Teratogenic Potential of Various Antidiarrheal Agents in New Zealand Rabbits[a]

Difenoxin	Dosage, mg/kg		
	0	2.5	10
Adult rabbit			
Pregnancy, %	80	90	90
Mortality, %	5	5	0
Litter			
Mean litter size	4.8	6.3	4.1
Average weight at birth, g	43.4	38.7	35.3
Live fetuses, %	82.8	84.1	53.0
Dead fetuses, %	0	0	0
Resorbed fetuses, %	17.2	15.9	47.0
Abnormalities	+[b]	+[b]	+[b]

Loperamide	Dosage, mg/kg			
	0	5	20	40
Adult rabbit				
Pregnancy, %	70	60	70	80
Mortality, %	20	10	15	60
Litter				
Mean litter size	6.5	5.4	5.3	5.3
Average weight at birth, g	40.9	41.4	38.1	34.1
Live fetuses, %	98.6	95.2	89.2	87.0
Dead fetuses, %	0	0	0	4.3
Resorbed fetuses, %	1.4	4.8	10.8	8.7
Abnormalities	+[b]	0	0	+[b]

Fluperamide	Dosage, mg/kg			
	0	1.25	5	20
Adult rabbit				
Pregnancy, %	70	75	70	80
Mortality, %	0	0	0	65
Litter				
Mean litter size	4.1	3.9	5.3	3.7
Average weight at birth, g	41.1	40.6	37.3	33.7
Live fetuses, %	85.1	75.3	86.9	56.4
Dead fetuses, %	0	0	1.2	0
Resorbed fetuses, %	14.9	24.7	11.9	43.6
Abnormalities	0	+[b]	+[b]	0

[a] Treatment period: day 6 through day 18 of pregnancy.
[b] Abnormalities of the type commonly encountered in control fetuses of the same New Zealand strain.

TABLE 47

Pregnancies and Litter Data of Wistar
Rats Receiving Various Antidiarrheal Agents [a]

Difenoxin	Dosage, mg/kg				
	0	0.16	2.5	20	80
Adult rat					
Pregnancy, %	90	85	80	90	73
Mortality, %	0	0	0	0	25
Litter					
Mean litter size	11.1	11.0	10.6	8.9	8.5
Average weight at birth, g	5.8	5.9	6.2	6.1	5.9
Live fetuses, %	93.5	92.0	93.5	78.8	30.9
Dead fetuses, %	6.5	8.0	6.5	21.2	69.1
Survival rate of weaning, %	41.2	30.2	13.3	4.0	0
Abnormalities	+[b]	0	0	0	0

Loperamide	Dosage, mg/kg			
	0	2.5	10	40
Adult rat				
Pregnancy, %	95	95	100	95
Mortality, %	0	0	5	0
Litter				
Mean litter size	9.8	11.2	11.7	9.6
Average weight at birth, g	5.9	6.0	5.9	5.5
Live fetuses, %	91.5	95.5	98.5	92.7
Dead fetuses, %	8.5	4.5	1.5	7.3
Survival rate of weaning, %	79.6	90.6	71.0	13.8
Abnormalities	0	0	0	0

[a] Period covering the final one-third of gestation throughout lactation to weaning, 3 weeks after delivery.

[b] Abnormalities of the type commonly encountered in control fetuses of the same Wistar substrain.

4.3.3.3. Perinatal and Postnatal Toxicity

The results of these studies are presented in Table 47. In the difenoxin study five animals out of 20 died at 80 mg/kg and at the same high dose a slight decrease in the percentage of pregnancies occurred. Litter size, weight at birth, and the percentage of live and dead fetuses of the 0.16 and 2.5 mg/kg dosage groups were comparable with the control group. At 20 and 80 mg/kg, litter size and number of live fetuses decreased. Decreased survival rate during the postnatal period was noted with increasing dosages and considered to be related to lack of maternal care. No abnormalities were noted among the experimental pups.

In the loperamide study there was no difference between the control group and the various dosage groups with regard to mortality rate, pregnancy rate, duration of gestation, litter size, weight at birth, and percentage of live and dead fetuses. No abnormalities were noted among the offspring of the various experimental groups. As a result of decreased food consumption of the dams in the 40 mg/kg dosed group, a decrease of fetal weight gain and survival rate was noted in this group at the time of weaning. No abnormalities were noted among the experimental pups.

4.4. SUMMARY

Diphenoxylate, fetoxylate, difenoxin, loperamide, and fluperamide have been reported to be useful therapeutic agents for the treatment of diarrhea in man. Our safety evaluation studies in a variety of laboratory animals indicated that these compounds are extremely well tolerated.

The acute oral toxicity of diphenoxylate, fetoxylate, difenoxin, loperamide, and fluperamide was evaluated in mice, rats, guinea-pigs, and dogs. The safety margins, i.e., the ratio of the lethal dose to the antidiarrheal dose, were extremely high (>800) for all five compounds. The subacute and chronic oral toxicity of diphenoxylate, fetoxylate, difenoxin, loperamide, and fluperamide were investigated in rats and dogs and all five compounds were found to be very safe substances. Oral administration of doses exceeding several times the pharmacologically active doses over prolonged periods of time (up to 18 months in rats and 12 months in dogs) were well tolerated and did not cause significant abnormalities as observed by clinical examination, clinical pathology, gross pathology, and histopathology. In rats and rabbits the compounds were devoid of embryotoxicity, teratogenicity, and of effects on male and female fertility as evidenced by the studies on the reproductive processes carried out in rats and rabbits.

REFERENCES

Arunlakshana, O. and Schild, H. O. (1959). Some quantitative uses of drug antagonists. Brit. J. Pharmacol. 14, 48-58.

Banwell, J. G. and Sherr, H. (1973). Effect of bacterial enterotoxins on the gastrointestinal tract. Gastroenterology 65, 467-477.

Bass, P., Kennedy, J. A., and Wiley, J. N. (1972). Measurement of fecal output in rats. Am. J. Digest. Diseases 10, 925-928.

Bass, P., Kennedy, J. A., Wiley, J. N., Villareal, J., and Butler, D. E. (1973). CI-750, a novel antidiarrheal agent, J. Pharmacol. Exp. Therap. 186, 183-198.

Bayliss, W. M. and Starling, E. H. (1899). The movements and innervation of the small intestine, J. Physiol. (London) 24, 99-143.

Bennett, A., Eley, K. G., and Scholes, G. B. (1968a). Effects of prostaglandins E_1 and E_2 on human, guinea-pig and rat isolated small intestine. Brit. J. Pharmacol. 34, 630-638.

Bennett, A., Eley, K. G., and Scholes, G. B. (1968b). Effects of prostaglandins E_1 and E_2 on intestinal motility in the guinea-pig and rat. Brit. J. Pharmacol. 34, 639-647.

Bennett, A. and Misiewicz, J. J. (1973). Drugs used in treating disordered motility of the alimentary tract. In Pharmacology of Gastrointestinal Motility and Secretion, P. Holton (Ed.), Vol. II. Pergamon Press, New York, pp. 433-455.

Binder, H. J. (1973). Fecal fatty acids mediators of diarrhea, Gastroenterology 64, 847-850.

Black, J. W., Duncan, W. A. M., and Shanks, R. G. (1965). Comparison of some properties of pronethalol and propanolol. Brit. J. Pharmacol. 25, 577-591.

Bonnycastle, D. D. (1965). Cathartics and laxatives. In Drill's Pharmacology in Medicine, 3rd ed., J. R. Di Palma (Ed.). McGraw-Hill Book Co., New York.

Bortoff, A. (1972). Digestion: motility. Ann. Rev. Physiol. 34, 261-290.

Bright-Asare, P. and Binder, H. J. (1973). Stimulation of colonic secretion of water and electrolytes by hydroxy fatty acids. Gastroenterology 64, 81-88.

Butler, D. E., Meyer, R. F., Alexander, S. M., Bass, P., and Kennedy, J. A. (1973). Synthetic antidiarrheal agents. I. An approach to the separation of antidiarrheal activity from narcotic analgesic activity. J. Med. Chem. 16, 49-54.

Cash, R. A., Nalin, D. R., Forrest, J. N., and Abrutyn, E. (1970). Rapid correction of acidosis and dehydration of cholera with oral electrolyte and glucose solution. Lancet 2, 549-550.

Collier, H. O. J., Fieler, F. C., and Paris, S. K. (1948). A biological evaluation of the purgative activity of senna extracts, Quart. J. Pharm. Pharmac. 1, 252-259.

Daniel, E. E. (1973). A conceptual analysis of the pharmacology of gastrointestinal motility. In Pharmacology of Gastrointestinal Motility and Secretion. P. Holton (Ed.). Pergamon Press, New York, pp. 457-545.

De Coster, M., Kerremans, R., and Beckers, J. (1972). A comparative double-blind study of two antidiarrheals, difenoxin and loperamide. Tijdschr. Gastroenterol. 15, 337-342.

Demeulenaere, L., Verbeke, S., Muls, M., and Reyntjens, A. (1974). Loperamide: an open multicentre trial and a double-blind cross-over comparison with placebo in patients with chronic diarrhoea. Curr. Therap. Res. 16, 32-39.

Dom, J., Leyman, R., Schuermans, V., and Brugmans, J. (1974). Loperamide (R 18 553), a novel type of antidiarrheal agent. Part VIII. Clinical investigation. Use of a flexible dosage schedule in a double-blind comparison of loperamide with diphenoxylate in 614 patients suffering from acute diarrhea. Arzneimittel-Forsch. 24, 1660-1665.

Dupont, H. L. and Hornick, R. B. (1969). Diarrheal diseases. Disease-a-Month, July.

Dutta, N. K., Marker, P. H., and Roa, N. R. (1972). Berberine in toxin induced experimental cholera. Brit. J. Pharmacol. 44, 153-159.

Eichenwald, H. F. and McCracken, G. H. (1970). Acute diarrheal disease. Med. Clin. North Am. 54, 443-453.

Fingl, E. (1970). Cathartics and laxatives. In The Pharmacological Basis of Therapeutics, 4th ed., Goodman, L. S. and Gilman, A. (Eds.). MacMillan, New York.

Finkelstein, R. A., Norris, H. J., and Dutta, N. V. (1964). Pathogenesis of experimental cholera in infant rabbits. I. Observations on the intra intestinal infection and experimental cholera produced by cell-free products. J. Infect. Diseases 144, 203-216.

Finney, D. J. (1962). Probit Analysis, Cambridge University Press, Cambridge, pp. 236-254.

Fontaine, J., Van Nueten, J. M., and Janssen, P. A. J. (1973). Analysis of the peristaltic reflex in vitro: effects of some antagonists. Arch. Intern. Pharmacodyn. Therap. 203, 396-399.

Fontaine, J., Van Nueten, J. M., and Reuse, J. J. (1976). Effects of the prostaglandins E_1 and E_2 on the peristaltic reflex in vitro; interaction with indomethacin. Submitted for publication.

Fontaine, J. and Van Nueten, J. M. (1976). Characterization of some parameters in the analysis of the peristaltic reflex of guinea-pig ileum in vitro. In preparation.

Forth, W., Rummel, W., and Baldauf, J. (1966). Wasser- und Elektrolytbewegung am Dünn- und Dickdarm unter dem Einfluss von Laxantien, ein Beitrag zur Klärung ihrer Wirkungsmechanismen. Arch. Exp. Pharm. Pathol. 254, 18-32.

Frigo, G. M., Torsoli, A., Lecchini, S., Falaschi, C. F., and Crema, A. (1972). Recent advances in the pharmacology of peristalsis. Arch. Intern. Pharmacodyn. Therap. 196 (suppl.), 9-24.

Geiger, E. (1940). Bioassay of senna leaves and the fluid extract of senna U.S.P. J. Am. Pharm. Assoc. 29, 148-183.

Geivers, H., Van Nueten, J. M., Leeuws, M., Reneman, R. S. (1974). The determination of small volume displacements in experiments on isolated tissues using an ultrasonic transittime technique. In Cardiovascular Applications of Ultrasound, R. S. Reneman (Ed.). North Holland Publishing Co., Amsterdam, pp. 162-169.

Goodman, L. S. and Gilman, A. (1965). In The Pharmacological Basis of Therapeutics 3rd ed., p. 271. McMillan, New York.

Gordon, J. E. (1968). Weanling diarrhea. Interaction of Nutrition and Infection, Scrimshaw, Taylor, and Gordon (Eds.). Geneva, WHO Monograph No. 57.

Green, M. W., King, C. G., and Beal, G. D. (1936). The constituents in cascara sagrada extract. II. A method of bioassay. J. Am. Pharm. Assoc. 25, 107-110.

Heykants, J., Brugmans, J., and Verhaegen, H. (1972b). Difenoxin (R 15 403), the active metabolite of diphenoxylate (R 1132). Part 6: Absorption, excretion and metabolism in man, Arzneimittel-Forsch. 22, 529-531.

Heykants, J. J. P., Lewi, P. J., and Janssen, P. A. J. (1972a). Difenoxin (R 15 403), the active metabolite of diphenoxylate (R 1132). Part 4: Distribution in the rat of diphenoxylate and difenoxin. Arzneimittel-Forsch. 22, 520-526.

Iwao, I. and Terada, Y. (1962). On the mechanism of diarrhea due to castor oil. Japan. J. Pharmacol. 12, 137-145.

Janssen, P. A. J. and Jageneau, A. H. (1957). A new series of potent analgesics: Dextro 2:2-diphenyl-3-methyl-4-morpholino-butyrylpyrrolidine and related amides. Part I. Chemical structure and pharmacological activity. J. Pharm. Pharmacol. 9, 381-400.

Janssen, P. A. J., Jageneau, A. H., Van Proosdij-Hartzema, E. G., and De Jongh, D. K. (1958). The pharmacology of a new potent analgesic, R 951 2[N-(4-carbethoxy-4-phenyl)-piperidinol]-propiophenone HCl. Acta Physiol. Pharmacol. Neerlandica 7, 373-402.

Janssen, P. A. J., Jageneau, A. H. M., Demoen, P. J. A., Van de Westeringh, C., Raeymaekers, A. H. M., Wouters, M. S. T., Sanczuk, S., Hermans, B. K. F., and Loomans, J. L. M. (1959a). Compounds related to pethidine. I. Mannich bases derived from norpethidine and acetophenones. J. Med. Chem. 1, 105-120.

Janssen, P. A. J., Jagenau, A. H., and Huygens, J. (1959b). Synthetic anti-diarrheal agents. I. Some pharmacological properties of R 1132 and related compounds. J. Med. Chem. 1, 299-308.

Janssen, P. A. J., Jageneau, A. H. M., Demoen, P. J. A., Van De Westeringh, C., De Canniere, J. H. M., Raeymaekers, A. H. M., Wouters, M. S. J., Sanczuk, S., and Hermans, B. K. F. (1959c). Compounds related to pethidine. II. Mannich bases derived from various esters of 4-carboxy-4-phenyl-piperidine and acetophenones, J. Med. Chem. 1, 309-317.

Janssen, P. A. J. (1961). Vergleichende pharmakologische Daten über sechs neue basische 4'-fluorobutyrophenon Derivate: Haloperidol, Haloanison, Triperidol, Methylperidid, Haloperidid, und Dipiperon. Arzneimittel-Forsch. 11, 819-824, 932-938.

Janssen, P. A. J. (1961). Piritramide (R 3365), a potent analgesic with unusual chemical structure. J. Pharm. Pharmacol. 13, 513-530.

Janssen, P. A. J., Niemegeers, C. J. E., and Dony, J. G. H. (1963a). The inhibitory effect of fentanyl (R 42 63) and other morphine-like analgesics on the warm water induced tail withdrawal reflex in rats. Arzneimittel-Forsch. 13, 502-507.

Janssen, P. A. J., Niemegeers, C. J. E., Schellekens, K. H. L., Verbruggen, F. J., and Van Nueten, J. M. (1963b). The pharmacology of dehydrobenzperidol, a new potent and short acting neuroleptic agent chemically related to haloperidol. Arzneimittel-Forsch. 13, 205-211.

Janssen, P. A. J., Niemegeers, C. J. E., Schellekens, K. H. L., Dresse, A., Lenaerts, F. M., Pinchard, A., Schaper, W. K. A., Van Nueten, J. M. and Verbruggen, F. J. (1968). Pimozide, a chemically novel highly potent and orally long-acting neuroleptic drug. Part I. The comparative pharmacology of pimozide, haloperidol, and chlorpromazine. Arzneimittel-Forsch. 18, 261-279.

Janssen, P. A. J., Niemegeers, C. J. E., Schellekens, K. H. L., Lenaerts, F. M., Verbruggen, F. J., Van Nueten, J. M., and Schaper, W. K. A. (1970a). The pharmacology of penfluridol (R 16 341), a new potent and orally long-acting neuroleptic drug. Europ. J. Pharmacol. 11, 139-154.

Janssen, P. A. J., Niemegeers, C. J. E., Schellekens, K. H. L., Lenaerts, F. M., Verbruggen, F. J., Van Nueten, J. M., Marsboom, R. H. M., Hérin, V. V., and Schaper, W. K. A. (1970b). The pharmacology of fluspirilene (R 6218), a potent, long-acting and injectable neuroleptic drug. Arzneimittel-Forsch. 20, 1689-1698.

Janssen, P. A. J., Niemegeers, C. J. E., Schellekens, K. H. L., Demoen, P., Lenaerts, F. M., Van Nueten, J. M., Van Wijngaarden, I., and Brugmans, J. (1971). Benzetimide and its optical isomers. Arzneimittel-Forsch. 21, 1365-1373.

Janssen, P. A. J., Niemegeers, C. J. E., Schellekens, K. H. L., Marsboom, R. H. M., Hérin, V. V., and Amery, W. K. P. (1971a). Bezitramide (R 4945), a new potent and orally long-acting analgesic compound. Arzneimittel-Forsch. 21, 862-867.

Karim, A., Garden, G., and Trager, W. (1971). Biotransformation of diphenoxylate in rat and dog, J. Pharmacol. Exp. Therap. 177, 546-555.

Karim, A., Ranney, R. E., Evensen, K. L., and Clark, M. L. (1972). Pharmacokinetics and metabolism of diphenoxylate in man. Clin. Pharmacol. Therap. 13, 407-419.

Kimberg, D. V., Field, M., Johnson, V., Henderson, A., and Gershon, E. (1971). Stimulation of intestinal mucosal adenyl cyclase by cholera enterotoxin and prostaglandins. J. Clin. Invest. 50, 1218-1230.

Kosterlitz, H. W. and Robinson, J. A. (1957). Inhibition of the peristaltic reflex in the isolated guinea-pig ileum. J. Physiol. (London), 136, 249-262.

Kosterlitz, H. W. and Lees, G. M. (1964). Pharmacological analysis of intrinsic intestinal reflexes. Pharmacol. Rev. 16, 301-339.

Kottegoda, S. R. (1969). An analysis of possible nervous mechanisms involved in peristaltic reflex. J. Physiol. (London), 200, 687-712.

Kottegoda, S. R. (1970). Peristalsis of the small intestine. In Smooth Muscle, E. Bülbring, A. F. Brading, A. W. Jones, and T. Tomita (Eds.). Edward Arnold, London, pp. 525-541.

Krueger, H., Eddy, N. B., and Sumwalt, M. (1941). Public Health Reports, Suppl. No. 165. U.S. Govt. Print. Off., Washington, D.C.

Lee, Y., Sanner, J. H., and Dobrin, E. I. (1972). The antidiarrheal activity of S.C.-26100 in experimental animals. Fed. Proc. 31, 1658.

Lin, T. M., Benslay, D. N., Ensminger, P. W., and Nash, J. F. (1967). Experimental production of diarrhea and its prevention by malethamer in monkeys. Arch. Intern. Pharmacodyn. 169, 147-161.

Litchfield, J. T. and Wilcoxon, F. (1949). Simplified method of evaluating dose-effect experiments. J. Pharmacol. Exp. Therap. 96, 99-113.

Loewe, S. (1939). Bioassays of laxatives on monkeys (Rhesus) and on lower mammalians (dye meal methods). J. Am. Pharm. Assoc. 28, 427-432.

Lou, T. C. (1949). The biological assay of vegetable purgatives. Part I. Senna leaf and fruit and their preparations. J. Pharm. Pharmacol. 1, 673-682.

Low-Beer, T. S. and Read, A. E. (1971). Progress report. Diarrhea: mechanisms and treatment. Gut 12, 1021-1036.

Macht, D. I. and Barba-Gose, J. (1931). Two new methods for pharmacological comparison of insoluble purgatives. J. Am. Pharm. Assoc. Sci. Ed. 20, 558-564.

Maenza, R. M., Powell, D. W., Plotkin, G. R., Formal, S. B., Jervis, H. R., and Sprinz, H. (1970). Experimental diarrhea: Salmonella enterocolitis in the rat. J. Infect. Diseases, 121, 475-485.

Magnus, R. (1906). Die stopfende Wirkung des Morphins. Arch. Ges. Physiol. 115, 316.

Magnus, R. (1908). Die stopfende Wirkung des Morphins. Arch. Ges. Physiol. 122, 210.

Marazzi-Aberti, E. and Turba, C. (1966). α-Isopropyl-α-(2-dimethylaminoethyl)-1-naphtyl acetamide (Naphthypramide, D.A. 992): a new anti-inflammatory agent. 1. Anti-inflammatory activity and acute toxicity. Arch. Intern. Pharmacodyn. 162, 378-396.

Marsboom, R. and Van Ravestyn, C. (1971). Effect of benzetimide (R 4929) on ruminal and intestinal motility in sheep. Brit. Vet. J. 127, 264-270.

Marsboom, R., Temmerman, R., and Symoens, J. (1973). The effect of benzetimide on intestinal motility in pigs. Vet. Rec. 93, 382-384.

Marsboom, R. (1974). Personal communication.

Masri, M. S., Goldblatt, L. A., De Eds, F., and Kohler, G. O. (1962). Relation of cathartic activity to structural modifications of ricinoleic acid of castor oil. J. Pharm. Sci. 51, 999-1002.

McCarty, D. A., Chen, G. M., Kaump, D. H., Potter, D., Holappa, K. K., and Ensor, C. (1965). The pharmacologic and toxicologic evaluation of the ganglionic blocking agent dibutadiamin. Arch. Intern. Pharmacodyn. 154, 263-282.

McMurdoch, H. (1971). Antibiotics in the management of disease of the gut. Practitioner 206, 5-11.

Meyer, H. (1890). Über den wirksamen Bestandteil des Ricinusöls. Arch. Exp. Pathol. Pharmakol. 28, 145-152.

Niemegeers, C. J. E., Lenaerts, F. M., and Janssen, P. A. J. (1972). Difenoxin (R 15403), the active metabolite of diphenoxylate (R 1132). Part II. Difenoxin, a potent, orally active and safe antidiarrheal agent in rats. Arzneimittel-Forsch. 22, 516-518.

Niemegeers, C. J. E. and Janssen, P. A. J. (1974a). Bromoperidol, a new neuroleptic of the butyrophenone series. Comparative pharmacology of bromoperidol and haloperidol. Arzneimittel-Forsch. 24, 45-52.

Niemegeers, C. J. E., Van Nueten, J. M., and Janssen, P. A. J. (1974b). Azaperone, a sedative neuroleptic of the butyrophenone series with pronounced anti-agressive and anti-shock activity in animals. Arzneimittel-Forsch. 24, 1798-1806.

Niemegeers, C. J. E., Lenaerts, F. M., and Janssen, P. A. J. (1974c). Loperamide (R 18 553) a novel type of antidiarrheal agent. Part I. In vivo pharmacology and acute toxicity. Comparison with morphine, codeine, diphenoxylate, and difenoxin. Arzneimittel-Forsch. 24, 1633-1636.

Niemegeers, C. J. E., Lenaerts, F. M., and Janssen, P. A. J. (1974d). Loperamide (R 18 553) a novel type of antidiarrheal agent: Part II. In vivo parenteral pharmacology and acute toxicity in mice. Comparison with morphine, codeine, and diphenoxylate. Arzneimittel-Forsch. 24, 1636-1641.

Nilsson, F. and Johansson, H. (1973). A double isotope technique for the evaluation of drug action on gastric evacuation and small bowel propulsion studied in the rat. Gut 14, 475-477.

Paton, W. D. M. (1955). The action of morphine and related substances. The response of the guinea-pig ileum to electrical stimulation by coaxial electrodes. J. Physiol. (London) 127, 40-41 P.

Paton, W. D. M. and Zar, M. A. (1968). The origin of acetylcholine released from guinea-pig intestine and longitudinal muscle strips. J. Physiol. (London) 194, 13-33.

Phillips, S. F. (1972). Diarrhea: a current view of the pathology. Gastroenterology 63, 495-518.

Phillips, R. A., Love, A. H. G., Mitchell, T. G., and Neptune, E. M. (1965). Cathartics and the sodium pump. Nature 206, 1367-1368.

Powell, D. W., Plotkin, G. R., Maenza, R. M., Solberg, L. I., Catlin, D. H., and Formal, S. B. (1971a). Experimental diarrhea. I. Intestinal water and electrolytic transport in rat Salmonella enterocolitis. Gastroenterology 60, 1053-1064.

Powell, D. W., Plotkin, G. R., Solberg, L. I., Catlin, D. H., Maenza, R. M., and Formal, S. B. (1971b). Experimental diarrhea. II. Glucose stimulated sodium and water transport in rat Salmonella enterocolitis. Gastroenterology 60, 1065-1075.

Powell, D. W., Solberg, L. I., Plotkin, G. R., Catlin, D. H., Maenza, R. M., and Formal, S. B. (1971c). Experimental diarrhea. III. Bicarbonate transport in rat Salmonella enterocolitis. Gastroenterology 60, 1076-1086.

Purdon, R. A. and Bass, P. (1973). Gastric and intestinal transit in rats measured by a radioactive test meal. Gastroenterology 64, 968-970.

Rakatansky, H. and Kirsner, J. B. (1974). Drugs for gastrointestinal diseases. In Drugs of Choice, W. Modell (Ed.). C. V. Mosby Co., St. Louis, pp. 295-320.

Read, A. E. (1971). Anti-diarrheal agents. Practitioner 206, 69-76.

Reynell, P. C. and Spray, G. H. (1958). Chemical gastroenteritis in the rat. Gastroenterology 34, 867-873.

Rubens, R., Verhaegen, H., Brugmans, J., and Schuermans, V. (1972). Difenoxin (R 15 403), the active metabolite of diphenoxylate (R 1132). Part 5: Clinical comparison of difenoxin and diphenoxylate in volunteers and in patients with chronic diarrhea. Double-blind crossover assessments. Arzneimittel-Forsch. 22, 526-529.

Sanner, J. H. (1972). Dibenzoxazepine hydrazides as prostaglandin antagonists. Intra-Sci. Chem. Rept. 6, 1-9.

Schmid, W. (1952). Zum Wirkungsmechanismus diatetischer und medikamentoser Darmmittel. Arzneimittel-Forsch. 2, 6-20.

Schuermans, V., Van Lommel, R., Dom, J., and Brugmans, J. (1974). Loperamide (R 18 553), a novel type of antidiarrheal agent. Part VI. Clinical pharmacology. Placebo-controlled comparison of the constipating activity and safety of loperamide, diphenoxylate and codeine in normal volunteers. Arzneimittel-Forsch. 24, 1653-1657.

Stokbroekx, R. A., Vandenberk, J., Van Heertum, A. H. M. T., van Laar, G. M. L. W., Van der Aa, M. J. M. C., Van Bever, W. F. M., and Janssen, P. A. J. (1973). Synthetic antidiarrheal agents. 2,2-Diphenyl-4-(4′-aryl-4′-hydroxypiperidino)butyramides. J. Med. Chem. 16, 782-786.

Travell, J. (1954). Pharmacology of stimulant laxatives. Ann. N.Y. Acad. Sci. 58, 416-425.

Trendelenburg, P. (1917). Physiologische und pharmakologische Versuche über die Dünndarmperistaltik. Arch. Exp. Pathol. Pharmakol. 81, 55-129.

Tsurumi, K., Hayashi, M., Hibino, R., and Fujimura, H. (1969). Testing method for cathartic agents in mice. Nippon Yakurigaku Zasshi 65, 643-648.

Van Nueten, J. M. (1968). The effect of diphenoxylate on the peristaltic reflex of the guinea-pig ileum. Arch. Int. Pharmacodyn. Therap. 171, 243-245.

Van Nueten, J. M. and Janssen, P. A. J. (1972). Difenoxin (R 15 403), the active metabolite of diphenoxylate (R 1132). Part 3: Inhibition of the peristaltic activity of the guinea-pig ileum in vitro. Arzneimittel-Forsch. 22, 518-520.

Van Nueten, J. M., Geivers, H., Fontaine, J., and Janssen, P. A. J. (1973). An improved method for studying peristalsis in the isolated guinea-pig ileum. Arch. Int. Pharmacodyn. Therap. 203, 411-414.

Van Nueten, J. M., Janssen, P. A. J., and Fontaine, J. (1974). Loperamide (R 18 553), a novel type of antidiarrheal agent. Part III. In vitro studies on the peristaltic reflex and other experiments on isolated tissues. Arzneimittel-Forsch. 24, 1641-1645.

Van Nueten, J. M., Fontaine, J., and Janssen, P. A. J. (1976). Analysis of the effects of loperamide (R 18 553) on the peristaltic reflex of the isolated guinea-pig ileum. In preparation.

Van Rossum, J. M. (1963). Cumulative dose-response curves. II. Technique for the making of dose-response curves in isolated organs and the evaluation of drug parameters. Arch. Intern. Pharmacodyn. Therap. 143, 299-330.

van Wijngaarden, I. and Soudijn, W. (1972). Difenoxin (R 15 403), the active metabolite of diphenoxylate (R 1132). Part 1: The excretion and metabolism in rats of difenoxin, the pharmacologically active metabolite of the antidiarrheal agent diphenoxylate. Arzneimittel-Forsch. 22, 513-516.

Verhaegen, H., De Cree, J., and Schuermans, V. (1974). Loperamide (R 18 553), a novel type of antidiarrheal agent. Part VII. Clinical investigation. Efficacy and safety of loperamide in patients with severe chronic diarrhea. Arzneimittel-Forsch. 24, 1657-1660.

Watson, W. C. and Gordon, R. S. (1962). Studies on the digestion, absorption and metabolism of castor oil. Biochem. Pharmacol. 11, 229-236.

Watson, W. C., Gordon, R. S., Karman, A., and Jover, A. (1963). The absorption and excretion of castor oil in man. J. Pharm. Pharmacol. 15, 183-188.

Williams, E. M. V. and Streeten, O. H. P. (1950). The action of morphine, pethidine, and amidone upon the intestinal motility of conscious dogs. Brit. J. Pharmacol. 5, 584-603.

Winkelstein, A. (1961). Symptomatic treatment of diarrhea with diphenoxylate. Am. J. Gastroenterol. 36, 692-697.

CHAPTER V

MODERN ANTIDIARRHEALS IN MEDICAL PRACTICE

André Reyntjens and Harbans Lal

V.1. INTRODUCTION

Diarrhea is one of the most common symptoms the general practitioner is called upon to treat. Certainly the internist and gastroenterologist, as well as the pediatrician, may see an inordinately large percentage of patients in his practice with this affliction. Diarrhea is often a source of considerable inconvenience to the patient and in severe cases may lead to serious and possibly life-threatening situations, involving dehydration, electrolyte imbalance, and protein loss. Although investigation of the underlying cause of diarrhea should be carried out at an early stage, this may often not be feasible or prove successful. Often as not, etiology reveals a past or present clinical condition, for which no causal treatment may be available. In all these cases, symptomatic antidiarrheal therapy may be urgently indicated to relieve the patients' discomfort and also to prevent subsequent systemic effects.

Besides diet, rest, and rehydration, which are still the mainstays of palliative treatment, many pharmacological agents have been tried in the past. Some of these act on the intestinal contents, while others may provide a type of barricade between intestinal contents and the intestinal wall. The latter group of drugs comprises absorbent, astringent, and softening and "coating" medications, such as kaolin, activated charcoal, and aluminum and bismuth salts. Their therapeutic value, however, was seriously questioned 20 yr ago (Bonnycastle, 1958). The more reliable, more widely used agents act within the intestinal wall, such as the anticholinergic drugs together with the opium derivatives. However, unlike the intestine of certain animal species, the human intestine is not very responsive to anticholinergic drugs and these compounds, when used alone, are often not effective against hyperperistalsis. These agents almost invariably produce the well-known anticholinergic side-effects in exchange for questionable control of the diarrheal syndrome. The opium derivatives, on the other hand, do effectively control the hyperperistaltic movements of the intestines and, when combined with the anticholinergics, provide the most effective symptomatic antidiarrheals available to date. One obvious drawback of the opium derivatives has been their undesirable CNS effects such as dullness and their potential addictiveness (Cayer and Sohner, 1961; Barowsky and Schwartz, 1962; Hock, 1961; Winkelstein, 1961).

The search for new therapeutic agents and compounds with a much more specific effect on the intestine (i.e., without significant morphine-like CNS action) has been the most important goal in the symptomatic treatment of diarrhea. In our clinical judgment, the recently synthesized compound loperamide fulfills this goal, while the older compounds diphenoxylate and its active metabolite diphenoxine only approach it. This chapter on the therapeutics of modern antidiarrheals in medical practice is therefore limited to these three specific and effective compounds (loperamide, diphenoxylate, and diphenoxine). We shall consider their therapeutic use for the symptomatic treatment of diarrhea in adults and children, and in addition review the data on their use under other circumstances, such as the control of intestinal motility and the use of diphenoxylate in the detoxification regimen for the treatment of heroin addicts.

We have adopted the arbitrary distinction between acute and chronic diarrhea because of the wide differences in the therapeutic approaches and evaluation methods in these two groups.

Diphenoxylate with atropine* was first marketed in 1960 both in Europe and in the United States. It is now widely available world-wide under a variety of tradenames (Reasec, Lomotil, Retardin, Diarsed). Diphenoxine, the metabolite of diphenoxylate, has recently been introduced in Europe and is under consideration for marketing in the United States. Loperamide was marketed in Europe in 1974 under the tradename Imodium. It is expected to be available soon in the United States. If not otherwise mentioned the formulations of the drugs under discussion are as follows:

Diphenoxylate*: each tablet contains   2.5 mg diphenoxylate HCl plus
                                        0.025 mg atropine sulfate

---

*For the sake of clarity, and only within this chapter, the clinical use of the term "diphenoxylate" refers to the product which contains diphenoxylate and atropine, and not simply diphenoxylate alone. The reader is advised to always think of these two chemical moieties together when the term "diphenoxylate" is used, especially when a clinical situation is involved.

	pediatric formulations:	drops, the contents of one tablet in 1 ml (25 drops); syrup; the contents of one tablet in 5 ml
Diphenoxine:	each tablet contains	0.5 mg diphenoxine HCl plus 0.025 mg atropine sulfate
Loperamide:	each capsule contains	2 mg loperamide HCl

V.2. SYMPTOMATIC TREATMENT OF ACUTE DIARRHEA IN CLINICAL PRACTICE

2.1. THE NEED IN THERAPY

It is a widespread clinical practice to treat acute diarrhea with antibacterial agents often before or even without bacteriological examination of stools, on the assumption that the condition is due to bacterial infection. The overwhelming evidence, however, indicates that many of the most common forms of acute diarrhea may be nonbacterial. A case in point may be the frequently encountered "travelers' diarrhea," known by a variety of names in different parts of the world. Even in the case of an infectious diarrhea, the question arises as to how frequently the responsible pathogen would be a virus or other microorganisms, which are not responsive to the commonly prescribed antibiotics. Apart from the cases where the laboratory examination (or an epidemic condition) gives a clear-cut indication for a specific anti-infective, such as infections due to amebiasis, shigella, or salmonella, it would appear that antibacterials as a group offer a far less important range of application than prescribing habits would suggest (Arabehety et al., 1964; Cohen et al., 1967; Eichenwald and McCracken, 1970; Low-Beer and Read, 1971; Moffet et al., 1968; Raby and Shooman, 1967; Ramsay, 1968; Rutgeerts, 1973). On the other hand, effective symptomatic antidiarrheals consequently have a wide applicability, either before the etiology can be determined, or when no causal treatment is available, simply because they provide symptomatic relief.

The objective of symptomatic treatment with antidiarrheal drugs is to reduce the loss of water and electrolytes and, by doing that, to allow patients to recover, regain their strength and resume their normal activities. The three antidiarrheals mentioned above perform this task very well.

2.2. THERAPEUTIC EVALUATION

When organizing the therapeutic evaluation of an antidiarrheal agent, we must consider that frequently acute diarrhea is a self-limiting disease, which may spontaneously regress in hours or within a day or two. Clinical trials in acute diarrhea are complicated by the reluctance of the investigator to use placebos and the paucity of acute diarrhea patients available for follow-up, especially when the trial patients are obtained from a university clinic. Some practical and successful designs for the clinical evaluation of loperamide have been developed and are described below (see Sect. 2.5).

2.3. DIPHENOXYLATE

Diphenoxylate was shown to provide rapid relief of symptoms in acute diarrhea with an average daily dosage of 20 mg (15-40 mg) in 74 to 93% of the patients treated (Dziuba, 1961; Hock, 1961; Van Derstappen and Vandenbroucke, 1961). Twelve hours after initiation of treatment, 41% of the patients no longer presented with increased stool frequency. This percentage increased to 68% at 24 hr, to 80% at 2 days, and to 90.5% at 3 days (Murphy, 1968). In another study, diphenoxylate proved at least as effective as codeine sulfate, providing a return to normal stool frequency within 3 days in 84% of the patients (Bond et al., 1966).

2.4. DIPHENOXINE

We have found diphenoxine, the active metabolite of diphenoxylate, to be at least as effective as the latter in the treatment of acute diarrhea. From a theoretical potency standpoint, diphenoxine may be considered to be five times as potent as diphenoxylate, but from a clinical standpoint this is not realistic. In other words, the same number of tablets is used to treat the typical acute diarrhea case with both compounds, but with diphenoxine the tablets contain only one fifth of the active ingredient.

2.5. LOPERAMIDE

Loperamide is a new drug and, until recently, has been in an investigational status in many countries including the United States. In 1974 it became available for sale in Europe and South America. However, while the number of studies available are somewhat limited, the number of patients in these clinical trials is substantial.

2.5.1. Patient Profile

Data are available from more than 1400 subjects who participated in six separate clinical studies. One study was controlled by a placebo group; diphenoxylate was used as comparison in three studies; one study used an "open" design, and in the remaining study, loperamide was compared with placebo, diphenoxylate, and mexaform.

2.5.2. Dosage

Generally, in these acute studies, subjects were given two capsules initially, followed by one capsule after each unformed stool until diarrheal was cont rolled or until a maximum of eight capsules had been consumed each day. In two studies, two capsules of the test drug were administered initially followed by one capsule of diphenoxylate or other known antidiarrheal preparation after each unformed stool.

2.5.3. Course of Therapy

Since in most cases, acute diarrhea is self-limiting, the test compound was administered in most studies for 3 days; in one study the test drug was given for 7 days. In two studies the subjects took two initial capsules of loperamide or the appropriate double-blind medication, followed by one capsule of diphenoxylate or other antidiarrheal medication after each unformed stool.

2.5.4. Results Summarized

The overall results indicate that both diphenoxylate and loperamide were effective in controlling acute diarrhea in all of the patients treated, and both drugs were significantly superior to placebo. However, loperamide was effective in a mean total dose of 7.71 mg(less than four capsules) while diphenoxylate was effective in a mean total dose of 12.4 mg (five capsules). Thus on milligram for milligram basis, it appears that loperamide is more effective than diphenoxylate. This difference is statistically significant (see Table 1).

2.5.5. Results Analyzed

Zelveder (1975) investigated loperamide in a double-blind, placebo-controlled trial in 163 patients with acute diarrhea (141 patients completed

TABLE 1

Drug Doses Found Necessary to Control Acute Diarrhea

Drug	Number of patients	Mean dosage, mg in 72-hr period
Diphenoxylate	505	12.40
Loperamide	604	7.71

the study). Patients, randomly assigned to placebo or loperamide, received two 2-mg capsules of test drug. Starting $1\frac{1}{2}$ hr after capsule intake, all patients recorded stool frequency and consistency, side effects, and additional capsule intake. If diarrheic stools occurred during this 24-hr period, diphenoxylate capsules were administered following each loose stool.

At the end of the 24-hr period, 43 of the 71 loperamide patients (61%0 had not required additional therapy against 22 (31% of the placebo-treated patients). Of the placebo-treated group, 63 of the 70 patients (90%) recorded loose stools after 2 hr and required antidiarrheal therapy.

In the double-blind study of Dom et al. (1974), 614 patients with acute diarrhea were evaluated. Two to three capsules controlled diarrhea in 42% of the loperamide group as compared to only 26% in diphenoxylate group (see Table 2). Amery et al. (1975) evaluated the time of occurrence of the first unformed stool after administration of loperamide, mexaforme,* diphenoxylate, or placebo in a double-blind study of 213 patients. They reported that the first unformed stool occurred after a median time of 24 hr in patients treated with loperamide, 3 hr in the mexaforme group, and 2 hr in the diphenoxylate or placebo group. In evaluating the data of Amery et al. during the 72-hr treatment period, the mean number of stools pretherapy were 8.2 for the loperamide group and 7.9 for diphenoxylate group. However, posttherapy analysis (after 72 hr) showed that all patients were controlled with both drugs but the mean of stools for loperamide patients was 3.3 compared to 4.0 for diphenoxylate patients, and the mean total dosages were 9.0 mg of loperamide as compared to 14.0 mg for loperamide ($p = 0.001$). This difference was statistically significant. The effectiveness of loperamide was significantly greater ($p < 0.05$) than each of the other treatments used. Even 1 hr after medication, the number of subjects without recurrence of unformed stools was much higher than with placebo ($p < 0.05$) in only the loperamide group. Amery concluded that loperamide appeared to have a more rapid onset of action than the control agents.

---

*Trademark of a combination drug containing 400 mg cailquinol and 40 mg phanquone.

TABLE 2

Effectiveness of Diphenoxylate and Loperamide in Control of Acute Diarrhea

Drug	Experimental factors	Predrug	Day 1	Day 2	Day 3
Diphenoxylate	Number of patients	311	261	135	44
	Number of patients taking capsules	—	311	142	52
	Dosage, mg per patient[a]	—	10.8	5.3	4.3
	Number of unformed stools				
	Total	2433	760	280	75
	Mean	7.9	2.9	2.1	4.3
Loperamide	Number of patients	303	238	93	23
	Number of patients taking capsules	—	303	89	24
	Dosage, mg per patient[b]	—	7.8	3.4	3.0
	Number of unformed stools				
	Total	2493	620	163	40
	Mean	8.2	2.6	1.8	1.7

[a]Overall 14.0 mg for the 3-day period.
[b]Overall 9.0 mg for the 3-day period.

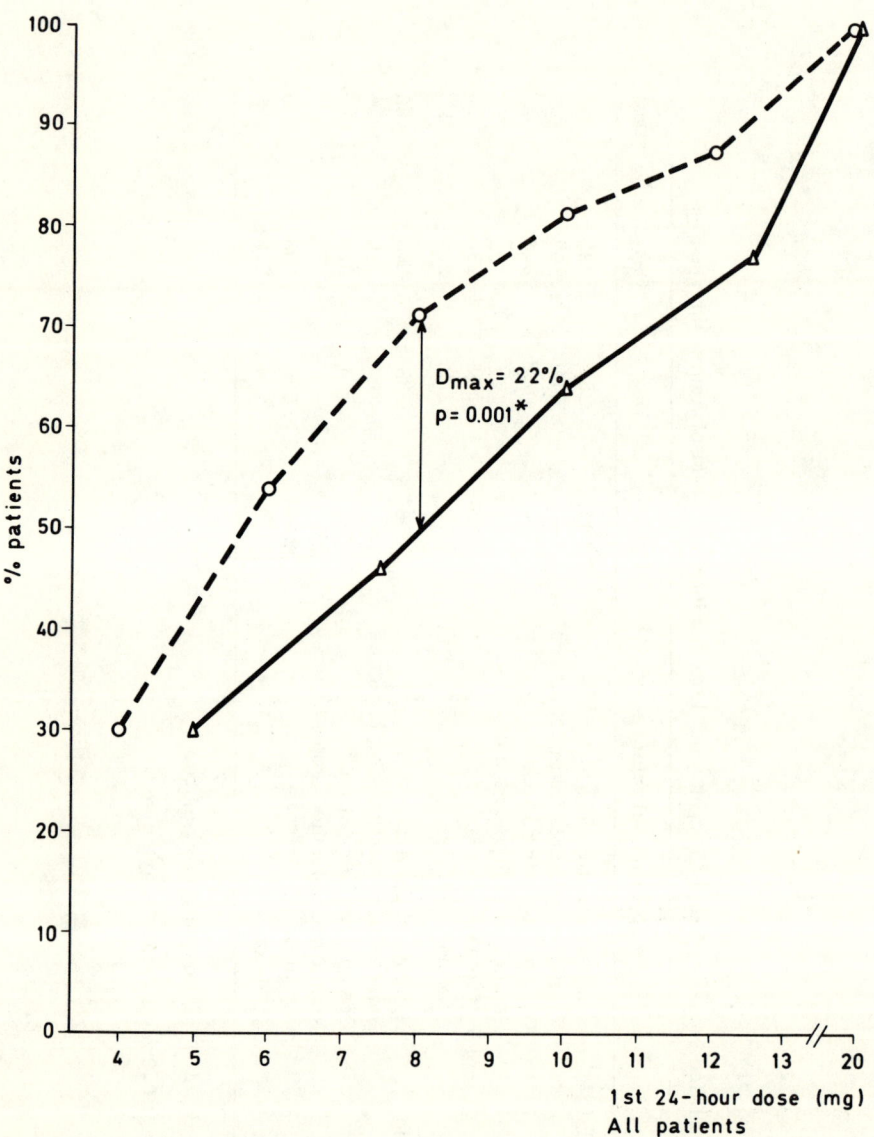

Fig. 1. Relative cumulative frequency distribution of the total doses used in the first 24-hr study period — overall results. *Kolmogorov-Smirnov two-sample test, one-tailed probability. O---O, loperamide; △——△, diphenoxylate.

Jancloes (1975) compared loperamide to diphenoxylate with regard to frequency and consistency of each stool, and related this to the number of capsules taken in a double-blind study with 46 patients. He found the number of unformed stools comparable in the loperamide and diphenoxylate group for day 1 and day 2, while on the 3rd day, there were five cases of unformed stools in the diphenoxylate group for each one case of unformed stool in the loperamide group.

With regard to stool consistency, loperamide was significantly better ($p < 0.001$) during day 1 and day 2. On day 3, in this study Vancloes found five diphenoxylate subjects with two liquid or eight loose stools for each loperamide case with one loose stool. The mean total dose of loperamide was 10.9 mg vs. 14.3 mg for diphenoxylate when taken over a 3-day period.

In the United States a double-blind comparison of loperamide with diphenoxylate was conducted in 340 patients with acute diarrhea. Patients with at least four liquid or soft stools during the 24 hr prior to treatment were allocated randomly to either loperamide or diphenoxylate. An initial dose of two 2-mg capsules of their double-blind medication was administered, and patients were instructed to take one capsule after each unformed stool during the 72-hr study period. The study recorded symptoms, time, and consistency of each motion (see Fig. 1).

Of 159 subjects treated with loperamide, 81% obtained relief within 24 to 36 hr, as opposed to 55% of the 181 subjects treated with diphenoxylate. The median dose of loperamide taken by these subjects during the 72-hr treatment period was 6 mg (three capsules) while the median dose of diphenoxylate was 10 mg (four capsules). This difference was statistically significant ($p < 0.025$). In both patient groups, stool frequency was decreased and stool consistency was improved. Improvement, however, occurred more rapidly with loperamide than with diphenoxylate. Loperamide was superior to diphenoxylate in reducing the frequency of bowel movements and stool consistency at lower doses. No major adverse effects were reported with either drug. Patient complaints were minor and self-limiting. These study results are in agreement with the European data previously discussed.

V.3. SYMPTOMATIC TREATMENT OF CHRONIC DIARRHEA

3.1. GENERAL COMMENTS

In cases of acute diarrhea symptomatic treatment is often instituted before establishing a precise diagnosis. Chronic diarrhea, on the other hand, occurs in a generally well-defined nosological framework. In many of the classified conditions the more or less specific treatment often falls short of arresting the diarrhea and therefore does not permit the patient to lead a normal life. Thus the proper treatment of chronic diarrhea with an adequate therapeutic regimen is paramount to the return of the patient to normal life.

Chronic diarrheas of various etiologies have been shown to be highly responsive to diphenoxylate, diphenoxine, and loperamide, with the possible exception of certain cases of ulcerative colitis, where the presence of diarrhea was questionable, i.e., in cases where the stools were actually mainly discharges of blood and pus.

3.2. DIPHENOXYLATE

Diphenoxylate has been used effectively as an antidiarrheal agent in treating various types of chronic diarrhea associated with Crohn's disease, ulcerative colitis, functional, postresection, and radiation diarrhea, and in tumors of the colon and irritable colon.

Table 3 presents the results obtained in 763 patients suffering chronic diarrhea, as reported in a number of clinical studies. (Barowsky and Sehwartz, 1962; Baufle et al., 1965; Camatte and Francois, 1963; Cayer and Sohmer, 1961; Dziuba, 1961; Gabriele and Moulinier, 1963; Goulston, 1973; Gürtler, 1965; Hock, 1961; Kasich, 1961; Lichstein, 1965; Machella, 1960; Manciaux et al., 1968; Merlo and Brower, 1960; Miotti, 1968; Moeller, 1965; Müller, 1967; Owens, 1965; Poirier and Poirier, 1961; Pourquier et al., 1963; Shärli, 1967; Valla, 1965; Van Derstappen and Vandenbroucke, 1961; Van Derstappen et al., 1960; Weingarten et al., 1961; Winkelstein, 1961.) The majority of the investigators used an initial dose of 10 mg (four tablets) of diphenoxylate until the diarrhea was improved, which generally took from a few days to a few weeks. Afterwards, an individually adapted maintenance dose was sought, which generally ranged from 5 to 15 mg (2 to 6 tablets). This maintenance dose may be lowered or may need to be increased for shorter or longer periods of time, depending on the evolution of the disease. It was observed in these studies that the chronic diarrhea patients themselves easily learned to adapt the dosage. The most convincing and satisfying results have been obtained in Crohn's disease, postresection diarrhea, and functional diarrhea.

3.3. DIPHENOXINE

A double-blind crossover placebo-controlled investigation established that diphenoxine was five times more potent than diphenoxylate in producing constipation in healthy volunteers (Rubens et al., 1972). This dose-response relationship between both drugs has been confirmed in other double-blind crossover studies. An early study (Hillerbrand, in preparation) tested 20

TABLE 3

Summary of Results Derived from Clinical Studies on 763 Patients with Chronic Diarrhea

Type of diarrhea	Patients treated	Excellent to good	Moderate to fair	Poor to absent	Comment
Regional ileitis	77	63	8	6	Including enteritis, ileitis, regional enteritis
Postsurgical diarrhea	158	126	18	19	Including vagotomy, gastrectomy, ileostomy, endostomy
Ulcerative colitis	132	90	11	31	
Functional diarrhea	198	160	18	20	Including malabsorption, dyspepsia steatorrhea, digestive insufficiency
Irritable colon	67	66	1	—	Including colitis mucosa, nervous diarrhea, spastic colitis
Diarrhea due to disorders of organs outside the gut	28	22	2	4	Including uremia, pancreatitis, livercirrhosis, hyperthyreosis
Diarrhea due to radiotherapy	87	81	6	—	
Carcinoma of the colon	16	12	—	4	
	763[a]	620[a]	59[a]	84[a]	

[a]Total

hospitalized patients with diarrhea resulting from X-ray therapy. Based on stool frequency and consistency, complete or marked improvement was noted in 14 of 17 diphenoxine treated patients (82%) and in 13 of 18 patients treated with diphenoxylate (72%). The median daily dose for both drugs was three tablets per day. Similar results were obtained in 14 patients with chronic diarrhea of various origins (Rubens et al., 1972). Complete relief or marked improvement was noted by 12 patients during both treatment periods. The median dose for both drugs was six tablets daily. In an open multicentric trial (Reyntjens, in preparation) 61 patients with chronic diarrhea of varying origins were treated for one month with 4 to 8 diphenoxine tablets daily. Of these 61 patients, 37 had previously been treated with diphenoxylate. Treatment with diphenoxine resulted in normal stools in 38 of the patients (62%), marked improvement in 17 patients (28%) and no improvement in 6 patients (10%).

3.4. LOPERAMIDE

3.4.1. Dosage

Clinical studies of loperamide for symptomatic control of chronic diarrhea used an individually adapted dosage regimen of two 2-mg capsules of loperamide as an initial daily dosage, followed by one capsule after each loose stool (maximum dosage eight capsules per day). The dosage was individually reduced until control (i.e., 1 or 2 formed stools daily) was achieved. Daily control was achieved with a dosage of three to four capsules in the majority of cases.

3.4.2. Patient and Study Profile

Twelve separate studies covering 368 subjects are available for analysis, reporting the effective use of loperamide in comparison to placebo or diphenoxylate in controlling chronic diarrhea. In seven of the studies placebo was employed for comparison, in four studies diphenoxylate, and one study was open in design. Diphenoxine was included in one study.

Initially, the subjects were required to discontinue their current antidiarrheal medication to permit a relapse, and pretherapy baselines were established. Open treatment with loperamide was then instituted with each subject being titrated individually to an optimum daily dose, which then was administered in one or two doses daily. Wherever specified, a double-blind crossover phase was then instituted. The crossover treatment was continued for a few days to a few weeks. Additional data or long-term follow up was then obtained with loperamide being administered in open design for 6 to 44 months. Table 4 presents the pretherapy diagnoses of the disease conditions

TABLE 4

Diagnosis Categories of Patients
Treated with Loperamide and Diphenoxylate
for Chronic Diarrhea

Diagnosis	Number of patients
Postsurgical[a]	87
Crohn's disease[b]	67
Functional etiology[c]	66
Colitis[d]	44
Ulcerative colitis[b]	39
Malabsorption states	31
Postradiotherapy	16
Carcinoma of colon	8
	358[e]

[a] Postvagotomy, gastrectomy, ileal or colonic resection with anastomosis, colostomy or ileostomy.

[b] Excluding surgical cases.

[c] Irritable colon syndrome, hyperperistalsis.

[d] Of inflammatory nature due to infections, granulomatons or unknown etiology.

[e] Total

causing the chronic diarrhea in the patients included in this review and analysis. In each procedure, the therapy was initiated by two capsules which were followed by one capsule after each loose stool up to a daily allowable maximum of five to eight capsules.

3.4.3. Results Summarized

The data of 12 separate studies demonstrate that loperamide is a highly effective drug in treating patients with chronic diarrhea. Loperamide effectively improved the consistency of stools and significantly reduced their frequency in patients with chronic diarrhea. Loperamide was shown to delay intestinal carmine transit time and also decrease fecal loss due to ileostomies and colostomies.

On a milligram for milligram basis, loperamide was more effective than diphenoxylate when the two drugs were used clinically in similar situations.

3.4.4. Results Analyzed

To provide further insight into the use of antidiarrheal drugs in chronic diarrhea we shall briefly review each of the 12 studies recently completed referred to above.

In the open phase of their study with loperamide, Mainquet and Fiasse (1975) demonstrated a reduction of stool frequency from 6 to 2 ($p < 0.006$) and median stool-consistency improvement from liquid to loose with loperamide ($p < 0.005$). In the double-blind phase of their study, loperamide was found to be highly superior to placebo ($p < 0.0001$) for both of the above parameters. In 18 subject pairs, median intestinal carmine transit time was 2.25 hr for placebo, in contrast to 4.6 hr for loperamide ($p < 0.005$). In 17 subject pairs with ileostomies, median daily fecal weights were decreased from 800 to 480 g with loperamide ($p < 0.0003$).

Tijtgat et al. (1975) evaluated 20 subjects with ileostomies who were treated with loperamide. Their fecal output was decreased by 22% as compared to pretherapy measurements. In a second study, during the initial open phase loperamide controlled chronic diarrhea in 11 of 15 patients (73%) with significant decreases in stool frequency ($p < 0.01$) and stool consistency ($p < 0.05$). In the subsequent (placebo-controlled double-blind) phase of this study, loperamide treated patients continued to show excellent control of their diarrheal condition while patients on placebo deteriorated with increased stool frequency ($p < 0.01$) and reduced consistency ($p < 0.05$). Fewer abdominal cramps were noted during use of loperamide.

In the open trial with loperamide in 109 outpatients with chronic diarrhea, Demulenaere et al. (1974) reported normalization of stools in 75 patients with an average daily dosage of 10 mg loperamide. In another 21 patients in the same study, the authors noted that overall treatment was effective in 90% of their patients. Before loperamide therapy, 68 patients complained of abdominal cramps, while only nine reported cramps with loperamide therapy. In 32 patients who were observed from 6 to 17 months while on loperamide therapy, similar improvements were noted without dosage increases, i.e., no tolerance developed to the antidiarrheal action of loperamide.

In a double-blind study by Demeulemere et al. (1976), placebo was used in control groups. Stool frequency and consistency was significantly improved ($p < 0.001$).

Chapaux (unpublished report) used loperamide in 12 patients with chronic diarrhea attributable to X-ray or radioisotope therapy. These patients had previously failed to respond to diphenoxylate. In 8 of 12 patients (67%), loperamide effectively controlled diarrhea. Stool consistency was improved from liquid to formed, abdominal cramps were reduced, and the number of stools were reduced to less than three per day.

Van Trappen (1975) reported satisfactory results with diphenoxylate and loperamide in their double-blind crossover study. In comparison with a drug-free interval, stool frequency and consistency improved significantly during treatment with loperamide ($p < 0.001$) as well as with diphenoxylate ($p < 0.006$). The improvement was significantly greater with loperamide. The average daily dosage of loperamide was 6.9 mg ($p < 0.001$) as compared to 17.7 mg for diphenoxylate, a significant difference.

De Coster et al. (1972) compared loperamide with diphenoxine in 20 surgical patients (intestinal resections). All patients were followed for up to 3 months. The 10 patients on loperamide showed marked improvement while only 3 of 10 patients on diphenoxine showed similar improvement.

Karg et al. (1975) reported complete or marked relief of diarrhea, based on stool frequency and consistency, in 14 of 16 loperamide treated patients (88%), as opposed to 9 of 16 diphenoxylate treated patients (56%0. The loperamide median daily dose was 6 mg while 12.5 mg was required with diphenoxylate. As with the Van Trappen study cited above, this difference in dosage levels was significant.

In a crossover study, Verhaegen (1975a) reported complete diarrheal relief in 6 of 10 patients (60%) and marked improvement in three of the remaining patients with both test drugs, loperamide and diphenoxylate. The optimum average daily dose was 10.2 mg for loperamide and 15 mg for diphenoxylate. Relief of diarrhea occurred in 5.67 days with loperamide and 8.11 days with diphenoxylate. The difference between the two time periods was statistically significant.

Hirschowitz (1975) completed a double-blind study in 22 patients using loperamide, and placebo as a control. In the initial one-month open phase of the study, a median daily dose of 6 mg of loperamide was effective in 17 of 22 cases (77%) in decreasing stool frequency from six to three bowel movements per day ($p < 0.001$); stool consistency was changed from watery to mushy ($p < 0.001$). During the double-blind phase of the study of those subjects who remained on loperamide, stool frequency was recorded as two bowel movements per day with stool consistency improved to soft. Subjects, however, who received placebo relapsed within a median of two weeks, had increased stool frequency to a median level of four daily movements, and significant changes in stool consistency to watery ($p < 0.02$). Loperamide treatment was resumed in these relapsed patients at a median dose of 8 mg/day. Control of the diarrhea was quickly achieved. In this group, 18 patients were observed for periods of up to 18 months, and no tolerance to the antidiarrheal effect of loperamide was noted.

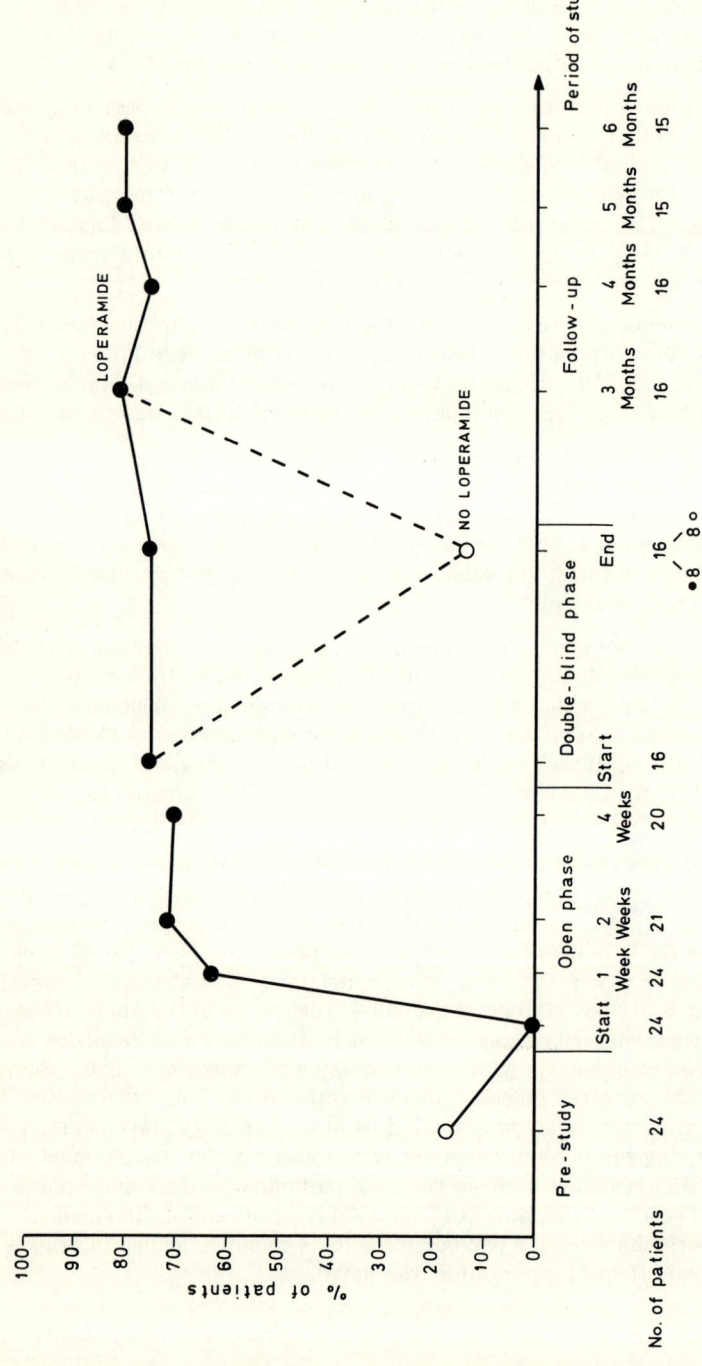

Fig. 2. Percent of patients with normal or soft stools after administration of loperamide.

Modern Antidiarrheals in Medical Practice 221

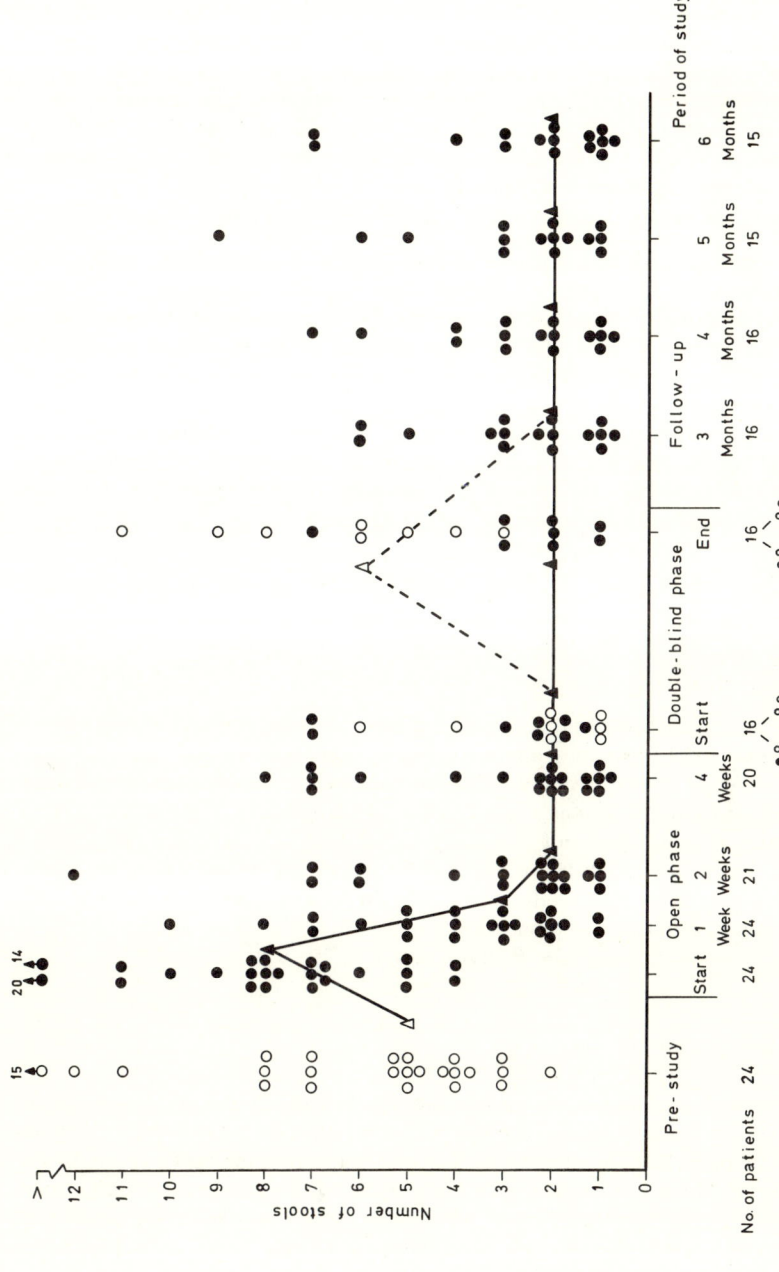

Fig. 3. Number of stools per day after administration of loperamide. ●, loperamide; ○, no loperamide; △, median; ▲, median.

Galambos (1975) completed a similar study in 24 patients. The design of the study is illustrated in Fig. 2. There was an excellent response of patients to loperamide during the 4-week open study. During the double-blind phase, loperamide patients continued to respond satisfactorily, but, as anticipated, placebo patients relapsed. When these placebo patients were reinstated on loperamide therapy they were successfully controlled at an average daily dosage of 8 mg. In the initial one-month open phase of the study a median dose of 8 mg of loperamide was effective in 18 of 24 cases (75%) in decreasing stool frequency from eight to two stools per day ($p < 0.0001$) and stool consistency changed from watery to soft ($p < 0.001$).

During the double-blind phase of this study of subjects who remained on loperamide, stool frequency was found to be a median of two per day with consistency improved from soft to normal after a median of 33 days of treatment. However, subjects who received placebo relapsed within a median of 4 days, had increased stool frequency to six per day with a consistency change from soft to watery. Resumption of loperamide treatment effectively controlled the diarrhea with a dose of 8 mg/day which produced a median of two bowel movements per day, and a change to a formed stool consistency was achieved (see Fig. 3). These patients have been followed for 18 months without any evidence whatsoever of drug tolerance.

In the study of Gordon et al. (1975), 51 patients were evaluated. The initial one-month open phase of the study utilized a median daily dosage of 6 mg of loperamide and was effective in 37 or 73% of the cases in decreasing stool frequency from six to two bowel movements per day ($p < 0.001$); stool consistency change from watery to soft ($p < 0.001$).

During the double-blind phase of the study of subjects remaining on loperamide, stool frequency and consistency remained essentially unchanged. However, subjects who received placebo relapsed within a median of 7 days, had increased stool frequency to a median of six per day ($p < 0.001$), and a consistency change from soft to watery ($p < 0.002$). Treatment was then resumed with loperamide (8-10 mg daily), and the diarrhea was controlled for up to 4 months with a median of two to three stools per day and a stool consistency fluctuating between watery and soft. (For a summary of the above-mentioned studies, see Sect. 3.4.3.)

3.4.5. Safety

In a number of studies, repeated hematological indices and serum analyses in over 500 subjects with chronic diarrhea have not demonstrated any trends towards abnormalities during loperamide therapy ranging up to 44 months in duration. No drug interaction with a multiplicity of concurrent medications was observed; urine, EKG, blood pressures, slit-lamp and clinical ophthalmological examinations have shown no adverse trends. The most frequent adverse experiences reported on therapy were primarily constipation (3%) which may be attributable to overdosage. Generally, other side effects such as nausea, abdominal pain, and flatulence in the order of 1%, and were of a minor and self-limiting nature.

V.4. PEDIATRIC USE OF MODERN ANTIDIARRHEALS

In the pediatric clinical situation, diphenoxylate is quite frequently prescribed for children. There are several published studies of pediatric use. In one study, the effect of diphenoxylate on the intestinal passage of food has been investigated in 10 neonates. The interval (transit time) between a meal containing a small amount of charcoal powder and the appearance of black stools was noted before and after diphenoxylate was given (0.62 mg daily). The intestinal passage of food after diphenoxylate is significantly slower than during the control period, (Shärli, 1967: Fig. 4).

In the same review, diphenoxylate was evaluated in seven children with congenital intestinal hypoplasia and provided, in all cases, a slowing of bowel peristalsis. The drug was well tolerated at doses varying from 0.62 mg twice daily for premature infants, to 0.62 four times daily for infants from 4 to 12 months old (Shärli, 1967).

Since chronic diarrhea (as opposed to acute) is a rather infrequent disease in children, it may be assumed that most prescriptions are for acute gastroenteritis. This condition is generally mild in nontropical areas, but may be very severe in tropical countries due to the potential for rapid and severe loss of water producing electrolyte imbalance.

In infants, diarrhea is frequently seen as a result of intolerance of the food, in particular to milk powders and commercial baby formulas; this diarrhea generally subsides with a change of the composition of the formula, but in many cases an antidiarrheal may be useful during the dietary adaptation process. Loperamide has been used with favorable results in a series of babies with such dietary problems (Lambrechts, in press), with a dosage regimen of 0.15 mg/kg body weight in two daily doses. The same dosage regimen as used in adults was also tried in children with acute diarrhea; the initial dose was 0.2 mg/kg, followed by 0.1 mg/kg after each unformed stool (Crivaro, in preparation).

The use of diphenoxylate, and presumably also diphenoxine in babies has been recently questioned (see Sec. 8).

In summary, the suggested dosage regimen for the pediatric use of antidiarrheals is as follows:

Diphenoxylate: 0.1 mg/kg body weight three times a day (in children under 2 yr this dosage should never be exceeded).

Loperamide: about 0.1 mg/kg body weight as a first dose, followed by 0.05 mg/kg body weight after each unformed stool.

V.5. INDICATIONS FOR DECREASING THE INTESTINAL MOTILITY IN SITUATIONS OTHER THAN DIARRHEA

Experiments performed in healthy volunteers have shown that a single dose of 10 mg of diphenoxylate has inhibited gastrointestinal motility for more than 6 hr. This effect (with a staggered dose of 40 mg) could be maintained more than 24 hr (Demeulenaere, 1958). The use of diphenoxylate in diarrhea, which is in a strict sense a manifestation of "hyperstaltism," is based upon this principle. In some cases, however, it may be necessary to reduce an otherwise normal intestinal motility and hence the number of bowel movements. Such is the case, for instance, in anal incontinence where the imminence of evacuation can neither be perceived nor postponed because of sphincteral obstruction or lack of sensitivity. Diphenoxylate reduces the number of evacuations to about one per day, thus providing the necessary "education of the intestine" and makes life bearable for these patients again (Vigoni, 1960). This use for diphenoxylate has found quite an unexpected application with the beginning of space flights. The operations to be performed during the flight require total freedom in movement and diphenoxylate was chosen to "assist in avoiding inflight defecation when necessary" (Berry, 1967).

V.6. THE USE OF DIPHENOXYLATE IN DETOXIFICATION OF HEROIN ADDICTS

Abstinence symptoms occurring at withdrawal from narcotics during detoxification treatment are generally suppressed by substituting strongly addictive drugs such as methadone. However, recent evidence suggests that these types of agents often possess their own addiction liability and thus the merits of this procedure have been questioned.

Diphenoxylate has very weak addictive properties, and moreover its very low solubility practically forbids its parenteral administration. Diphenoxylate was thus tried in several withdrawal programs and the experience to date, though limited, is promising. The doses used varied widely and depended on the level of addiction. In moderate addiction, daily doses ranging from 15 to 30 mg for 4 to 7 days proved to be sufficient (Glatt et al., 1970). In heavy users, by comparison, the treatment had to be far more drastic, with a total dose amounting to 260 mg in about 5 days (Goodman, 1968).

Diphenoxylate provides complete relief of autonomic and other physiological withdrawal symptoms, but the authors insist upon the necessary administration of sedatives and tranquilizers (barbiturates, phenothiazine, benzodiazepines) to overcome the anxiety reactions which might induce the patient to stop the treatment.

V.7. ABUSE POTENTIAL OF ANTIDIARRHEALS

As has been stated in previous sections, there is apparently no potential for abuse of the antidiarrheals, diphenoxylate and loperamide. Diphenoxylate has been on the market since 1960 and several billion doses have been administered. Reflective of its weak morphine-like activity, we have found no reports in the literature suggesting any abuse or addiction liability in the last 15 yr. It appears that the weak CNS action of diphenoxylate does not have any euphoric component to stimulate abuse. Rather its CNS effects may be dysphoric and act against its abuse.

With loperamide, the case may even be stronger from a pharmacological standpoint, although its newness prevents thorough clinical judgment which is possible with diphenoxylate. In all of the animal studies described in previous chapters, loperamide was shown to lack any morphine-like pharmacological action or CNS mediated narcotic-like subjective effect. No "dependence" on loperamide could be produced even with prolonged treatment of the rat and other species, and it showed aversive properties when offered to rats previously made addicted to narcotic drugs. In addition to the animal studies reported previously, and those mentioned here, studies were conducted in patients to determine any possible narcotic-like effects of loperamide.

Brugmans (1975) compared loperamide with diphenoxylate and codeine in placebo-controlled, double-blind studies in which these drugs were crossed-over in the same patients. Doses of loperamide as high as 16 mg did not produce any opiate-like euphoria nor any effect on pupil size. In addition, pupil size was not altered by 4 mg of naloxone given subcutaneously. In the same study, however, opiate-like effects were noticed with codeine and diphenoxylate. The pupil size remained unaffected by naloxone after loperamide treatment but were somewhat enlarged in diphenoxylate treated patients and even more enlarged in codeine treated patients. These data are illustrated in Fig. 4.

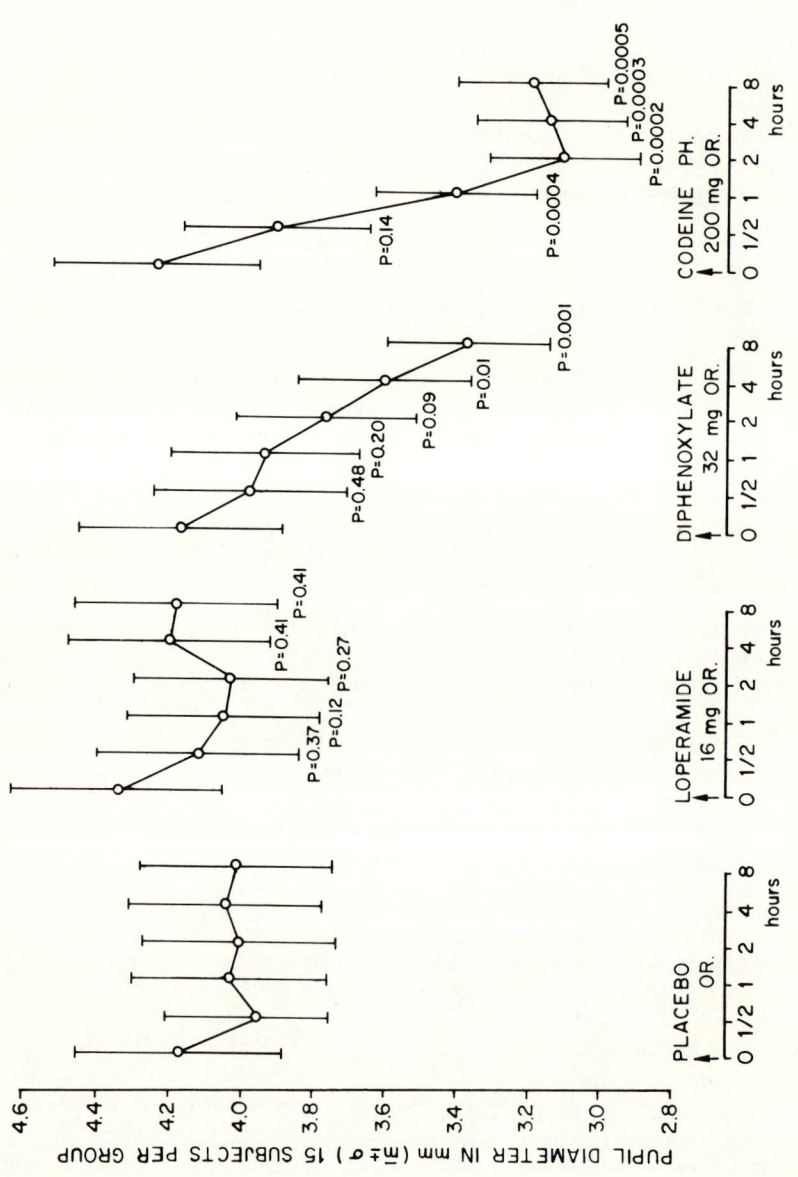

Fig. 4. Effect of antidiarrheals on pupil size.

In a study by Verhaegen (1975b), 10 subjects with chronic diarrhea were treated with loperamide for from 10 days up to 3 yr. Pupil dilation did not occur upon naloxone challenge. A similar study by Mainquet (1975) also produced negative results with loperamide. In this study, 20 subjects with chronic diarrhea were treated for an average of 18 months with an average daily dose of 6 mg of loperamide. Half of the subjects were injected subcutaneously with saline and the remaining 10 patients received 4 mg of naloxone. No significant difference of pupil size was observed between the two groups.

Since the naloxone challenge test is recognized as a sensitive indication of opiate activity and also for potential opiate abuse, we can conclude that loperamide is devoid of opiate-like action when used in either the acute or chronic situation.

Another characteristic of almost all narcotic drugs is that a rapid tolerance develops to their pharmacological actions. This is likewise not the case with loperamide. In the studies of Verhaegen (1975b), Mainquet and Fiasse (1975), and Reyntjens (in preparation) a total of 62 patients were given a median dose of loperamide (4-6 mg) for a period of 11 to 23 months. Analysis of their data established that the patients were controlled with these doses and that the dose levels did not have to be increased with time. On the contrary, after achieving initial control of the diarrhea, the doses of loperamide could often be reduced.

Therefore, based upon the extensive tests in animals, the lack of morphine-like subjective action in human patients, the negative results in naloxone challenge tests in patients, and absence of tolerance (i.e., the necessity to increase the dose) in the chronic clinical situation, it may be concluded that loperamide is devoid of any narcotic-like action and that no abuse potential exists with this drug.

V.8. SIDE EFFECTS AND SAFETY

As can be expected from the mechanism of action of diphenoxylate, diphenoxine, and loperamide, any dosage in excess of the individually adapted therapeutic dose for the control of the diarrhea may produce constipation. This "side effect" (merely an extension of the therapeutic effect) may, therefore, be easily controlled by adjustments of the dosage.

Side effects observed with diphenoxylate are generally mild, having only rarely caused the interruption of treatment. Nausea, somnolence, dryness of the mouth, and dizziness are the most frequently mentioned, the incidence being lower than 8% in 1220 patients as reported in the clinical studies reviewed above. It should be noted that many of the reported side effects may not be due to the antidiarrheal medication at all but rather to the diarrheal condition itself or to associated medications.

The experience with diphenoxine is more limited but the available data would suggest the same picture exists as for diphenoxylate.

By comparison, the side effects with loperamide are even less common than with diphenoxylate and diphenoxine. In the few studies where loperamide was compared with placebo no significant difference in side effects could be detected. Both diphenoxylate and loperamide have been prescribed in chronic diarrhea in combination with other drugs, such as tranquilizers, antidepressants, corticosteroids, antibiotics, and salazopyrine, and no incompatibility has been reported with either of these drugs.

A very important point for the clinician is the early recognition of the signs of intoxication with these agents so that supportive care may be initiated without any loss of time. The therapeutic procedures consist in endotracheal intubation and gastric lavage.

Induced emesis is not recommended since a rapid change in the respiratory neurological status will enhance the chance of aspiration and subsequent bronchic infection (Ginsburg and Moulinier, 1973; Henderson and Psaile, 1969). Naloxone is the vital factor in the treatment of respiratory depression. Its effect begins immediately after IV or IM injection. Pediatric doses of naloxone generally range from 5 to 10 $mg/1.73 \; m^2$ and the initial dose for neonates (younger than 6 months) amounts to 0.25 mg. Diphenoxylate has a prolonged action, while that of naloxone is quite short. Constant monitoring is thus necessary to avoid any chance of any potential recurrence of a respiratory depression.

However, special attention should be given to the potential hazards of overdosing diphenoxylate in babies and infants. It appears that children under 1-2 yr of age are much more sensitive to the effects of overdosing of diphenoxylate with its frequently prescribed associated atropine moiety, than are older children and the adults. While in the adult no cases of acute intoxication have been reported, several such cases in babies and infants have been reported in the literature, two of them with a fatal outcome. In most cases the overdosing had been accidental.

It has been suggested that diphenoxylate not be used in children under 2 yr of age and in several countries this suggestion has been embodied as a contraindication in the package insert. In other countries, the use of diphenoxylate in children is not considered a contraindication, provided the dosage scheme is strictly adhered to. This, of course, is an a-priori assumption in good clinical practice. In some cases, however, massive doses have been ingested; in others the dosage used was not greatly in excess of the therapeutic one.

In most intoxication situations the first symptoms are due to an atropine-like intoxication (flush, tachypnea, hyperthermia, lethargy, convulsions due to the hyperthermia) and may remain for 2-3 hr. About 30 min later the symptoms of a diphenoxylate intoxication may abruptly occur, i.e., hyperthermia, subsiding of the flush and depression of the CNS, and the most severe expression, which is the respiratory depression.

No significant haematological or biochemical changes have, however, been reported in patients, both children and adults, who received diphenoxylate, diphenoxine, or loperamide for prolonged periods of time (Van Derstappen and Vandenbroucke, 1961; Weingarten et al., 1961; Mainquet and Fiasse, 1975; Verhaegen, 1974).

REFERENCES

Amery, W. et al. (1975). A multicentric double-blind study in acute diarrhea comparing loperamide (R-18553) with the common anti-diarrheal agents and a placebo. NDA 17-690, Vol. 1.1, p. 02-00286.

Arabehety, J. J., Dolcini, H. A., and Stapler, N. H. (1964). Acción antidiarreica y antispasmodica del clorhidrato de difenoxilato (Lomotil). La Semana Medica 17, 563-566.

Barowsky, A. and Schwartz, S. A. (1962). Method for evaluating diphenoxylate hydrochloride. Comparison of its antidiarrheal effect with that of camphorated tincture of opium. J.A.M.A. 180, 1058-1061.

Baufle, G. H., Deschaseaux, P., and Hanhart, P. (1965). Essais cliniques d'un nouvel antidiarrhéique (Diarsed). J. Méd. Besançon 1, 313-317.

Berry, C. A. (1967). Space medicine in perspective. A critical review of the manned space program. J.A.M.A. 201, 232-241.

Bond, B., Brinckenhoff, W. C., Fishman, J., Hawker, P. G., Ison, L. J., McMichael, L. A., Silver, S. A., Stoll, L. J., and Williams, D. T. A. (1966). Treatment of diarrhoea with a synthetic compound. Practitioner 197, 815-817.

Bonnycastle, D. D. (1958). Catharics and Laxative. In Pharmacology in Medicine (2nd ed.), V. A. Drill (Ed.). McGraw-Hill Book Co., New York.

Brugmans, J. (1975). Pupillary constriction and mydriatic response to naloxone after single oral doses of codeine, diphenoxylate and loperamide in normal volunteers. NDA 17-690, Vol. 1.1, p. 02-00108.

Camatte, R. and François, G. F. (1963). Essais thérapeutiques du RO 1132 dans les diarrhées. Gaz. Hôp. 135, 89-95.

Cayer, D. and Sohmer, H. F. (1961). Long-term clinical studies with a new constipating drug, diphenoxylate hydrochloride. N. Caroline Med. J. 22.

Chapaux, J., Chapaux, R., and Royer, R. Action of loperamide in chronic diarrhoea following radiotherapy (in preparation).

Cohen, R., Kalser, M. H., Arteaga, I., Yawen, E., Frazier, D., Leite, C. A., Ahearn, D. G., and Roth, F. (1967). Microbial intestinal flora in acute diarrheal disease. J.A.M.A. 201, 835-840.

Crivaro, E. A. Evaluación de un nuevo antidiarreico, loperamide R 18 553 (in preparation).

De Coster, M., Kerremans, R., and Beckers, J. (1972). A comparative double blind study of two antidiarrhoeals, difenoxine and loperamide. Tijdschr. Gastroenterol. 15, 337-342.

Demeulenaere, L. (1958). Action du RO 1132 sur le transit gastro-intestinal. Acta Gastroenterol. Belg. 21, 674-680.

Demeulenaere, L., Verbeke, S., Muls, M., and Reyntjens, A. (1974). Loperamide: an open multicentric trial and a double-blind cross-over comparison with placebo in patients with chronic diarrhoea. Curr. Therap. Res. 16, 32-39.

Dom, J., Leyman, R., Schuermans, V., and Brugmans, J. (1974). Loperamide (18 553): A novel type of antidiarrheal agent. Part 8: clinical investigation; double-blind comparison of loperamide with diphenoxylate in a flexible dosage schedule for 614 patients with acute diarrhoea. Arzneimittel-Forsch. 24, 87-100.

Dziuba, K. (1961). Die Behandlung der akuten und chronischen Diarrhoe durch Hemmung der Magen- und Darmmotilitaet. Med. Welt 51, 2700-2703.

Eichenwald, H. F., McCracken, G. H., Jr. (1970). Acute diarrheal disease. Med. Clin. N. Am. 54, 443-453.

Gabriele, R. and Moulinier, R. (1963). Essais cliniques d'un nouvel anti-diarrhéique le RO 1132. Lyon Méd. 209, 1091.

Galambos, J. (1975). Long-term placebo controlled, double-blind evaluation of loperamide in the treatment of chronic diarrhea. NDA 17-690, Vol. 2.1, p. 1.

Ginsburg, C. M. (1973). Lomotil (diphenoxylate and atropine intoxication). Am. J. Diseases Children 125, 241-242.

Glatt, M. M., Lewis, D. M., and Wilson, D. T. (1970). An oral method of the withdrawal treatment of heroin dependence. A five years' study of a combination of diphenoxylate (Lomotil) and chlormethirazole (Heminevrier). Brit. J. Addict. 65, 237-243.

Goodman, A. L. (1968). Use of diphenoxylate hydrochloride in the withdrawal period of narcotic addiction, a preliminary report. South. Med. J. 61, 313-316.

Gordon, S. et al. (1975). A summary of five placebo controlled, double-blind studies of loperamide in the treatment of chronic diarrhea. NDA 17-690 Vol. 2.1, p. 18.

Goulston, R. (1973). Diagnosis and treatment of the irritable bowel syndrome. Drugs 6, 237-243.

Gürtler, J. (1965). Zur Behandlung von Nebenwirkungen der PAS-Therapie. Therap. Umschau 22, 611-613.

Henderson, W. and Psaila, A. (1969). Lomotil poisoning. Lancet 307, Feb.

Hillerbrand, P. Comparative double blind evaluation of difenoxine and diphenoxylate in the control of diarrhea associated with X-ray therapy (in preparation).

Hirschowitz, B. (1975). Long-term placebo controlled, double-blind evaluation of loperamide in the treatment of chronic diarrhea. NDA 17-690, Vol. 2.1, p. 9.

Hock, Ch. W. (1961). Relief of diarrhea with diphenoxylate hydrochloride (Lomotil). J. Med. Assoc. Georgia 50, 485-488.

Jancloes, M. (1975). Double blind, randomized, comparative study of loperamide and diphenoxylate in acute diarrhea. Clinical Research Report No. 35, Janssen Pharmaceutica, Belgium.

Karg, E. et al. (1975). Comparative study of loperamide and diphenoxylate in the control of chronic diarrhea resulting from radiotherapy according to a randomized cross-over, double-blind procedure. NDA 17-690, Vol. 1.1, p. 02-00222.

Kasich, A. M. (1961). Treatment of diarrhoea in irritable colon, including preliminary observation with a new antidiarrheal agent, diphenoxylate hydrochloride (Lomotil). Am. J. Gastroenterol. 35, 46-49.

Lambrechts. Le lopéramide dans le traitement des diarrhées aiguës du jeune enfant. To be published in Revue Med. Liège.

Lichstein, J. (1965). A clinical study of diphenoxylate in the treatment of diarrhea, Curr. Therap. Res. 7, 176-182.

Low-Beer, T. S. and Read, A. E. (1971). Diarrhoea: mechanisms and treatment. Gut 12, 1021-1036.

Machella, Th. E. (1960). Postsurgical problems of the gastrointestinal tract, gastric resection difficulties. J.A.M.A. 174, 1211-1217.

Mainguet, P. (1975). Effect of naloxone on pupil diameter after a long-term loperamide treatment for chronic diarrhea; a double-blind study. NDA 17-690, Vol. 1.1, p. 02-00116.

Mainguet, P. and Fiasse, R. (1975). Double-blind placebo-controlled study of loperamide in chronic diarrhea resulting from ileocolic lesions and/or resections. NDA 17-690, Vol. 1.1, p. 02-00174.

Manciaux, M., Thomas, R., and Toussaint, P. (1968). La place du RO 1132 dans le traitement des gastro-entérites infantiles. Ann. Méd. Nancy 7, 1015-1022.

Merlo, M. and Brower, Ch. (1960). The effect of diphenoxylate hydrochloride on diarrhea. Am. J. Gastroenterol. 34, 625-630.

Miotti, R. (1968). Anwendung der Peristaltikmoderators REASEC zur Therapie von Diarrhoen nach Roentgenbestrahlung oder Behandlung mit radioaktiven Isotopen, Schweiz. Med. Wochschr. 98, 761-763.

Moeller, H. C. (1965). Treatment of irritable colon. Mod. Treatm. 2, 988-1002.

Moffet, H. L., Schulenberger, H. K., and Burkholder, E. R. (1968). Epidermology and etiology of severe infantile diarrhoea. J. Pediat. 72, 1.

Müller, W. (1967). Über die Anwendung von Reasec in der Chirurgie. Praxis 56, 730-733.

Murphy, J. E. (1968). A comparison of antidiarrhoeal preparations in acute diarrhoea in general practice. Practitioner 200, 570-574.

Owens, F. J. (1965). Medical treatment of ulcerative colitis. Mod. Treatm. 2, 937-958.

Poirier, A. and Poirier, M. (1961). Un nouvel antidiarrhéique le RO 1132. Gaz. Méd. France 22, Nov.

Pourquier, H., Belotte, J., and Lamarque, J. L. (1963). Essai d'un nouvel antidiarrhéique. Le RO 1132 dans les diarrhées consécutives aux irradiations abdominales et pelviennes. J. Radiol. Electrol. 44, 647-648.

Puls, G. (1975). Double-blind, cross-over comparison of loperamide with diphenoxylate in the management of chronic diarrhea. NDA 17-690, Vol. 1.1, p. 02-00227.

Raby, M. B. and Shooman, H. (1967). The treatment of gastro-enteritis in general practice. A comparative trial of four combinations of diphenoxylate and neomycine, active and placebo. Clin. Trials J. 4, 803-809.

Ramsay, A. M. (1968). Acute infective diarrhoea. Brit. Med. J. 2, 347-350.

Reyntjens, A. A multicentric pilot-trial of difenoxine (R 15 403), a new antidiarrhoeal agent (in preparation).

Rubens, R., Verhaegen, H., Brugmans, J., and Schuermans, V. (1972). Difenoxine (R 15 403) the active metabolite of diphenoxylate (RO 1132). Part 5: Clinical comparison of difenoxine and diphenoxylate in volunteers and in patients with chronic diarrhoea. Double-blind cross-over assessments. Arzneimittel-Forsch. 22, 526-529.

Rutgeerts, L. (1973). Diarree. Tijdschr. Geneeskunde 12, 560-570.

Shärli, A. (1967). Zur Therapie von Resorptionstoerungen bei anatomische Verkürzungen und Hypoplasien des Intestinal Traktes mit Reasec (Diphenoxylat) beim Kinde. Schweiz. Med. Wochschr. 97, 288-290.

Tijtgat, G. et al. Loperamide in the symptomatic control of chronic diarrhea, double-blind, placebo controlled study. NDA 17-690, Vol. 1.1, p. 02-00241.

Valla, A. (1965). Le traitement des diarrhées chroniques. Considérations sur leur traitement symptomatique par le diphénoxylate. Rev. Méd. Normandes 7.

Van Derstappen, G. and Vandenbroucke, G. (1961). Behandlungsergebnisse mit Diphenoxylat bei 264 Fällen von Diarrhoe. Med. Klin. 56, 162-964.

Van Derstappen, G., Vantrappen, G., and Vandenbroucke, J. (1960). Longterm clinical studies with RO 1132. A new constipating drug. Gastroenterology 39, 725-729.

Vantrappen, G. (1975). A double-blind cross-over comparison of loperamide HCl with diphenoxylate HCl in the symptomatic treatment of chronic diarrhoea. NDA 17-690, Vol. 1.1, p. 92-00189.

Verhaegen, H. (1974). Longterm safety evaluation of loperamide treatment. Sec. 10, R 18 553/24, Jan. 1974.

Verhaegen, H. (1975a). Double-blind, cross-over comparison of loperamide and diphenoxylate in the treatment of chronic diarrhea. NDA 17-690, Vol. 1.1, p. 02-00161.

Verhaegen, H. (1975b). Mydriatic response to naloxone in patients with chronic diarrhea treated with loperamide for up to 18 months. NDA 17-690, Vol. 1.1, p. 02-00113.

Vigoni, M. (1960). Traitement de l'incontinence anale. Acta Chir. Belg. 59, 139-148.

Weingarten, B., Weiss, J., and Simon, M. (1961). A clinical evaluation of a new antidiarrheal agent. Am. J. Gastroenterol. 35, 628-633.

Winkelstein, A. (1961). Symptomatic treatment of diarrhea with diphenoxylate. Am. J. Gastroenterol. 36, 692-697.

Zelvelder, W. G. (1975). A double-blind placebo controlled trial of loperamide in acute diarrhea. NDA 17-690, Vol. 1.1, p. 02-00261.

CHAPTER VI

THE ABUSE POTENTIAL OF MODERN ANTIDIARRHEALS

VI.1. FACTS AND FALACIES OF ADDICTION LIABILITY AND ABUSE POTENTIAL

Harbans Lal

1.1. HISTORICAL BACKGROUND

For centuries poppy extracts and opium preparations have been employed in the clinical control of diarrhea. Although in most countries, these preparations have been replaced by more specific synthetic drugs, their use is still prevalent in many developing countries. Because of this strong tradition of association between morphine and antidiarrheal chemotherapy, it has been widely believed that, like morphine, other antidiarrheal drugs have the risk of being abused. This suspicion is further supported by the fact that earlier synthetic drugs for diarrhea were derived from structural modifications of pethidine, a synthetic morphine-like narcotic.

Nevertheless, the most widely used synthetic antidiarrheal drug, diphenoxylate, has to our knowledge never been abused. This drug has been available since 1960, and, as described in the previous chapter, nearly half a billion doses of diphenoxylate are currently sold every year. Any potential abuse should therefore have been apparent by this time, after 15 yr.

All new drugs must, of course, be carefully examined for any possible risk of abuse. This chapter has been written in order to discuss the factors which are believed to contribute to the abuse potentials of potent chemical compounds. We will illustrate the predictive procedures used in order to give the reader a greater insight into this problem.

1.2. ESSENTIALS OF DRUG ABUSE

Drug abuse is defined as the self-administration of any drug in a manner which deviates from approved medical practice and from accepted social patterns of use in a given society. It is known to develop as a result of interaction between drug action, the personality of the subject, and his social environment.

Careful examination of the abuse characteristics of morphine-like narcotics clearly suggests that, apart from the pharmacological properties of these drugs, customs and forms of availability have greatly influenced their abuse. Indeed all narcotics with similar pharmacological properties are not abused to the same extent. In Western countries there is a predominance of heroin abuse, but in many other countries abuse of morphine is more prevalent. A certain segment of society is known to abuse only synthetic narcotics.

For the evaluation of abuse potential of a synthetic new drug, it is necessary to consider at least three important aspects. The first is the pharmacological action of the drug, then the actual and acquired (learned) mental perception of the drug actions, and finally the social attitudes toward abuse of that type of drug. An analysis of the socioeconomical factors that influence drug abuse is beyond the scope of this book. We will therefore limit our discussion to the major pharmacological and psychological factors that determine the possibility of abuse. Various pharmacological characteristics must be present before a drug can be considered as being a subject of abuse possibility. However, it should be pointed out that most of these factors are still speculative. There are not enough experimental data available to state with certainty exactly what determines the abuse liability of a chemical agent. Most of the factors which have been considered important by many investigators and many regulatory agencies are discussed below. Results obtained with experimental animals are described in section VI.2. These data will be briefly mentioned in order to put them in their proper perspective with regard to human drug abuse.

1.2.1. Psychoactive Properties

Today it is widely acceptable that there are specific effects of psychoactive drugs on the central nervous system (CNS) which play a primary role in the initiation and, possibly, in the continuation of drug abuse. Such effects are common to all types of drugs which have been abused. To date, not enough is known to define this CNS activity precisely. It is said to be some sort of euphoric effect which is described as a feeling of satisfaction or a "high". Euphoria produced with opioids is considered to be a subjective state of "unusual well being" that is incommensurate with objective reality (Wikler, 1974). Another property of such euphoria is that it produces a psychic drive to experience pleasure and avoid discomfort that requires periodic or continuous administration of the drug. According to an internationally recognized authority in the field of drug abuse (Eddy et al., 1970), "this mental state is the most powerful of all the factors involved in chronic intoxication with psychotrophic drugs, and with certain types of drugs it may be the only factor involved, even in most intense craving and perpetuation of compulsive abuse." It should be mentioned here that the opposite of drug induced euphoria is also true. A number of CNS active drugs produce dysphoric effects in such a manner that their abuse is resisted. A great deal of work has been done in order to measure narcotic euphoria objectively. Even though many of these investigations are still in progress several features of that euphoria have been described. They can be explained in terms of certain pharmacological characteristics of the CNS drugs which have been abused.

1.2.1.1. Perception Strength

The most basic requirement for a drug to produce an euphoric effect seems to be that this drug must cause a CNS action which can be clearly perceived by the subject. It is reasonable to assume that if the CNS effect of a drug cannot reach the perception threshold, that this effect cannot be regarded as euphoric or dysphoric. Once the CNS effect of a drug is readily perceived, the second most important effect of the drug leading to abuse, is that its CNS action is identified with that of opiate-like euphoria. According to Frazer et al. (1961) "if one were to select, on the basis of single doses, the most important single subjective response identifying a drug as being subject to morphine-like abuse probably this measure would be whether the former opiate addicts identify this drug as an opiate."

Several criteria for identifying the critical morphine-like effects of drugs being investigated for abuse potential have been developed. Some of the criteria have been applied to antidiarrheal drugs and will therefore be described here.

Overt behavior: The opiate-like drugs produce a wide variety of CNS effects. However, for the purpose of preclinical evaluation, the CNS effects of these drugs are recognized as weak excitement in mice and cats, catatonia in rats, and changes in respiration, pupil size, and electroencephalography in higher orders of animals. Of course, analgesia is the most important CNS effect of opiate-like drugs. The CNS effects of narcotic analgesics are readily distinguished from CNS effects of other drugs by the use of narcotic antagonists. It has been demonstrated that narcotic antagonists specifically block the action of narcotic drugs, and tolerance to the antagonistic potency of these drugs does not develop. Various CNS effects of antidiarrheal drugs have been described in Sect. IV.1 and will not be elaborated upon here. It suffices to mention that the morphine-like CNS activity of modern antidiarrheal drugs is considerably diminished. Diphenoxylate and difenoxin are devoid of any CNS activity at therapeutic doses and produce only mild CNS effects at higher doses. Loperamide is completely devoid of any CNS activity at all tolerated doses. Only at lethal doses can depression and ataxia be seen in experimental animals.

Behavioral discrimination of central effects: As explained above, the central effects of narcotic analgesics must be perceivable by the subject. This perception is experimentally evaluated by appropriate discrimination tests.

As laboratory animals cannot speak, other indications must be found. To accomplish this a number of procedures have been developed in which behavioral responses are analyzed in order to determine whether the subject can discriminate the specific CNS effect of a drug. In the laboratory many species of animals have been employed for these tasks. However, because of its ease in handling and easy availability, the rat has been the animal of choice in these investigations.

Usually animals are trained to make two (or more) types of response: to obtain a reward, to avoid punishment, or both. After initial learning of the responses, the discrimination training is begun. On certain days the animals are injected with CNS active drugs while on other days they are injected with placebo. After each injection they are then trained to choose only one of the responses they have previously learned and the "feeling" caused by drug injection is made the only basis for determining which response is selected. The correct choice of response is rewarded by food and the alternate incorrect choice is followed by nonreward or punishment. Active drugs produce physiological effects which form distinctive stimuli that can be discriminated from one another and from the placebo. Discrimination becomes evident after several days of training when the subject becomes "experienced" in recognizing different drug effects. Once the differential response has been well established, these animals can be used to test the euphoric effects of new drugs. When a novel drug is tested with these animals, the choice of the drug or placebo response made by the animal, measures whether the new dose of a drug is experienced by the animal as being similar to the familiar drug feeling or similar to placebo treatment.

It was originally thought that potent effects of drugs on peripheral systems (such as autonomic effects) would confuse the interpretation of the results obtained from these discrimination tests. However, several experiments conducted to study this question indicate that, in the case of almost all the drugs of abuse studied, the discrimination response of the trained animal was based entirely upon the central effects of the drugs. For example, rats trained to discriminate amphetamine from placebo gave placebo responses when hydroxyamphetamine was used as a test drug (Roffman and

Lal, 1972). Similarly, methylscopolamine was "recognized" as placebo by the rats trained to discriminate scopolamine from placebo. Both hydroxyamphetamine and methylscopolamine produce pronounced peripheral effects. However, they are devoid of CNS actions since the blood-brain barrier prevents them from penetrating into CNS structures. In general, whenever a drug with both CNS and peripheral effects is employed for discrimination training, only discrimination of CNS effects is learned.

Advantage has been taken of these experiments to detect the morphine-like subjective effects, or lack of them, associated with many new drugs. These data have recently been reviewed by Rosecrane et al. (1975), who concluded that "discrimination-stimulus effect of drugs in animals is somewhat analogous to the perceptual and subjective effects of drugs in man." According to Overton (1973), pioneer psychologist in this field, who introduced the concept of discrimination learning, discrimination techniques have produced very consistent and interpretable results. Apart from the reliability of these tests, there is the fact that, in discrimination testing, the subjective effects of morphine-like effects are being assessed through the "opinion" of trained animals who may be considered as "experienced" drug takers. It is well known that experienced drug abusers can discriminate very well between "good" and "bad" because they have learned discrimination through hit-and-miss experience during extended periods when they obtained their drug supplies from street dealers who are often unreliable.

Morphine-like drugs are capable of producing CNS stimuli which can be readily discriminated by experimental animals. For the purpose of testing whether antidiarrheal drugs would produce morphine-like CNS effects, two groups of rats were trained to discriminate between narcotic and placebo effect. One group learned to press one bar when injected with fentanyl and to press another bar when injected with placebo. The second group was trained to press one bar when injected with morphine sulfate and another bar when injected with placebo. In each group, half the animals pressed the bar on the right side of the cage as the drug bar and the bar on the left side as the placebo bar. The other half of the rats in each group was required to select the left bar as drug bar and the right bar as placebo bar. Such counterbalancing was necessary to avoid interference of any natural preference in rats for one side of the cage or the other. No clue other than the particular "feelings" produced by the drug or placebo injection was provided to select the correct bar. The correct selection was rewarded by food for every ten bar presses, while ten incorrect bar presses were punished by nonreward to hungry rats. After all the rats had learned and sufficiently practiced the drug-placebo discrimination, they were given several novel drugs for testing.

It was found that the rats pushed the drug bar whenever they were tested with an injection of morphine, methadone, fentanyl, dextromoramide, and phenoperidine. Similarly, they pressed the placebo bar whenever they were injected with saline, apomorphine, amphetamine, haloperidol, or loperamide. In the case of loperamide, doses as high as 100 times the effective antidiarrheal dose were recognized as placebo by our well-trained rats. Diphenoxylate was recognized as a narcotic when given in very high doses. Mere antidiarrheal doses of diphenoxylate were identified as placebo. On the basis of previous experience with this type of tests it is safe to conclude that loperamide (in any dose) does not produce any morphine-like subjective effects that can be recognized by subjects experienced in identifying narcotics.

It is interesting to note that for diphenoxylate similar data from human experiments, somewhat comparable to the rat test just described, are available. Frazer and his co-workers at the National Institute of Mental Health, Drug Addiction Center in Lexington (1961) selected eight veteran narcotic addicts, who were trained to differentiate subjectively between placebo and active drug in a well-controlled experimental setting. In addition, the subjects could also differentiate between different doses of the same drug and between structurally different narcotic drugs.

The eight subjects were given narcotics or placebo for 18-20 days during which time reliable discrimination was established. They were then given test compounds and their responses were recorded. The subjects reliably recognized all narcotic drugs as morphine-like compounds but only less than 25% recognized pharmacological doses of diphenoxylate as producing any subjective effects.

1.2.1.2. The Quality of Euphoric Effects

Beyond the mere perception of the subjective effects of psychoactive drugs, the quality of euphoria produced by these drugs is critical in determining whether a drug will be widely abused. Narcotic drugs produce subjective effects which are unpleasant in the beginning but which are soon experienced as pleasant and desirable. The effects of cocaine-like drugs are always perceived as pleasant while the subjective effects of amphetamine are both pleasant and aversive, depending upon the dose and other conditions of administration. Drugs which do not produce pleasant subjective effects are not abused. Neuroleptics, such as chlorpromazine and haloperidol, are centrally active drugs but are known to produce either no subjective effects or aversive feelings. Therefore, their abuse has never been reported. On the contrary, patients on prolonged neuroleptic therapy do not even ask for continuation of the medication as would be expected from patients who are experienced with drugs producing morphine-like euphoric effects. As mentioned above, diphenoxylate, at therapeutic dose levels, and loperamide, at any dose level, do not produce CNS related effects. In experimental situations when large doses of diphenoxylate were intentionally administered to produce subjectively detectable effects in human subjects, these effects were disliked by the experienced addicts (Frazer et al., 1961), suggesting that diphenoxylate and also loperamide have no euphoric effects. High doses of diphenoxylate and loperamide have not been tested in human subjects for this purpose. However, from several clinical experiences one can safely infer that they do not produce morphine-like euphoric effects in patients treated for diarrhea.

Loperamide has been tested in experimental animals to determine whether these animals would choose to ingest loperamide solutions under any condition. In these experiments, loperamide was mixed with saccharin and given in drinking water to laboratory rats. Saccharin was used to mask the taste. It was found that rats readily ingested the loperamide solution if that was the only source of fluid available. However, when an alternate source of drinking water was provided, they always drank the water which did not contain loperamide. Another group of rats was forced to drink loperamide solutions mixed with saccharin for several weeks. After that period, these rats were given a choice between a loperamide-solution and a loperamide-free solution. Both solutions contained saccharin. The rats always drank only the loperamide-free solution. This type of experiment suggests that there is little chance of rats or other animals orally abusing loperamide irrespective of whether or not they had had prior experience with this drug.

1.2.2. Tolerance

Tolerance is a basic mechanism which is employed by a wide variety of biological systems as a mechanism of survival, when confronted either with unfamiliar chemicals or with newer concentrations of familiar chemicals. Tolerance to numerous chemical structures can be demonstrated in unicellular organisms as well as in highly complex living systems such as man.

Although tolerance is not limited to addiction-producing drugs, the narcotic drugs are notorious for producing marked tolerance. Also, in the case of narcotics, production of tolerance is an important factor in contributing toward the establishment of narcotic dependence and abuse. Because of tolerance, larger and larger quantities of a narcotic must be consumed to obtain the same degree of pharmacological effect. This permits exposure of the nervous system to ever-increasing drug concentrations which leads to the development of physical dependence. Because of this relationship between tolerance and physical dependence in the case of narcotic drugs, tolerance characteristics have been taken in the past as a means of evaluating the physical dependence properties of each new drug.

To the best of our knowledge no direct experiment on the development of tolerance to antidiarrheal drugs has been reported. However, there have been many situations in which such drugs have been administered for prolonged periods.

In toxicity studies the drugs are given to animals for several months. Similarly, the antidiarrheal drugs are administered for several weeks in order to control chronic diarrhea. Perusal of those data reveals that neither in animals nor in human subjects, is tolerance to the specific antidiarrheal drugs present. No necessity for increasing doses for clinical effectiveness in chronic patients has been reported. If tolerance does not develop, the likelihood of larger quantities being ingested is very slight. Therefore, even if there were addicting antidiarrheal drugs, no physical dependence is anticipated. Our conclusions are further supported by extensive field trials, in which no physical dependence was reported even after about five years of clinical use.

There are no reports whatsoever on addiction in patients currently using antidiarrheal drugs, though they have been used by millions of patients throughout the world.

1.2.3. Physical Dependence

Because of numerous complexities associated with the phenomenon of physical dependence, no single definition of it is available. However, most investigators consider physical dependence as an altered physiological state which consists of a latent hyperexcitability of the CNS. It is produced by the frequent and prolonged administration of certain drugs. Physical dependence is manifested subjectively and objectively as the abstinence syndrome (withdrawal illness) upon abrupt termination of the particular drug or upon the administration of an antagonist.

Physical dependence on morphine and meperidine-like drugs has long been recognized as a unique pharmacological phenomenon. Until recently, the ability of these drugs to produce physical dependence has always been considered to be the most crucial factor in predicting their abuse potential. However, in recent years several investigators have questioned the emphasis on physical dependence per se. Rather, they offered evidence to show, that it is the direct pharmacological effect of a drug which plays a primary role in the initiation of drug abuse common to many types of drugs. This pharmacological effect is such that under this influence a subject develops a psychological desire to reexperience these effects after his first trial or first few trials of drug use. The latter aspect of the drug effects is described as a reinforcement of drug-seeking behavior. The reinforcing effects of a drug have been more widely related to the drug abuse of many classes of drugs, while physical dependence has primarily contributed to the continuous abuse of narcotic drugs.

Narcotic withdrawal is a very aversive and unpleasant experience. Avoidance of this state is the main reason why experienced addicts continue to abuse narcotic drugs. Once physically dependent, a subject will often be a life long of abuser of narcotic drugs. These subjects consider consumption of narcotics as the assurance for the continued avoidance of withdrawal discomforts as well as other anxieties of life.

1.2.3.1. Procedures Employed to Determine Physical Dependence

Conventionally there are two principal approaches which have been employed to predict the dependence liability of new drugs.

Single-dose suppression: The test drug is evaluated for its ability to suppress abstinence signs in morphine-dependent animals. The test is generally qualitative in nature but more elaborate designs for quantification are feasible. This procedure cannot be considered as reliable in predicting the dependence liability of all drugs, but is valuable in predicting the abuse potential of narcotics. If a drug can suppress the discomforts of narcotic withdrawal it is liable to be abused by addicts for the same purpose. It is not reliable in predicting dependence liability per se, since suppression of withdrawal symptoms can be achieved by drugs which provide symptomatic relief through quite unrelated mechanisms. Haloperidol, atropine, p-chloro-amphetamine, clonidine, Valium, and barbiturates are examples of drugs which are useful in the acute suppression of narcotic withdrawal without themselves being narcotic drugs.

Establishment of physical dependence: Direct determination of the ability of a drug to produce physical dependence when administered chronically to mice, rats, guinea pigs, dogs, monkeys, or human subjects is a more reliable technique for predicting dependence liability. Usually, the drug is administered in the highest tolerated doses for several days, and the physical dependence is determined by the intensity of withdrawal symptoms.

The full description of procedures employed to produce physical dependence and to measure withdrawal syndromes is too extensive to cover in this book. Moreover, several monographs are available for consultation. However, in order to acquaint the reader with this field a brief description of the procedures used in mice and rats is included.

Addiction in mice: Even though mice are considered unreliable subjects for the study of narcotic addiction, they are often employed for reasons of convenience and economy. Physical dependence in mice is produced either by repeated injections of narcotic drugs or by the subcutaneous implantation of a pellet of morphine base. After a few days, withdrawal can be observed upon removal of the pellet, but much more dramatic effects are elicited by using naloxone-precipitated withdrawal. The abstinence syndrome in mice includes defecation, urination, sniffing, increased motor activity, tremors, and jumping. The jumping response after naloxone has been extensively used as an index for estimating the degree of dependence owing to the ease of measurement.

It may be remembered that the jumping syndrome, as a measure of addiction, was recommended primarily on the basis of the empirical observation that narcotic antagonists elicit jumping response in mice which have been pretreated with large doses of narcotic drugs. However, it must be pointed out that jumping is not specifically associated with narcotic-drug administration. Many drugs not related to narcotic analgesics are also known to elicit jumping in mice.

Koppanyi et al. (1970) reported jumping in mice treated with a convulsant barbiturate. Jumping in rats is produced when desipramine is administered after treatment with drugs of the tetrabenazine group (Sulser et al., 1964; Matussek and Linsmayer, 1968).

Weissman (1973) reported mouse jumping with α-naphthyloxyacetic acid treatment and rat jumping after the administration of either amphetamine and tetrabenazine (Weissman, 1967), or intravenous apomorphine (Weissman, 1971). Collier et al. (1974) reported rat jumping after administration of theophyllin and naloxone, without any treatment with narcotics.

Recently, we have seen jumping of high frequency following injections of amphetamine and levo-dopa. With these drugs mice show reliable and intense jumping which can be blocked with neuroleptic drugs, such as pimozide. We also noticed that in some mice, jumping is elicited by injection of haloxone (a narcotic antagonist often employed to elicit jumping in addicted mice) without any pretreatment with narcotics. Naloxone also increases the jumping produced by lower doses of amphetamine and levo-dopa. Narcotic drugs are known to enhance certain direct effects of naloxone (Van Nueten and Lal, 1974).

In the light of these observations, mouse jumping cannot be taken as reliable index of addiction liability. However, since some data with antidiarrheal drugs in mice are available, they are mentioned here.

In a reported study, mice were given 10 intraperitoneal injections over a period of 4 days; the last injection was followed by naloxone. Jumping was seen in mice treated with morphine, diphenoxylate, or loperamide. In the case of morphine, a dose 4 to 10 times higher than that causing inhibition of gastrointestinal tract motility was sufficient. With diphenoxylate, doses 30 to 150 times higher were necessary. With loperamide, jumping was seen only with doses which were within the lethal dose-range, i.e., 70 to 300 times higher than the dose which blocks gastric motility. If mouse jumping is considered as a test for narcotic drugs, these data indicate that with antidiarrheal drugs positive signs can only be produced when near-lethal doses are administered.

Addiction in rats: The rat has been extensively employed to study physical dependence on narcotic drugs. In addition to the ease with which dependence is produced in the rat, the withdrawal syndrome exhibited by the rat is consistent, reliable, and can be objectively measured. It may be brought about either by administering narcotic antagonists or by abrupt termination of chronic narcotics.

The withdrawal syndrome in the rat can be divided into two phases known as early or primary abstinence and protracted abstinence. The early syndrome is usually taken for the preclinical screening of the drugs used for the development of physical dependence.

The rat can be made physically dependent on narcotics by (1) repeated administration of narcotic drugs; (2) implantation of pellets from which a drug is continuously released; (3) intravenous infusion of a narcotic; and (4) administration of orally active narcotics in drinking water. Withdrawal symptoms include decrease in food and fluid consumption, increased urination, defecation and locomotor activity, loss of body weight, hypothermia, sleep disturbances shown by EEG, ptosis, jumping, writhing, piloerection, aggression, "wet-dog" shakes (intense shaking movement of the body which resembles the shaking movements made by a dog when it emerges from water), irritability on handling, and enhanced catecholamine excretion.

To our knowledge there are no published reports of studies on the addiction liability of diphenoxylate in animals. However, according to a personal communication received from Eddy (1959) large doses of diphenoxylate may produce narcotic dependence in experimental monkeys and suppress the symptoms of narcotic withdrawal.

In human studies Frazer and Isbell (1961) observed no morphine-like acute effects or development of addiction when therapeutic doses of diphenoxylate were employed. However, it was possible to provoke mild morphine-like symptoms if doses were increased to 188 mg daily (about 90 times the therapeutic dose). Even with high doses the intensity of physical dependence was not greater than that observed with codeine, which produces only weak physical dependence.

Since loperamide is an orally active drug and since its penetration into the brain after oral administration has been shown, an investigation was conducted to determine whether withdrawal symptoms could be observed after prolonged oral administration of loperamide to rats.

In this experiment, loperamide treatment was compared with fentanyl treatment in order to avoid drawing the wrong conclusions from a purely negative experiment. Rats were given drug solutions in drinking water. One group received fentanyl while the other group received loperamide. Saccharin was used to mask the taste. Drug solutions were the only fluid available for drinking. Drug concentrations were gradually increased, as is normal in drug-dependence experiments. In about 2 weeks, the rats were drinking total fluid containing more than 16 mg/kg of fentanyl every day and more than 40 mg/kg of loperamide every day. After they had ingested those drugs in such high concentrations for a week, drug solutions were replaced by saccharin solutions. During these days of withdrawal, typical narcotic withdrawal symptoms were observed in fentanyl-treated rats. They included significant decrease in food and fluid intake, loss of body weight, occurrence of "wet-dog" shakes, and aggression. None of these symptoms were observed in the rats of the loperamide group. Rats treated with loperamide consumed normal amounts of food and fluid and showed normal weight gain. It should be remembered that loperamide was consumed in daily doses that were 300 times higher than the pharmacologically active doses of this drug. It is therefore clear that loperamide is a nonaddicting drug.

1.2.4. Properties that Reinforce Drug-seeking Behavior

Drug-seeking behavior has been extensively analyzed by behavioural scientists. It is believed that drug-seeking behavior should be considered as all types of behavior under influence of psychological factors. To understand this mode of analyzing abuse, an understanding of the concept of reinforcement is necessary.

Behavior is believed to be maintained by the quality and quantity of its consequences. These consequences have been called "reinforcers." Therefore, reinforcers are those consequences of behavior which control the rate of occurrence of a particular pattern of behavior. Reinforcers are classified as either positive or negative, depending upon the manner in which they exert control over behavior. Positive reinforcers increase the rate of the behavioral response which precedes them. Negative reinforcers increase the rate of the response which precedes their postponement or absence. For example, if a rat pushes a bar which produces food, the food will be considered a positive reinforcer. However, if the same rat pushes the same bar to keep his cage unlighted because absence of pressing will turn a bright light on, the bright light is then a negative reinforcer. In this case avoidance of the bright light (a negative response) prompted the rat's action.

Reinforcers do not necessarily follow every behavioral response. Sometimes reinforcers are presented only after several responses. Such chains of responding can be maintained more efficiently when conditioned reinforcers are available after each response. A conditioned reinforcer is a previously neutral event which acquires the property of a reinforcer through repeated pairing with unconditioned reinforcers. For example, candy is usually a positive reinforcer for a child. A child will emit responses such as running to the candy man's car. The car can become a conditioned reinforcer because the very sight of it will make the child run towards it even though the car itself is not consumed. It is only associated with the availability of consumable candy. In a closely related manner, neutral events (stimuli) can also set an occasion for behavior to occur or not to occur. For example, if positive reinforcers are produced by responses only when another environmental circumstance is present, not only this circumstance will come to function as a conditioned reinforcer but will also set an occasion for the responses to occur for positive reinforcement. When previously neutral events prompt the occurrence or nonoccurrence of behavior, those events are referred to as discriminative stimuli. For example, if a bell is attached to the candy man's car, after a few times, the sound of bell will cause the child to run towards the car, even when the car itself is still out of sight. It is therefore clear that behavior responses can often be acquired even when the primary reinforcers do not directly follow the action taken. In such cases conditioned reinforcers and discriminative stimuli will maintain behavior for varying lengths of time.

1.2.4. Drugs as Reinforcers

Drugs which have frequently been abused are also shown to produce a special type of effect on the CNS, so that the frequency of administration of that drug is increased. This effect of a drug has been described in many ways and is also stated as being consistent with the idea that it constitutes a reinforcement.

Self-administration (abuse) of a drug is reinforced by the CNS effect of that drug and the act of self-administration is increased in frequency. Eventually, a subject so experienced becomes compulsive about it and begins to seek the drug for abuse even when high cost or other penalties for such behavior are imposed.

Most information on the reinforcing properties of drugs was only obtained recently, when it was established that laboratory animals can be trained to self-administer a whole variety of drugs. In these experiments, laboratory animals are implanted with an intravenous or intraarterial cannula attached to a source of drug solution. The animals are trained to push a lever which activates an electronic delivery system. Thus a known quantity of a drug in aqueous solution is delivered directly into the blood stream, whenever the lever is pushed.

It was found that a whole variety of laboratory animals ranging from rats to primates learn to self-administer drugs, often without becoming physically dependent. Most work has been done with opiates, but self-administration of synthetic narcotics, barbiturates, amphetamines, and cocaine has been demonstrated. Whereas drugs of the above types are self-administered, another class of drugs such as haloperidol are rejected and even serve as negative reinforcers. If the animals with implanted cannula are given solutions of haloperidol, self-administration of haloperidol is not acquired. Rather, drugs of the haloperidol type inhibit self-administration of other positively reinforcing drugs. It has been demonstrated that morphine self-administering rats cease to be so when they are administered haloperidol. In addition, if haloperidol is added to the solution of narcotic drugs, the self-administration of narcotic drugs ceases. This experimental observation has a clinical parallel in that no preparation which contains a narcotic drug in combination with a neuroleptic, has ever been reported to be abused. Furthermore, haloperidol has been reported to block drug craving in heroin addicts (Karkalis and Lal, 1973).

Morphine-like drugs are initially not reinforcing. However, after a few experiences with these drugs, the subject learns to perceive the reinforcing effects and self-administration is initiated. In low concentrations, the drug is then continuously abused. Once the abuse behavior has been established, several other factors (psychological and pharmacological) contribute to the frequency and extent of the abuse. Among the pharmacological factors are induced degree of tolerance and physical dependence. The psychological factors include the relationship between the efforts and the availability of drugs, the quality of subjective effects (euphoria), and strength of environmental circumstances which serve as conditional as well as discriminative stimuli.

1.2.4.2. Antidiarrheal Drugs

Antidiarrheal drugs have not been extensively studied in self-administration experiments because they are almost insoluble in aqueous media. For injection of a drug directly into blood stream, one needs an aqueous solution of that drug because only water can serve as a vehicle to transport the drug from a syringe via the systemic circulation to critical brain areas. If the drugs are insoluble in water, as all the modern antidiarrheals are, self-administration is not likely, on that account alone.

In a few experiments, in which training of animals for self-administration of diphenoxylate or loperamide was attempted, either by dissolving those drugs in water to their maximum solubility, or by providing suspensions for intragastric self-administration, no self-administration was obtained. This was true whether the laboratory animals used for those trials were completely untrained animals or were previously experienced in self-administration or morphine solutions. They include both rats and monkeys. The latter can even be trained to self-administer intragastric injections of morphine. But these monkeys did not self-administer stabilized suspensions of diphenoxylate even intragastrically. On the contrary, it was recently observed that loperamide ingestion was aversive to rats.

The rats were forced to drink saccharin solutions containing either loperamide or fentanyl, a potent analgesic drug which is effective orally. Since no other fluid was available for drinking, these rats readily ingested the only available fluid irrespective of whether it contained loperamide or fentanyl. After several days of forced drinking, the rats were given a choice between a saccharin solution and a saccharin solution containing the drug. It was found that the rats only selected solutions without loperamide irrespective of what was contained in the alternate solution. If the alternate solution contained fentanyl, it was preferred to those containing only saccharin or saccharin and loperamide. If the choice between saccharin and saccharin-loperamide was presented, the former was chosen.

Another group of rats was trained to select fentanyl solution from two available saccharin solutions. After the fentanyl preference and self-administration of fentanyl solution (orally) was clearly established, those rats were given the usual choice between two saccharin solutions except that loperamide replaced fentanyl in one of them. After several days of presentation, the rats did not drink the loperamide solution but always preferred the saccharin solution without drug. Such aversion was seen confirming their previous history of selecting drug-free saccharin solution. These data, although not conclusive since the solutions were not administered systemically, nevertheless, suggest that subjects even chronically accustomed to narcotic drugs are not likely to voluntarily self-administer loperamide.

In the case of diphenoxylate there is evidence of aversion from human experiments.

Frazer (1974) reported experiments performed at the National Institute of Mental Health, Narcotic Research Center at Lexington, Ky., where patients were trained to perceive the "likeable" effects of narcotic drugs. After several days of training, the subjects were given different drugs on certain days, interspersed with days of placebo treatment, and their reaction to the drug was evaluated by means of a questionaire. After administration of narcotic drugs, the subjects answered "yes" to the question, "would you like to take (the drug) daily?." On other trials, the same subjects were given diphenoxylate and were asked the same question. This time these subjects answered either "No," or "Don't care," suggesting that all narcotic experienced subjects who had previously established their liking for taking narcotics daily, specifically did not like the subjective effects of diphenoxylate and chose not to ask it for daily consumption. Such observations present strong evidence that the subjective effects following diphenoxylate, if any, are aversive even for experienced abusers of narcotic drugs.

1.2.4.4. Negative Reinforcing Properties During Withdrawal

It is now well accepted that once physical dependence to narcotic drugs is established, self-administration (abuse) of narcotic-like drugs is continued by an addict, in order to prevent or terminate the abstinence syndrome. Thus the withdrawal syndrome serves as a negative reinforcer. Drug-seeking behavior is strengthened by the postponement or termination of an already begun withdrawal syndrome. In this case, all drugs which either postpone narcotic withdrawal or reduce its intensity will be abused by addicts. Because of these observations it is believed that physical dependence provides a strong motivational state that maintains drug-seeking behavior. There are many experimental data to support this view in the case of self-administration or abuse of narcotic drugs.

As described previously, even established narcotic addicts found diphenoxylate to be an aversive rather than a reinforcing drug. There are experiments with rats in which similar findings were reported with the use of loperamide. In these experiments rats were made physically dependent on fentanyl. After the dependence was established, as evidenced from the withdrawal syndrome, and preference for fentanyl solutions for ingestion was achieved, the rats were given a choice between pure saccharin solutions and saccharin solutions containing loperamide. The solution not containing loperamide was always the only one consumed.

It is well known that gastrointestinal disturbances such as diarrhea and the resulting dehydration are among the prominent symptoms of narcotic withdrawal. Antidiarrheal drugs, being potent inhibitors of excited intestinal motility, are expected to provide some relief. In spite of this expected relief, the antidiarrheal drugs were not desired by the addicted subjects. Therefore, it seems that the aversion associated with the consumption of these drugs is rather strong.

1.3. SUMMARY

Determination of the abuse potentials of any drug is difficult. Factors which determine whether a drug will be abused or not are complex and not very well understood. The evidence reviewed in this section was obtained from experiments performed in mice, rats, monkeys, and human volunteers.

From the available information it is clear that known antidiarrheal drugs, i.e., diphenoxylate, difenoxin, and loperamide, do not show abuse potential. They are not soluble in aqueous media and their organic solutions are very irritating. Therefore, they cannot be sold for systemic injections by illicit means. Diphenoxylate and difenoxin produce only very weak subjective effects and the subjective effects obtained with high doses are aversive in nature. In addition, loperamide, the most recent antidiarrheal, is not addicting, is free of any perceivable subjective effects and is therefore considered to be completely free of abuse potentials.

VI.2. EXPERIMENTAL APPROACH TO THE EVALUATION OF DRUG-ABUSE LIABILITY

Francis Colpaert, Albert Wauquier, Harbans Lal, and Carlos Niemegeers

2.1. GENERAL CONSIDERATIONS

In the preceding section it was shown that diphenoxylate is a specific antidiarrheal agent, in that it effectively blocks diarrhea at doses far below those needed to produce central narcotic effects.

During the past 15 yr diphenoxylate has been extensively used and despite world-wide application, not a single case of its abuse has been reported. Thus, the mere ability of a drug to produce central narcotic effects is not a sufficient condition for abuse. Another requirement obviously may be, that the drug should function at doses devoid of side-effects sufficiently aversive to antagonize or even abolish pleasurable stimuli and, thereby, drug-seeking behavior.

Detailed knowledge of the possibility of abusing a new drug is undoubtedly extremely important. As already described here, even nearly toxic doses of the new drug, loperamide, fail to induce analgesia in rats and are devoid of any morphine-like behavioral effects in mice. These facts strongly suggest that loperamide does not produce the specific central actions shared by narcotic drugs. As their central effects most probably constitute the first prerequisite for the abuse potential of narcotic drugs, the above suggestion would imply that loperamide has no abuse potential. Indeed, the dissociation between possible narcotic and antidiarrheal effects is even greater in loperamide than in diphenoxylate.

The experimental evaluation of drug-abuse liability is designed to assess to what extent a particular drug would share the various central actions produced by representative drugs, known to be either potentially addictive or actually abused in humans. This research is also concerned with the specific qualitative-subjective stimuli associated with central drug actions.

In the laboratory of Janssen Pharmaceutica, a number of experiments are being performed to evaluate, among other things, possible central narcotic actions and associated subjective stimuli of newly synthetized drugs. This section briefly describes four experimental procedures and reports some original data on loperamide, as compared with narcotic analgesics.

2.2. NALOXONE-PRECIPITATED JUMPING IN MICE

Chronically administered morphine, upon discontinuation of the drug and subsequent naloxone injection, reliably induces jumping in mice (Saelens et al., 1971). In the following experiments the ability of diphenoxylate and loperamide to produce this behavior was compared to that of morphine.

Male white mice of a Swiss substrain and weighing 25 ± 1 g were used; the animals had free access to food and water. Morphine (5, 10, 20, 40, 80, 160, and 320 mg/kg), diphenoxylate (1.25, 2.50, 5, 10, 20, 40, and 80 mg/kg), and loperamide (0.31, 0.63, 1.25, 2.50, 5, 10 and 20 mg/kg) were studied.

All mice received 10 intraperitoneal injections over a period of 4 days (on Monday at 8 a.m. and 4 p.m., on Tuesday and Wednesday at 8 a.m., 12 a.m., and 4 p.m., and on Thursday at 8 a.m., and 12 a.m.). One hour later (at 1 p.m. on Thursday), the mice were intraperitoneally injected with 5 mg/kg naloxone and individually transferred into 1-liter glass jars. The number of jumps (all four paws at once off the bottom surface) was counted over a 15-min period immediately following the naloxone injection.

For each experiment, groups of four mice were used; three mice received a dose of one of the three compounds under investigation and one received saline. After each injection the incidence of Straub-tail, abnormal behavioral phenomena and mortality were also noted.

In 63 control mice, treated intraperitoneally with saline, naloxone-precipitated jumping was evident in four (6.3%); two mice jumped five times, one mouse 10 times, and one mouse 14 times.

The number of jumps for different dose levels of morphine, diphenoxylate, and loperamide is given in Table 1. Typical morphine-like behavioral effects, i.e., compulsive circling behavior, crouched appearance with Straub tail and arched back were observed with morphine at 10 mg/kg and above and, to a lesser extent, with diphenoxylate at 20 mg/kg and higher. Sedation, tremors, and ataxia were observed with loperamide at 10 mg/kg. Three daily injections of 160 mg/kg of morphine and 10 mg/kg of loperamide were lethal in three out of nine mice. Three daily 320 mg/kg morphine injections were lethal in seven out of nine mice; three injections of 20 mg/kg loperamide were lethal in all mice. Diphenoxylate was atoxic at the highest dose tested, i.e., 80 mg/kg.

With morphine, naloxone-precipitated jumping was dose-related and started at a total dose of 50.0 mg/kg. With diphenoxylate, jumping was observed at 100 mg/kg and higher. With loperamide, jumping was observed only at near toxic (50.0 mg/kg) and toxic (100 mg/kg) dose levels.

Thus, central behavioral effects were pronounced after intraperitoneal injections of morphine. To a lesser extent, morphine-like behavior was observed with high doses of diphenoxylate. However, the behavioral phenomena with loperamide, such as sedation and ataxia, are not narcotic-like but, instead, are rather reminiscent of neuroleptic drug overdosage.

Toxicity data for the three compounds are consistent with similar data presented elsewhere in this book (IV,4).

When comparing inhibition of gastrointestinal motility with naloxone-precipitated jumping, it is observed that jumping with morphine is precipitated in mice receiving a total dose of 50 mg/kg, i.e., a dose four to ten times higher than the acute dose producing inhibition of gastrointestinal motility; ED_{50} = 8.10 (5.16 - 12.7) mg/kg. With diphenoxylate, a dose of 100 mg/kg is needed, i.e., 30 to 150 times higher than the gastrointestinal motility blocking dose; ED_{50} = 1.49 (0.64 - 3.46) mg/kg. With loperamide, jumping is precipitated only at subtoxic dose levels, at least 70 to 300 times higher than the dose blocking gastrointestinal motility; 0.31 (0.17 - 0.71) mg/kg.

In conclusion, the ability of chronically administered morphine to produce jumping in mice subsequently treated with naloxone, is also evident in diphenoxylate. However, in relation to its respective antidiarrheal activity, much higher doses of diphenoxylate are required. This ability may also exist to some extent in loperamide but only if subtoxic or toxic doses are given.

2.3. NARCOTIC-WITHDRAWAL SYMPTOMS IN RATS

The following experiment was performed to determine whether loperamide would cause physical dependence such as is produced by narcotics after chronic administration. Physical dependence was demonstrated in a group of rats forced to ingest fentanyl chronically; specific narcotic-withdrawal symptoms were elicited in these animals upon discontinuation of the drug. Loperamide failed to produce similar withdrawal symptoms.

Twelve male albino rats, weighing 250-275 g were housed in individual cages and given drug solution in drinking water. One group of six rats was given fentanyl while the other group was given loperamide. Saccharin (0.2 mg/ml) was used to mask the taste of these drugs. The drug solutions were the only fluid available for drinking. Food was freely available.

The drug concentrations were gradually increased, as is conventionally done in drug-dependence experiments. The starting fentanyl concentration of 0.0083 mg/ml was increased on alternate days to 0.0167, 0.05, 0.0667, 0.0883, 0.1, 0.1167, and 0.133 mg/ml.

The concentration of loperamide was increased in the same way, but the final concentration was 0.333 mg/ml. During weekends, concentrations were not increased and the Friday concentration was maintained. The rats were maintained on the highest concentration of each drug for one week before

TABLE 1

Number of Naloxone-precipitated Jumps in Mice Treated with

Number of mice	Morphine, (total amount, mg/kg)						
	50	100	200	400	800	1,600	3,200
1	0	0	0	2	1	2	12
2	0	0	0	6	2	7	108
3	0	0	0	9	14	11	D_3
4	0	0	12	11	16	14	D_3
5	0	1	12	15	22	31	D_4
6	0	3	13	26	24	48	D_4
7	4	3	27	28	32	D_5	D_5
8	4	13	73	35	37	D_6	D_8
9	14	18	75	94	54	D_6	D_8
Median	0	1	12	15	22	—	—

[a] Aqueous micronized suspensions.
[b] Aqueous solution with 10% propylene glycol.
[c] D = dead and number of injections received.

Various Doses of Morphine, Diphenoxylate, and Loperamide

Diphenoxylate (total amount, mg/kg)							Loperamide (total amount, mg/kg)						
12.5	25.0	50.0	100	200^a	400^a	800^a	3.13	6.25	12.5	25.0	50.0	100	200^b
0	0	0	0	0	0	0	0	0	0	0	0	1	D_2^c
0	0	0	0	1	5	0	0	0	0	0	0	10	D_3
0	0	0	0	2	7	0	0	0	0	0	0	15	D_3
0	0	0	0	6	11	11	0	0	0	0	0	15	D_3
0	0	0	0	12	20	14	0	0	0	0	0	47	D_3
0	0	0	1	12	25	30	0	0	0	0	6	73	D_3
0	0	0	1	17	26	55	0	0	0	0	9	D_2	D_4
0	9	2	5	38	42	60	0	1	0	0	15	D_7	D_4
2	46	12	13	152	159	90	0	2	15	5	35	D_8	D_5
0	0	0	0	12	20	14	0	0	0	0	0	—	—

withdrawal. During three days of withdrawal a drug-free saccharin solution was provided for drinking. Withdrawal symptoms were measured once daily for 3 days.

The data summarized in Table 2 demonstrate the occurrence of typical narcotic-withdrawal symptoms in fentanyl-treated rats. They included significant decrease in food and fluid consumption, loss of body weight, the occurrence of "wet dog" shakes and aggression when rats of the same group were placed together. None of these symptoms were observed in the rats of the loperamide group. These rats consumed normal amounts of food and fluid and consequently demonstrated normal weight gain. No aggression was evident, "wet dog" shakes were negligible.

TABLE 2

Withdrawal Symptoms after Chronic Administration of Fentanyl and Loperamide

Symptoms	Time after withdrawal, hr	Fentanyl withdrawal	Loperamide withdrawal
Cumulative change[a] in body weight, g	24	-29 ± 5.3	+16 ± 2.0
	48	-22 ± 6.4	+13 ± 3.8
	72	-13 ± 6.8	+14 ± 4.3
Daily fluid intake, ml	24	15 ± 1.4	37 ± 2.4
	48	26 ± 2.6	35 ± 3.7
	72	34 ± 1.7	43 ± 4.2
Daily food consumption, g	24	17 ± 0.76	25 ± 1.3
	48	21 ± 0.97	26 ± 1.3
	72	26 ± 1.6	29 ± 2.4
"Wet dog" shakes[b] per 30 min	24	8.9 ± 1.7	1.6 ± 0.35
	48	6.2 ± 1.5	1.3 ± 0.39
	72	5.7 ± 1.0	1.2 ± 0.34
Aggression[c]	24	6/6	0/6
	48	6/6	0/6
	72	6/6	0/6

[a] Symbols (-) and (+) denote loss or gain of body weight, respectively.

[b] Sudden shaking movements of the rat body which resemble the movements exhibited by a dog drenched in water.

[c] Aggression (vocalization, attacks, biting) shown within 2 min of placing two rats together. Ratio shows number of groups showing aggression vs number of groups tested.

Thus, the prolonged oral ingestion of high fentanyl concentrations reliably produces physical dependence as evidenced by the predictable occurrence of narcotic-withdrawal symptoms upon discontinuation of the drug. Chronic oral ingestion of loperamide, at concentrations 300 times its pharmacologically active dose, does not produce similar withdrawal symptoms.

2.4. NARCOTIC PREFERENCE TEST IN RATS

Experimentally naive rats, when given the choice, apparently prefer to ingest saccharin solutions to fentanyl solutions. However, a reliable preference for fentanyl to saccharin can be developed upon chronic forced consumption of fentanyl solutions.

The present investigation also showed that there is an initial preference for saccharin to loperamide solutions in naive rats, and that forced consumption of drug solution for several weeks does not reverse this preference. Moreover, fentanyl experienced rats showed aversion to loperamide solution.

Male albino rats weighing 250-275 g were housed in individual cages and given a saccharin solution (0.2 mg/ml) to drink. Food was freely available. On the side opposite to the saccharin bottle, there was another bottle which was left empty. In order to prevent possible position preferences, the positions of saccharin and empty bottles were switched every second on third day.

After 4 days of habituation to the new cages and the drinking arrangement, either loperamide or fentanyl was added to the drinking fluid. The initial concentration of 0.0083 mg/ml was increased every second day except during week-ends, when the Friday concentration was continued. The increasing concentrations were 0.0083, 0.0161, 0.0333, 0.05, 0.0667, 0.0833, 0.1, 0.1167, and 0.133 mg/ml. The highest concentration was given for 6 days before preference tests were started.

During the preference test, the rats were offered the choice between saccharin solutions with or without drug. For this purpose, the second bottle was filled with a saccharin solution, while the first bottle contained the same drug as before. Rats that had been forced to drink fentanyl solution and now clearly showed a preference for fentanyl were then switched to a choice between saccharin and loperamide.

Data given in Tables 3 and 4 show a clear preference of rats for fentanyl over saccharin. These rats learned to consume fentanyl, irrespective of the position of the bottle. When loperamide was substituted for fentanyl, the animals abandoned their preference for the drug-bottle and started drinking only from the bottle that contained the saccharin solution without the drug.

Both the preference for fentanyl and the aversion to loperamide were highly reliable as they were seen day after day, and persisted after the positions of the bottles had been switched. The averaged data are illustrated in Fig. 1.

TABLE 3

Aversion from Low Loperamide Concentrations in Rats Preferring Fentanyl; Fluid Intake, ml

Experimental procedure		Rat 1		Rat 2		Rat 3		Rat 4		Rat 5	
		D[a]	S[b]	D	S	D	S	D	S	D	S
	F[c]	4	5	48	8	24	8	56	5	6	11
	F	4	30	42	1	46	12	50	2	35	22
	F	45	0	34	8	34	0	48	3	41	5
	F	48	5	50	7	62	5	49	0	43	2
Position switch											
	F[d]	184	9	205	28	165	15	113	55	180	41
	F	51	1	18	8	40	5	35	13	61	13
	F	64	2	55	6	75	3	34	27	34	11
	F	50	2	64	15	56	5	33	25	1	48
	F	49	3	43	6	48	4	32	25	81	10
Position switch											
	F[d]	192	2	211	39	179	9	97	68	134	56
	L[e]	3	32	3	5	7	7	4	27	5	57
	L	2	35	5	48	10	10	0	36	1	58
	L	2	42	5	28	32	6	2	54	1	42
	L	2	46	4	32	30	12	3	65	1	48
Position switch											
	F[d]	178	10	118	65	166	13	3	159	161	24

[a]D = Saccharin solution with drug. [b]S = Saccharin solution without drug. [c]F = Fentanyl concentration = 0.0333 mg/ml. [d]Total fluid intake on three successive weekend days. [e]L = Loperamide concentration = 0.0333 mg/ml.

Abuse: Evaluation

TABLE 4

Aversion from High Concentrations of Loperamide in Rats Preferring Fentanyl; Fluid Intake, ml

Experimental procedure		Rat 1		Rat 2		Rat 3		Rat 4		Rat 5	
		D^a	S^b	D	S	D	S	D	S	D	S
	F^c	10	3	5	13	28	14	3	1	7	3
	F	43	12	33	7	49	5	31	12	30	6
	F	24	14	63	10	26	5	72	3	55	6
	F	107	8	55	5	64	5	54	3	66	1
Position switch											
	F^d	116	82	147	68	194	3	170	29	136	35
	F	75	5	54	6	77	5	31	3	50	15
	F	85	2	47	3	62	11	69	2	53	6
	F	74	13	50	6	85	4	69	3	59	4
	F	65	14	57	0	58	1	56	0	58	7
Position switch											
	F^d	191	30	182	8	189	30	230	5	163	18
	L^e	2	10	3	18	2	19	3	1	5	23
	L	2	44	7	39	1	47	5	22	21	37
	L	0	51	0	45	1	41	8	46	6	57
	L	3	51	3	46	5	53	9	35	5	59
Position switch											
	L^d	5	182	2	174	3	169	49	95	14	171

^{a}D = Saccharin solution with drug. ^{b}S = Saccharin solution without drug. ^{c}F = Fentanyl concentration = 0.033 mg/ml. ^{d}Total fluid intake on three successive weekend days. ^{e}L = Loperamide concentration = 0.133 mg/ml.

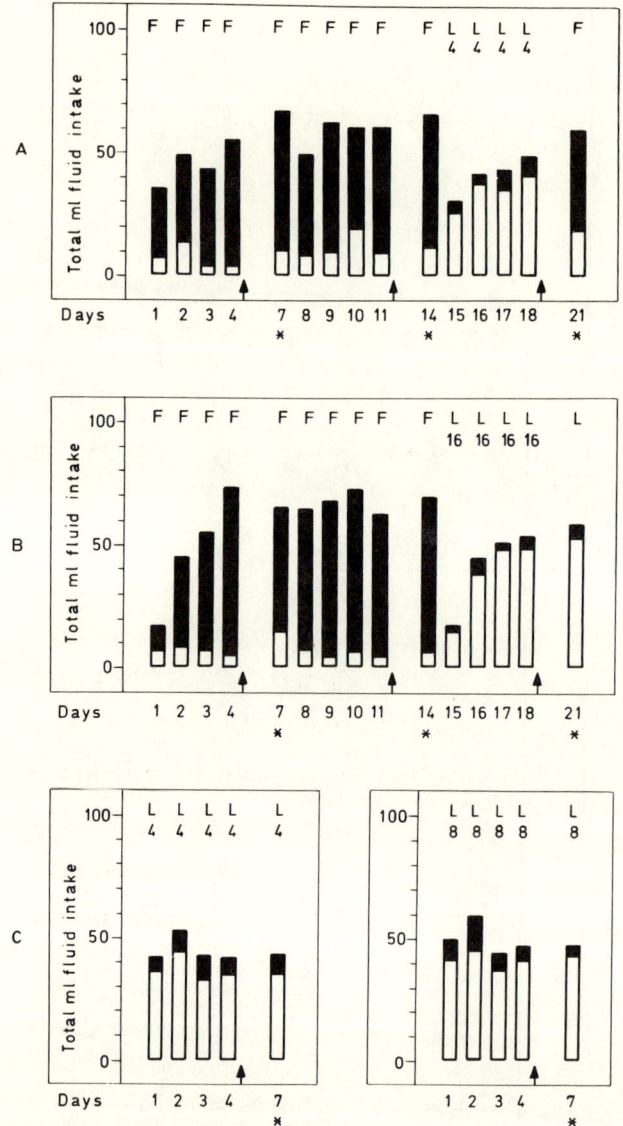

Fig. 1. Mean quantities of fluid intake during preference tests. ■, saccharin solution plus drug; □, saccharin solution alone; F, fentanyl; L_4, loperamide (0.0333 mg/ml); L_{15}, loperamide (0.133 mg/ml); A and B, after forced fentanyl consumption; C, after forced loperamide consumption; X, mean daily fluid intake during weekends; ↑, position of bottles switched.

TABLE 5

Loperamide Aversion after Prolonged Loperamide Intake; Fluid Intake, ml

Experimental procedure	Rat 1		Rat 2		Rat 3		Rat 4		Rat 5		Rat 6		Rat 7	
	D[a]	S[b]	D	S	D	S	D	S	D	S	D	S	D	S
Loperamide, 0.0333 mg/ml	0	52	1	39	24	10	9	29	1	47	7	40	1	39
	1	57	1	48	40	3	8	39	1	50	1	56	4	58
	2	42	1	44	39	1	24	9	1	42	1	44	0	45
	1	41	1	38	29	1	12	31	1	42	3	47	2	41
Position switch	5	153	2	119	102	26	40	86	1	112	1	153	28	80
Loperamide, 0.0667 mg/ml	5	40	2	52	2	48	28	29	11	28	13	43	2	42
	12	42	12	56	3	57	13	53	14	43	32	12	16	48
	2	43	2	43	0	37	0	51	10	41	26	16	8	27
	3	50	3	47	2	43	4	56	9	28	8	31	7	35
Position switch	3	137	7	129	0	133	4	170	20	121	14	123	28	104

[a] D = Saccharin solution with drug.
[b] S = Saccharin solution without drug.

All of the rats forced to drink loperamide survived, and no overt abnormalities were found in them, even after ingestion of the drug at doses roughly equal to 100 times the ED_{50} for antidiarrheal effect. When these animals were given the choice between loperamide-saccharin and saccharin alone, they readily abandoned the bottle to which they were previously habituated and began to drink from the bottle that did not contain loperamide (see Table 5). This active aversion to loperamide was long-lasting and reliable, as it was still obvious after about two weeks of preference tests and after regular switching of the position of the bottles. The mean quantities of fluid taken from each bottle are illustrated in Fig. 1.

Thus it is demonstrated that rats given prolonged experience with a potent narcotic in doses that are known to cause physical dependence soon learn to voluntarily ingest solutions containing that narcotic. In that respect they resemble human addicts, who after experience with heroin-like drugs choose to ingest narcotic drugs, even when a drug-free alternative is available. Experienced addicts are known to detect the euphoric effects of narcotics with great precision.

Our "narcotic-experienced" rats showed aversion to loperamide, suggesting that this substance was not perceived as a narcotic. On the contrary, loperamide was found to produce aversive stimuli. It should be added, however, that whereas the preference for fentanyl also appeared from the higher fluid intake, the aversion to loperamide was not so marked that it would substantially diminish the fluid intake in the period of forced drinking.

2.5. DISCRIMINATION LEARNING IN RATS

Morphine has been shown to produce a discriminative stimulus (DS) that controls operant behavior (Belleville, 1964; Gianutsos and Lal, 1975; Hill et al., 1971). Thus, an animal can be trained to make a specific response after the administration of morphine and to make an alternative response following solvent injection. It is therefore suggested that the DS produced by morphine and, if so, by othernarcotics, provides an original and direct means of investigating the central-subjective effects elicited by narcotic drugs.

Ten male Wistar rats (210 ± 10 g) were used in these experiments. They were housed in standard animal test cages, fitted with two levers, a food cup, and a house light; the experiments were programmed by solid-state logic modules.

After initial shaping, rats were trained to lever press 10 times for each food pellet (FR 10). According to whether the animal was injected SC (t-30 min) with 0.04 mg/kg fentanyl or solvent (1 ml/100 g) it was required to press either the one ("fentanyl lever," FL) or the opposite ("solvent lever," SL) lever, respectively, in order to get reinforcement. Responses on the incorrect lever were inconsequential. In five rats, the left lever was assigned to be the "fentanyl lever," the right lever being the "solvent lever." In another five rats, the assignments were opposite, i.e., the solvent lever on the left and the fentanyl lever on the right. The number of responses made on the incorrect lever before obtaining the first food pellet (and, thus, before having made 10 correct responses) was recorded. Sessions lasted for 15 min each. Daily sessions were given on 5 consecutive days a week. Injections were programmed according to two weekly alternating sequences. During one week, the sequence was fentanyl-solvent-solvent-fentanyl-fentanyl; during the other it was solvent-fentanyl-fentanyl-solvent-solvent. Training criterion was reached when the number of incorrect responses, made before the first 10 correct responses, did not exceed 2 on at least 5 consecutive training sessions.

Testing then proceeded as follows: On Wednesdays, the well-trained rat was injected with the test compound; on the remaining days, the usual training procedure was continued. On introducing the rat into the test cage, the experimenter noticed on which of two levers the animal first made a total of 10 responses; this lever was subsequently referred to as the "selected lever." Once this choice was established (that is, 10 responses being made on one of both levers), the rat obtained a first food pellet; further reinforcement was made contingent upon pressing the selected lever. Drugs, doses, routes, time of administration, and test results are briefly summarized in Table 6.

From the data on solvent and fentanyl days it is clear that the 10 rats used in these experiments were highly trained to emit responses on either the "solvent" or the "fentanyl" lever according to the drug administered. It should be stressed, that the presence or absence of (central) stimuli produced by the injection preceding testing were the exclusive basis on which the rat was to select the lever. Thus, the training dose (0.04 mg/kg SC) of fentanyl consistently made the animals press the "fentanyl lever;" the reverse is true for the solvent injection. Similarly, the oral dose of 1.25 mg/kg fentanyl induced the same lever selection as the subcutaneous standard dose.

As is shown in Table 6, the injection of all other narcotics (morphine, phenoperidine, piritramide) was generalized with the fentanyl cue. Diphenoxylate at a large dose (20 mg/kg oral) also elicited this cue. Despite the severe response inhibition (up to 67%) produced, the SC (5 mg/kg) and oral (10, 20, and 40 mg/kg) administration of loperamide consistently made the animals select the "saline lever."

Following adequate training, rats were found to respond highly predictably when injected with fentanyl; alternative responses occurred when saline was given.

Appropriate oral doses of fentanyl and SC doses of other narcotic analgesics produced the same cue which, apparently, made the rats select the "fentanyl lever." This cue can therefore be considered to be the narcotic

TABLE 6
Test Results Obtained in the Discrimination Learning Procedure

Compound	Dose, mg/kg	Route	Time, min	Animals tested	Animals selecting		Responses, %, on		Total responses as a percent of solvent performance
					SL[a]	FL[b]	SL[a]	FL[b]	
Solvent	—	SC	30	10	10	0	99.6	0.40	—
Fentanyl	0.04	SC	30	10	0	10	0.90	99.1	82.0
Morphine	10.0	SC	30	5	0	5	0.50	99.5	43.78
Piritramide	5.00	SC	30	5	0	5	0.30	99.7	91.80
Phenoperidine	0.31	SC	30	5	0	5	2.30	97.7	105.2
Loperamide	5.00	SC	30	5	5	0	95.0	5.00	34.52
Fentanyl	1.25	Oral	60	5	0	5	6.3	93.7	118.9
Diphenoxylate	20.0	Oral	60	5	0	5	0.7	99.3	106.44
Loperamide	10.0	Oral	60	5	5	0	99.9	0.10	84.93
Loperamide	20.0	Oral	60	5	5	0	99.5	0.50	64.66
Loperamide	40.0	Oral	60	5	5	0	99.4	0.60	33.34

[a]Solvent lever.
[b]Fentanyl lever.

cue, that is, the subjectively experienced stimulus associated with the central actions of narcotic drugs. The generality of the latter statement is convincingly supported by recent research in this field (Barry, 1974; Gianutsos and Lal, 1975). Diphenoxylate may produce this cue provided the dose is sufficiently high.

Most relevant to the experimental approach of drug-abuse liability is the finding that loperamide at oral doses up to 40 mg/kg does not produce the narcotic cue. We preferred not to expose these valuable rats to still higher doses of loperamide, since toxicity might occur at 80 mg/kg.

A dose-related response inhibition is found following increasing oral doses of loperamide. It may therefore be concluded that, whatever (central?) action of loperamide might cause this inhibition, this action is definitely not associated with the occurrence of subjective stimuli similar to that induced by narcotic drugs.

2.6. SUMMARY

Sect. VI.2 is concerned with the significant problem of drug-abuse liability. An experimental approach is proposed, and a number of procedures are described that enable us to assess a drug's possible central narcotic actions as well as associated subjective stimuli.

Four recent investigations in this field are summarized. Unlike fentanyl, morphine, and other narcotic drugs, loperamide, upon chronic administration, does not produce naloxone-precipitated jumping in mice or narcotic-withdrawal symptoms in rats; no preference for loperamide can be experimentally established despite the enormous doses that are chronically applied. Also, loperamide cannot substitute for fentanyl in rats with a learned preference for narcotics. Initial differences in taste-qualities of loperamide and fentanyl are excluded as a possible explanation of the findings.

Finally, the discrimination-learning procedure provides the most direct and conclusive evidence of the inability of loperamide to induce subjective stimuli specifically associated with the central action produced by all narcotic drugs tested. Because of the absence of those subjective stimuli, no motivation exists that would promote abuse of loperamide. From these experiments, it is concluded that loperamide does not possess abuse potentials.

REFERENCES

Barry, H. (1974). Classification of drugs according to their discriminable effects in rats. Fed. Proc. 33, 1814-1824.

Belleville, R. E. (1964). Control of behavior by drug-produced internal stimuli. Psychopharmacologia 5, 95-105.

Collier, H. O. J., Francis, D. L., Henderson, G., and Schneider, C. (1974). Quasi morphine-abstinence syndrome. Nature 249, 471-473.

Eddy, N. B. (1959). Chemical structure and action of morphine-like analgesics and related substances. Chem. Ind. 1462-1469.

Eddy, N. B., Friebel, H., Hahn, K. J., and Hallach, H. (1968). Codeine and its alternates for pain and cough relief. Part I: Codeine, exclusive of its antitussive action. Bull. World Health Org. 38, 673-641.

Eddy, N. B., Friebel, H., Hahn, K. J., and Hallach, H. (1969a). Codeine and its alternates for pain and cough relief. Part II: Alternatives for pain relief. Bull. World Health Org. 40, 1-53.

Eddy, N. B., Friebel, H., Hahn, K. J., and Hallach, H. (1969b). Codeine and its alternates for pain and cough relief. Part III: Antitussive action of codeine mechanism, methodology, and evaluation. Bull. World Health Org. 40, 425-454.

Eddy, N. B., Friebel, H., Hahn, K. J., and Hallach, H. (1969c). Codeine and its alternates for pain and cough relief. Part IV: Potential alternates for cough relief. Bull. World Health Org. 40, 639-719.

Eddy, N. B., Hallach, H., Isabell, H., and Seevers, M. H. (1970). Drug dependence: its significance and characteristics. In Drug Abuse, Data and Debate, P. H. Blaeky (Ed.). Thomas, Springfield

Frazer, H. F. and Isbel, H. (1961). Human pharmacology and addictiveness of ethyl 1-(3-cyano-3,3-phenylpropyl)-4-phenyl-4-piperidinecarboxylate hydrochloride (R 1132, diphenoxylate). Bull. Narcotics UN Dept. Social Affairs 13, 29-43.

Frazer, H. F., Van Horn, G. D., Martin, W. R., Wolbach, A. B., and Isabell, H. (1961). Methods for evaluating addiction liability. (A) Attitude of opiate addicts towards opiate-like drugs, (B) A short-term direct addiction test. J. Pharmacol. Exp. Therap. 133, 371-387.

Frazer, H. F. (1974). Certain theoretical and practical considerations involved in evaluating the overall abuse potential of opiate agonists and antagonists. In Advances in Biochemical Psychopharmacology, vol. 8, Narcotic Antagonists, M. C. Braude, L. S. Harris, E. L. May, I. P. Smith, and J. E. Villarreal (Eds.). Raven Press, New York, pp. 439-453.

Gianutsos, G. and Lal, H. (1975). Effect of loperamide, halperidol, and methadone in rats trained to discriminate morphine from saline. Psychopharmacologia 41, 267-270.

Hill, H. E., Jones, B. E., and Bell, E. C. (1971). State-dependent control of discrimination by morphine and pentobarbital. Psychopharmacologia 22, 305-313.

Karkalas, J. and Lal, H. (1973). A comparison of haloperidol with methadone in blocking heroin withdrawal symptoms. Intern. Pharmacopsychiat. 8, 248-251.

Koppanyi, T., Maling, H. M., Saul, W., and Brodie, B. B. (1970). Jumping activity induced by sodium 5-(1,3-dimethyl-1-butyl)-5-ethylbarbiturate, I. The role of the sympathetic nervous system. J. Pharmacol. Exp. Therap. 172, 170-179.

Matuszek, N. and Linsmayer, M. (1968). The effect of lithium and amphetamine on desmethylimipramine-Ro-5-1284 induced motor hyperactivity. Life Sci. 7, 371-375.

Overton, D. (1973). State dependent learning produced by addicting drugs. In Opiate Addiction: Origin and Treatment, S. Fischer and A. M. Friedman (Eds.). B. H. Winston and Sons, Washington, D.C., pp. 61-75.

Roffman, M. and Lal, H. (1972). Role of brain amines in learning associated with amphetamine state. Psychopharmacologia 25, 195-204.

Rosecrane, J. (1975). Discriminative-stimuli associated with narcotic drugs. In Neurobiology of Drug Addiction, Vol. 1, Futura Publishing Co. (forthcoming).

Saelens, J. K., Granat, F. R., and Sawyer, W. K. (1971). The mouse jumping test. A simple screening method to estimate the physical dependence capacity of analgesics. Arch. Intern. Pharmacodyn. 190, 213-218.

Sulser, F., Bickel, M. H., and Brodie, B. B. (1964). The action of desmethylimipramine in counteracting sedation and cholinergic effects of reserpine-like drugs. J. Pharmacol. Exp. Therap. 144, 321-330.

Van Nueten, J. M. and Lal, H. (1974). Naloxone-induced facilitation of contractions, spontaneous activity and tolerance to morphine in ileum of morphine-dependent guinea pigs. Arch. Intern. Pharmacodyn. 208, 378-382.

Weissman, A. (1967). Jumping behaviour in rats. Evidence for a desmethylimipramide-like action of amphetamine. Fed. Proc. 26, 738.

Weissman, A. (1971). Cliff jumping in rats after intravenous treatment with apomorphine. Psychopharmacologia 21, 60-65.

Weissman, A. (1973). Jumping in mice elicited by α-naphthyloxyacetic acid. J. Pharmacol. Exp. Therap. 184, 11-17.

CHAPTER VII

CONCLUSION

Willem Van Bever

Diarrhea may be caused by neoplasm, protozoa, bacteria, molds, viruses, drugs, allergies, radiation, vitamin deficiencies, and other specific agents. Effective specific therapy is highly desirable, but unfortunately often unavailable. However, the antidiarrheal drugs described in this book have made it possible to provide adequate and effective symptomatic relief of diarrhea, no matter what may have caused it. Once diarrhea is under control many pathophysiological processes correct themselves. In other cases, more specific therapy, if available, can be applied with greater ease and effectiveness.

For many years, opium, morphine, codeine, and their congeners have been the drugs of choice for symptomatic treatment of diarrhea. However, this group of drugs has the disadvantage, especially upon prolonged use, of possessing narcotic and dependence liabilities. Systematic study of the correlations between analgesic and constipating activity of several hundreds of analgesically active compounds has revealed the possibility of synthesizing analgesic-type compounds, devoid of analgesic action, but behaving as highly active inhibitors of gastrointestinal propulsion and defecation.

Excellent separation between analgesic and antidiarrheal properties was achieved in 1958 with a series of ester derivatives of 1-(3-cyano-3,3-diphenylpropyl-4-phenyl-4-piperidinecarboxylic acid. Diphenoxylate, butoxylate, and fetoxylate are representatives of this class of synthetic antidiarrheal agents. Their active metabolite difenoxin, the corresponding acid, was subsequently synthesized and found to be five times more active than the parent diphenoxylate. Numerous attempts to improve diphenoxylate, by chemical modification of its structure, were unsuccessful. However, simultaneous replacement of the cyano group by an amide and of the carboxyl substituent on the piperidine ring by an hydroxyl function gave rise to a novel class of antidiarrheal agents, the derivatives of 4-aryl-4-hydroxy-α,α-diphenyl-1-piperidinebutanamides. Loperamide and fluperamide are representatives of this class and are both characterized by a nearly perfect separation of analgesic and antidiarrheal activity.

In experimental animals the castor-oil test was found to reliably detect antidiarrheal drug activity. The test furthermore allowed accurate measurement of the duration of action and was suitable for the screening of large numbers of compounds. The RAS idea, expressed as the ratio of the oral ED_{50} value in the tail-withdrawal test over the oral ED_{50} value for one hour protection in the castor-oil test, proved to be an effective measure for the dissociation between antidiarrheal and analgesic actions in rats. Diphenoxylate and difenoxin were found to be effective antidiarrheals with relative antidiarrheal specificities of 85 and 102, respectively. Butoxylate and fetoxylate, although somewhat less potent than diphenoxylate, have relative antidiarrheal specificities of 105 and more than 376, respectively. Loperamide and fluperamide, however, have a considerably longer duration of action and have been shown to possess relative antidiarrheal specificities of greater than 1000 and greater than 600, respectively. Subsequent investigations in mice, in order to study comparatively the inhibition of gastrointestinal motility and narcotic behavioral effects, confirmed loperamide as the prototype of a novel class of antidiarrheal agents characterized by the complete absence of narcotic-like central effects even at subtoxic dose levels.

The effects of diphenoxylate, difenoxin, and loperamide on various isolated tissues were studied. All three substances inhibit the peristaltic reflex response of the isolated guinea-pig ileum. The response of the same tissue to coaxial stimulation and to nicotine was inhibited at the same low doses. The inhibition of peristaltic reflex is very specific and may account for the decrease of intestinal hypermotility. Loperamide effects are rapid in onset and of long duration, while difenoxin effects are fast, but of short duration. Diphenoxylate is slow but long acting. The antidiarrheal activity of these compounds is produced by local action on the intestinal wall. The compounds may interact locally with cholinergic as well as with noncholinergic mechanisms and with the intramural ganglia of Auerbach.

The distribution and pharmacokinetics of diphenoxylate, difenoxin, and loperamide were studied in rats, dogs, and men. Blood, brain, and liver levels were determined in rats as a function of time. Metabolism and excretion were studied in rats and men. Difenoxin was found to be the active metabolite of diphenoxylate. The largest amounts of all three drugs were found in the gastrointestinal tract. The pharmacokinetic properties of diphenoxylate, difenoxin, and loperamide were in agreement with their pharmacological activity.

The acute oral toxicity of diphenoxylate, fetoxylate, difenoxin, loperamide, and fluperamide was evaluated in mice, rats, guinea-pigs, and dogs. The safety margins, i.e., the ratio of the lethal dose over the antidiarrheal dose, were extremely high (> 800) for all five compounds. The

Conclusion

subacute and chronic oral toxicity of diphenoxylate, fetoxylate, difenoxin, loperamide, and fluperamide were investigated in rats and dogs. All five compounds were found to be very safe. Oral administration of doses exceeding several times the pharmacologically active dose over prolonged periods of time (up to 18 months in rats and 12 months in dogs) were well tolerated and did not cause significant abnormalities as observed by clinical examination, clinical pathology, gross pathology, or histopathology. In rats and rabbits the compounds were devoid of embryotoxicity, teratogenicity, and of effects on male and female fertility, as evidenced by the studies on reproductive processes made on rats and rabbits.

The therapeutic use of diphenoxylate, difenoxin, and loperamide in medical practice has been discussed. All three compounds provide rapid relief of symptoms in acute and chronic diarrhea of varying etiology. The control of other conditions, such as intestinal motility has also been reviewed. Side-effects during diphenoxylate or difenoxin administration are uncommon and generally mild. With loperamide the side-effects are still more uncommon. However, special attention should be given to the hazards of overdosing diphenoxylate in babies and children. Diphenoxylate has been available in Europe and the United States since 1960. Loperamide was introduced in Europe in 1974 and difenoxin will also become available in Europe in 1975.

From the information available it is clear that diphenoxylate, difenoxin, and loperamide do not show abuse potential. They are virtually insoluble in aqueous media and their organic solutions are very irritating. Diphenoxylate and difenoxin produce only very weak subjective effects, which at high doses are aversive in nature. In addition, the most recent antidiarrheal, loperamide is not addicting, is free of any perceivable subjective effects, and is therefore considered to be devoid of abuse potential. This statement is further substantiated by four recent investigations directed towards the assessment of possible narcotic actions as well as associated subjective stimuli.

At present, diphenoxylate has been used in medical practice for nearly fifteen years. All evidence, accumulated over these years, points towards the conclusion that this drug represents a major improvement over the use of opium and congeners in the symptomatic treatment of diarrhea. However, intensive research in the area of synthetic antidiarrheals has led to the development of a novel series of antidiarrheal agents of which loperamide is the prototype. Extensive pharmacological investigation and four years of clinical experience with loperamide indicate a significant improvement in comparison with diphenoxylate.

Consequently future research in the field of antidiarrheals will undoubtedly be directed toward further elucidation and understanding of the mechanism of action of loperamide and possibly toward its further improvement.

AUTHOR INDEX

Underlined numbers give the pages on which the complete references are listed.

A

Abrutyn, E., 73, <u>196</u>
Admiral, P. V., 49, <u>62</u>
Ahearn, D. G., 207, <u>230</u>
Alexander, S. M., 23, <u>61</u>, 67, <u>195</u>
Amery, W. K. P., 49, <u>62</u>, <u>199</u>, <u>229</u>
Arabehety, J. J., 207, <u>229</u>
Arteaga, I., 207, <u>230</u>
Arunlakshana, O., 120, <u>195</u>
Attenburrow, J., 28, <u>61</u>

B

Baldauf, J., 70, <u>197</u>
Banwell, J. G., 67, 70, <u>195</u>
Barba-Gose, J., 66, <u>200</u>
Barowsky, A., 206, 214, <u>229</u>
Barry, H., 265, <u>265</u>
Bass, P., 23, 54, <u>61</u>, <u>62</u>, 67, <u>195</u>, <u>202</u>
Baufle, G. H., 214, <u>229</u>
Bayliss, W. M., <u>195</u>
Beal, G. D., 67, <u>197</u>
Beckers, J., 132, <u>196</u>, 219, <u>230</u>
Bell, E. C., 262, <u>266</u>
Belleville, R. E., 262, <u>265</u>
Belotte, J., 214, <u>232</u>
Bennett, A., 114, 115, <u>195</u>
Benslay, D. N., 67, 69, <u>199</u>
Berry, C. A., 224, <u>229</u>
Bickel, M. H., 244, <u>267</u>
Binder, H. J., 69, 70, <u>195</u>
Black, J. W., 119, <u>195</u>
Bockmühl, M., 27, <u>61</u>
Bond, B, 208, <u>229</u>
Bonnycastle, D. D., 69, <u>195</u>, 205, <u>229</u>
Bortoff, A., 114, <u>195</u>
Bosker, J. T., 49, <u>62</u>
Briggs, F. B., 23, <u>61</u>
Bright-Asare, P., 69, <u>195</u>
Brinckenhoff, W. C., 208, <u>229</u>
Brodie, B. B., 244, <u>266</u>, <u>267</u>
Brower, Ch., 214, <u>232</u>
Brugmans, J., 67, 68, 75, 115, 132, 138, 139, 142, 145, 148, 153, <u>196</u>, <u>197</u>, <u>199</u>, <u>202</u>, 210, 214, 216, 225, <u>230</u>, <u>233</u>
Burkholder, E. R., 207, <u>232</u>
Butler, D. E., 23, 54, <u>61</u>, 67, <u>195</u>

C

Camatte, R., 214, 230
Carabateas, P. M., 23, 61
Cash, R. A., 73, 196
Catlin, D. H., 67, 201
Cayer, D., 206, 214, 230
Chapaux, J., 230
Chapaux, R., 230
Chen, G. M., 66, 200
Cignarella, G., 30, 63
Clark, M. L., 132, 136, 137, 153, 199
Claude, C. L., 23, 61
Cohen, R., 207, 230
Collier, H. O. J., 66, 196, 244, 266
Craig, P. N., 28, 61
Crema, A., 114, 197
Crivaro, E. A., 230
Crul, J. F., 49, 62

D

Daniel, E. E., 114, 196
De Canniere, J. H. M., 66, 113, 198
De Coster, M., 132, 196, 219, 230
De Cree, J., 203
De Eds, F., 68, 200
De Jongh, D. K., 66, 67, 198
Demeulenaere, L., 132, 196, 218, 224, 230
Demoen, P. J. A., 66, 67, 68, 75, 113, 198, 199
Deschaseaux, P., 214, 229
Dobrin, E. I., 66, 67, 68, 199
Dolcini, H. A., 207, 229
Dom, J., 196, 202, 210, 230
Dony, J. G. H., 62, 67, 75, 198
Dresse, A., 67, 118, 198
Duncan, W. A. M., 119, 195
Dupont, H. L., 73, 74, 196
Dupre, D. J., 27, 61
Dutta, N. K., 67, 196
Dutta, N. V., 67, 196
Dziuba, K., 208, 214, 230

E

Eddy, N. B., 66, 101, 113, 199, 245, 266
Ehrhart, G., 27, 61
Eichenwald, H. F., 73, 196, 207, 230
Eisleb, O., 24, 27, 61
Eley, K. G., 115, 195
Elks, J., 27, 28, 61
Ensminger, P. W., 67, 69, 199
Ensor, C., 66, 200
Evans, R. M., 27, 61
Evensen, K. L., 132, 136, 151, 153, 199

F

Falaschi, C. F., 114, 197
Fiasse, R., 227, 232
Field, M., 70, 199
Fieler, F. C., 66, 196
Fingl, E., 69, 196
Finkelstein, R. A., 67, 196
Finney, D. J., 73, 196
Fishman, J., 208, 229
Fontaine, J., 115, 116, 119, 131, 196, 197, 203
Formal, S. B., 67, 200, 201
Forrest, J. N., 73, 196
Forth, W., 70, 197
Fothergill, G. A., 23, 62
Francis, D. L., 244, 266
François, G. F., 214, 230
Frazer, H. F., 237, 240, 241, 245, 249, 266
Frazier, D., 207, 230
Friebel, H., 266
Frigo, G. M., 114, 197
Fujimura, H., 67, 202

G

Gabriele, R., 214, 230
Galambos, J., 222, 230
Garden, G., 147, 148, 150, 151, 199

Geiga, E., 67, 197
Geivers, H., 115, 116, 197, 203
Gershon, E., 70, 199
Gianutsos, G., 262, 265, 266
Gilman, A., 74, 197
Ginsburg, C. M., 231
Glatt, M. M., 225, 231
Goldblatt, L. A., 68, 200
Goodman, A. L., 225, 231
Goodman, L. S., 74, 197
Gordon, J. E., 73, 197
Gordon, R. S., 69, 203
Gordon, S., 222, 231
Goulston, R., 214, 231
Granat, F. R., 254, 267
Green, M. W., 67, 197
Gürtler, J., 214, 231

H

Hahn, K. J., 266
Hallach, H., 266
Hanhart, P., 214, 229
Hawker, P. G., 208, 229
Hayashi, M., 67, 202
Hems, B. A., 27, 28, 61
Henderson, A., 70, 199
Henderson, G., 244, 266
Henderson, W., 231
Herin, V. V., 49, 62, 67, 199
Hermans, B. K. F., 29, 61, 66, 113, 198
Heykants, J. J., 132, 138, 142, 145, 148, 153, 197
Hibino, R., 67, 202
Hill, H. E., 262, 266
Hillebrand, P., 231
Hirschowitz, B., 219, 231
Hock, Ch. W., 206, 208, 214, 231
Holappa, K. K., 66, 200
Horn, G. D., 237, 245, 266
Hornick, R. B., 73, 74, 196
Huygens, J., 23, 49, 52, 54, 62, 66, 67, 113, 198

I

Isbell, H., 237, 240, 241, 245, 266
Ison, L. J., 208, 229
Iwao, I., 67, 69, 197

J

Jageneau, A. H., 23, 49, 52, 54, 62, 66, 67, 74, 113, 197, 198
Jancloes, M., 213, 231
Janssen, P. A. J., 23, 24, 29, 40, 49, 52, 53, 54, 61, 62, 63, 66, 67, 68, 74, 75, 113, 131, 132, 138, 139, 142, 145, 148, 153, 196, 197, 198, 199, 200, 201, 202, 203
Jervis, H. R., 67, 200
Johansson, H., 115, 201
Johnson, V., 70, 199
Jones, B. E., 262, 266
de Jongh, D. K., 24, 53, 62
Jover, A., 69, 203
Jullien, C., 23, 61

K

Kalser, M. H., 207, 230
Karg, E., 219, 231
Karim, A., 132, 136, 147, 148, 150, 151, 153, 199
Karman, A., 69, 203
Kasich, A. M., 214, 231
Kaump, D. H., 66, 200
Kennedy, J. A., 23, 54, 61, 62, 67, 195
Kerremans, R., 132, 196, 219, 230
Kimberg, D. V., 70, 199
King, C. G., 67, 197
Kirsner, J. B., 74, 202
Kohler, G. O., 68, 200
Koppanyi, T., 244, 266
Kosterlitz, H. W., 114, 131, 199
Kottegoda, S. R., 114, 131, 199
Krueger, H., 66, 101, 113, 199

L

van Laar, G. M. L. W., 23, 49, 63, 132, 202
Lal, H., 238, 244, 262, 265, 266, 267
Lamargue, J. L., 214, 232
Lambrechts, 231
Lands, A. M., 24, 62
Lecchini, S., 114, 197
Lee, Y., 66, 67, 68, 199
Lees, G. M., 114, 199
Leeuws, M., 116, 197
Leite, C. A., 207, 230
Lenaerts, F. M., 40, 63, 66, 67, 68, 75, 118, 131, 198, 199, 200, 201
Lewis, D. M., 225, 231
Lewis, P. J., 132, 138, 142, 145, 148, 153, 197
Leyman, R., 196, 210, 230
Lichstein, J., 214, 232
Lin, T. M., 67, 69, 199
Linsmayer, M., 244, 267
Litchfield, J. T., 102, 200
Loewe, S., 66, 67, 200
Loomans, J. M. L., 66, 113, 198
Lou, T. C., 66, 200
Love, A. H. G., 70, 201
Low-Beer, T. S., 73, 200, 207, 232

M

Machella, Th. E., 214, 232
Macht, D. I., 66, 200
Maenza, R. M., 67, 200, 201
Magnus, R., 200
Mainguet, P., 218, 227, 232
Makosza, M., 27, 62
Maling, H. M., 244, 266
Manciaux, M., 214, 232
Manoury, P. M., 23, 61
Marker, P. H., 67, 196
Marsboom, R. H. M., 49, 62, 67, 199, 200

Masri, M. S., 68, 200
Matussek, N., 244, 267
McCarty, D. A., 66, 200
McCracken, G. H., Jr., 73, 196, 207, 230
McMichael, L. A., 208, 229
McMurdoch, H., 74, 200
Merlo, M., 214, 232
Mervyn, J. M., 23, 62
Meyer, H., 200
Meyer, R. F., 23, 61, 67, 195
Miotti, R., 214, 232
Misiewicz, J. J., 114, 195
Mitchell, T. G., 70, 201
Moeller, H. C., 214, 232
Moffet, H. L., 207, 232
Moulinier, R., 214, 230
Müller, W., 214, 232
Muls, M., 132, 196, 218, 230
Murphy, J. E., 208, 232

N

Nalin, D. R., 73, 196
Nash, J. F., 67, 69, 199
Neptune, E. M., 70, 201
Neveu, C., 30, 63
Niemegeers, C. J. E., 23, 40, 49, 62, 63, 66, 67, 68, 75, 118, 131, 198, 199, 200, 201
Nilsson, F., 115, 201
Norris, H. J., 67, 196

O

Overton, D., 267
Owens, F. J., 214, 232

P

Pagliarini, G., 30, 63
Paris, S. K., 66, 196
Paton, W. D. M., 119, 129, 131, 201
Pearce, C., 49, 62
Phillips, S. F., 70, 201

Author Index

Pinchard, A., 67, 118, <u>198</u>
Plotkin, G. R., 67, <u>200</u>, <u>201</u>
Poirier, A., 214, <u>232</u>
Poirier, M., 214, <u>232</u>
Potter, D., 66, <u>200</u>
Pourquier, H., 214, <u>232</u>
Powell, D. W., 67, <u>200</u>, <u>201</u>
van Proozdy-Hartzema, E. G., 24, 53, <u>62</u>
Psaila, A., <u>231</u>
Puls, G., <u>233</u>
Purdon, R. A., 67, <u>202</u>

R

Raby, M. B., 207, <u>233</u>
Raeymaekers, A. H. M., 66, 113, <u>198</u>
Rakatansky, H., 74, <u>202</u>
Ramsay, A. M., 207, <u>233</u>
Ranney, R. E., 132, 136, 151, 153, <u>199</u>
Read, A. E., 73, 74, <u>200</u>, <u>202</u>, 207, <u>232</u>
Reneman, R. S., 116, <u>197</u>
Reuse, J. J., 115, <u>197</u>
Reynell, P. C., 69, <u>202</u>
Reyntjens, A., 132, <u>196</u>, 218, <u>230</u>, <u>233</u>
Roa, N. R., 67, <u>196</u>
Robinson, J. A., 131, <u>199</u>
Roffman, M., 238, <u>267</u>
Rosecrane, J., 239, <u>267</u>
Roth, F., 207, <u>230</u>
Royer, R., <u>230</u>
Rubens, R., 115, 132, 139, <u>202</u>, 214, 216, <u>233</u>
Rummel, W., 70, <u>197</u>
Rutgeerts, L., 207, <u>233</u>

S

Saelens, J. K., 254, <u>267</u>
Salmon-Legagneur, F., 30, <u>63</u>
Sanczuk, S., 66, 113, <u>198</u>
Sanner, J. H., 66, 67, 68, <u>199</u>, <u>202</u>

Saul, W., 244, <u>266</u>
Sawyer, W. K., 254, <u>267</u>
Schaper, W. K. A., 67, 118, <u>198</u>, <u>199</u>
Schaumann, O., 24, 27, <u>61</u>
Schellekens, K. H. L., 49, <u>62</u>, 67, 68, 75, 118, <u>198</u>, <u>199</u>
Scheurmans, V., 115, 132, <u>202</u>, <u>203</u>
Schild, H. O., 120, <u>195</u>
Schmid, W., 66, <u>202</u>
Schneider, C., 244, <u>266</u>
Scholes, G. B., 115, <u>195</u>
Schuermans, V., <u>196</u>, 210, 214, 216, <u>230</u>, <u>233</u>
Schulenberger, H. K., 207, <u>232</u>
Schwartz, S. A., 206, 214, <u>229</u>
Serafin, B., 27, <u>62</u>
Shanks, R. G., 119, <u>195</u>
Shärli, A., 214, 223, <u>233</u>
Sherr, H., 67, 70, <u>195</u>
Shooman, H., 207, <u>233</u>
Silver, S. A., 208, <u>229</u>
Simon, M., 214, <u>234</u>
Sohmer, H. F., 206, 214, <u>230</u>
Solberg, L. I., 67, <u>201</u>
Soudijn, W., 23, 24, <u>63</u>, 115, <u>132</u>, 153, <u>203</u>
Spencer, K. N., 27, 28, <u>61</u>
Spray, G. H., 69, <u>202</u>
Sprinz, H., 67, <u>200</u>
Stapler, N. H., 207, <u>229</u>
Starling, E. H., <u>195</u>
Stokbroekx, R. A., 23, 49, <u>62</u>, <u>63</u>, 132, <u>202</u>
Stoll, L. J., 208, <u>229</u>
Streeten, O. H. P., 67, <u>203</u>
Sulser, F., 244, <u>267</u>
Sumwalt, M., 66, 101, 113, <u>199</u>
Symoens, J., 67, <u>200</u>

T

Temmerman, R., 67, <u>200</u>
Testa, E., 30, <u>63</u>
Thomas, R., 214, <u>232</u>

Tijtgat, G. , 218, 233
Torsoli, A. , 114, 197
Toussaint, P. , 214, 232
Trager, W. , 147, 148, 150, 151, 199
Travell, J. , 202
Trendelenburg, P. , 202
Tsurumi, K. , 67, 202

V

Valla, A. , 214, 233
Van Bever, W. F. M. , 23, 49, 63, 132, 202
Vandenberk, J. , 23, 49, 62, 63, 132, 202
Vandenbroucke, G. , 208, 214, 233
Vander Aa, M. J. M. C. , 23, 49, 63, 132, 202
Van Derstappen, G. , 208, 214, 233
Van de Westerlingh, C. , 66, 113, 198
Van Heertum, A. H. M. T. , 23, 49, 63, 132, 202
Van Lommel, R. , 202
Van Martin, W. R. , 237, 245, 266
Van Nueten, J. M. , 67, 68, 75, 115, 116, 118, 119, 131, 139, 196, 197, 198, 199, 201, 202, 203, 244, 267
Van Proosdij-Hartzema, E. G. , 66, 67, 198
Van Ravestyn, C. , 67, 200
Van Rossum, J. M. , 118, 203
Vantrappen, G. , 214, 219, 233
Van Wijngaardens, I. , 67, 68, 75, 115, 132, 153, 199, 203
Verbeje, S. , 132, 196

Verbeke, S. , 218, 230
Verbruggen, F. J. , 67, 75, 118, 198, 199
Verhaegen, H. , 115, 132, 138, 139, 142, 145, 148, 153, 197, 202, 203, 214, 216, 219, 227, 233, 234
Verhoeven, H. , 29, 61
Vigoni, M. , 224, 234
Villareal, J. , 23, 54, 61, 67, 195

W

Watson, W. C. , 69, 203
Weingarten, B. , 214, 234
Weiss, J. , 214, 234
Weissman, A. , 244, 267
van Wijngaarden, I. , 23, 24, 63
Wilcoxon, F. , 102, 200
Wiley, J. N. , 23, 54, 61, 62, 67, 195
Williams, D. T. A. , 208, 229
Williams, E. M. V. , 67, 203
Wilson, D. T. , 225, 231
Winkelstein, A. , 115, 203, 206, 214, 234
Wolbach, A. B. , 237, 245, 266
Wouters, M. S. T. , 66, 113, 198

Y

Yawen, E. , 207, 230

Z

Zar, M. A. , 119, 129, 131, 201
Zegveld, C. , 49, 62
Zelvelder, W. G. , 210, 234

SUBJECT INDEX

A

Absorption
 antidiarrheal, 133
 electrolytes, 11
 sodium, 11
 water, 11
Abuse potential, 225
 essential characteristics, 235
 experimental approaches, 251
Acetylcholine release, 129
Acute diarrhea, 207
Acute toxicity, 155, 166
Addiction, 235, 241, 243, 245, 251
Amphetamine, 238
Anal incontinence, 224
Anileridine
 behavioral morphine-like effects, 108
 castor-oil test, 77, 87
 tail-withdrawal test, 77, 87
Antidiarrheal activity
 castor-oil test, 68
 selected drugs, 51
 selection of method, 65
Apomorphine, 238
Artificially induced diarrhea, 67, 68

4-Aryl-4-hydroxy-α,α-diphenyl-1-piperidinebutanamides
 analytical data, 31
 antidiarrheal activity, 56
4-Aryl-4-hydroxy-3-methy-N,N-dimethyl-α,α-diphenyl-1-piperidinebutanamides
 analytical data, 34
 antidiarrheal activity, 59
4-Aryl-4-hydroxy-β or γ-methyl-α,α-diphenyl-1-piperidinebutanamides
 analytical data, 36
 antidiarrheal activity, 60
Auerbach's plexus, 8

B

$BaCl_2$-induced contractions, 129
Bacterial diarrhea, 14
Bacterial toxins, 12
Bezitramide
 castor-oil test, 77, 83
 tail-withdrawal test, 77, 83
Bile acids, 15
Bradykinine-induced contractions, 129

Butoxylate
  analytical data, 25
  castor-oil test, 50, 81, 96
  charcoal test, 51
  tail-withdrawal test, 81, 96

C

Castor oil
  test in rats, 68, 75
  metabolism, 69
Charcoal test, 67, 104
Chloridorrhea, 17
Chronic diarrhea, 213
Chronic toxicity, 155
Chronotropic effects, 119
CI-750, 23, 54
CNS-effects, 236
Coaxial stimulation, 119, 129
Codeine
  behavioral morphine-like effects, 108, 109, 110
  castor-oil test, 50, 77, 92
  charcoal test, 51, 104, 107
  tail-withdrawal test, 77, 92
Crohn's disease, 214
Cumulative dose technique, 118
1-(3-Cyano-3,3-diphenylpropyl)-4-phenyl-4-piperidine carboxylates
  analytical data, 25
  antidiarrheal activity, 50, 51

D

Dextromoramide, 53
  castor-oil test, 77, 85
  discrimination, 239
  tail-withdrawal test, 77, 85
Diarrhea, 7
  bacterial, 14
  causes, 13, 19
  hormonal and chemical factors, 16
  iatrogenic factors, 19
  osmotic factors, 13
  postvagotomy, 20
  symptoms, 7

Difenoximide, 23
Difenoxin
  absorption, 133
  acute diarrhea, 208
  acute toxicity, 166
  analytical data, 26, 40
  biotransformation, 147
  castor-oil test, 50, 77, 81, 95
  chronic diarrhea, 213
  chronic toxicity, 168
  clinical effects, 208, 214
  CNS-effects, 236, 250
  distribution, 142
  embryotoxicity, 187
  excretion, 145
  fertility, 187
  formulation, 206
  heart tissues, 128
  inhibition peristaltic reflex, 120
  interaction with response to electrical stimulation, 126
  interaction with various agonists, 126
  metabolism, 148
  perinatal toxicity, 192
  plasma levels, 133
  postnatal toxicity, 192
  safety margin, 166
  side effects, 227
  subacute toxicity, 156
  synthesis, 30
  tail-withdrawal test, 81, 95
  teratogenesis, 187
Diphenoxylate
  absorption, 133
  acute diarrhea, 207
  acute toxicity, 166
  analytical data, 25, 37
  behavioral morphine-like effects, 109, 110
  biotransformation, 147
  castor-oil test, 50, 72, 81, 97
  charcoal test, 51, 105, 107
  chronic diarrhea, 213
  chronic toxicity, 168
  clinical effects, 208, 214

Subject Index 281

[Diphenoxylate]
  CNS-effects, 237, 250, 254
  discrimination learning, 262
  distribution, 142
  embryotoxicity, 187
  excretion, 145
  formulation, 206
  heart tissues, 128
  inhibition peristaltic reflex, 120
  interaction with response to electrical stimulation, 126
  interaction with various agonists, 126
  metabolism, 147
  naloxone-precipitated jumping, 254
  pediatric use, 223
  plasma levels, 133
  safety margin, 166
  side-effects, 227
  subacute toxicity, 156
  synthesis, 23
  tail-withdrawal test, 81, 97
  teratogenesis, 187
  trade names, 37
  use during space flights, 224
  use in withdrawal programs 224
  world-wide use, 5
Discrimination of
  central effects, 238
  learning, 262
  stimulus, 238, 262
Dissociation
  antidiarrheal and analgesic activity, 74
  constipating and central effects, 101
Drug abuse, 235
Drug-seeking behavior, 246

E

Embryotoxicity, 159
Euphoria, 236
Euphoric effects, 240
Euphoric quality, 240
Excretion, 145

F

Fatty acids, 15
Fentanyl
  behavioral morphine-like effects, 108
  castor-oil test, 77, 84
  discrimination, 239
  discrimination learning, 262
  narcotic preference, 257
  physical dependence, 255
  tail-withdrawal test, 75, 84
Fertility, 158
Fetoxylate
  acute toxicity, 166
  analytical data, 26
  castor-oil test, 59, 81, 100
  chronic toxicity, 170
  safety margin, 167
  subacute toxicity, 168
  synthesis, 23
  tail-withdrawal test, 81, 100
Fluperamide
  acute toxicity, 166
  analytical data, 31
  castor-oil test, 56, 81, 98
  chronic toxicity, 183
  embryotoxicity, 187
  safety margin, 167
  subacute toxicity, 181
  synthesis, 23
  tail-withdrawal test, 56, 82, 98
  teratogenesis, 187
Functional diarrhea, 214

G

Gastrointestinal tract
  abnormal transport, 14
  absorption, 9
    bile acids, 15
    electrolytes, 11, 14
    fatty acids, 15
    malabsorption, 13
    mucosal disease, 12, 17
    osmolarity, 10

[Gastrointestinal tract]
  anatomy, 8
  chemical factors, 16
  clinical abnormalities, 19
  dysfunctions, 13
  functional abnormalities, 21
  humoral factors, 16
  metabolic diseases, 21
  motility, 9, 18
  physiology, 8
  resections, 20
  secretion, 9
  structural disease, 21
  transport disorders, 17

H

Haloperidol, 240
Histamine antagonism, 119
Humoral factors, 10, 16
5-Hydroxytryptamine antagonism, 131
Hypermotility, 18
Hypomotility, 18

I

Iatrogenic factors, 19
Intestinal secretion, 9, 12
Intoxication with antidiarrheals, 228
Intramural ganglia, 115
Isoprenaline-induced relaxation, 118
Isopropamide, 53

J

Jumping response, 244

L

Loperamide
  absorption, 141
  acute diarrhea, 208
  acute toxicity, 166
  analytical data, 31, 44

[Loperamide]
  behavioral morphine-like effects, 109, 110
  biotransformation, 154
  castor-oil test, 56, 82, 99
  charcoal test, 51, 106, 107
  chronic diarrhea, 216
  chronic toxicity, 177
  clinical studies, 208, 216
  CNS-effects, 237, 250, 254
  discrimination learning, 262
  distribution, 142
  embryotoxicity, 187
  excretion, 145
  fertility, 187
  formulation, 206
  heart tissues, 128
  inhibition peristaltic reflex, 120
  interaction response to electrical stimulation, 126
  interaction with various agonists, 126
  metabolism, 147
  naloxone-precipitated jumping, 254
  narcotic preference, 257
  pediatric use, 223
  perinatal toxicity, 192
  plasma levels, 133
  postnatal toxicity, 192
  safety margin, 166
  side-effects, 227
  subacute toxicity, 174
  synthesis, 28
  tail-withdrawal test, 81, 99
  teratogenesis, 187
  trade names, 44

M

Mechanism of action, 115
Meissner's plexus, 8
Metabolism, 132
Methadone
  behavioral morphine-like effects, 108

[Methadone]
  castor-oil test, 78, 88
  discrimination, 239
  tail-withdrawal test, 78, 88
Morphine
  abuse potential, 242
  behavioral morphine-like effects, 108, 109, 110
  castor-oil test, 50, 79, 91
  charcoal test, 51, 103, 107
  CNS-effects, 254
  discrimination, 239
  discrimination learning, 262
  naloxone-precipitated jumping, 254
  physical dependence, 242
  tail-withdrawal test, 79, 91
Motor factors, 18
Mouse jumping, 252
Mucosal disease, 12
Mucosal factors, 17

N

Naloxone jumping, 224, 254
Nervous diarrhea, 217
Nicotine-induced contractions, 131

O

Osmolarity, 10
Osmotic factors, 13
Overt behavior, 237
4-(1-Oxoalkyl)-4-phenyl-α,α-diphenyl-1-piperidinebutyronitriles
  analytical data, 25
  antidiarrheal activity, 50, 51

P

Papillary muscle, 119
Pediatric use of antidiarrheals, 223
Perception strength, 237
Perinatal toxicity, 160
Peristalsis
  induction, 116

[Peristalsis]
  inhibition, 116, 131
Pethidine
  behavioral morphine-like effects, 108
  castor-oil test, 80, 93
  tail-withdrawal test, 80, 93
Phenazocine
  behavioral morphine-like effects, 108
  castor-oil test, 78, 86
  tail-withdrawal test, 78, 86
Phenoperidine
  behavioral morphine-like effects, 108
  castor-oil test, 78, 89
  discrimination learning, 240, 263
  tail-withdrawal test, 78, 89
Physical dependence
  definition, 242
  determination, 243
  symptoms, 255
Physical properties, 37
  diphenoxine, 40
  diphenoxylate, 37
  loperamide, 44
Piritramide
  behavioral morphine-like effects, 108
  castor-oil test, 79, 90
  discrimination learning, 263
  tail-withdrawal test, 79, 90
Postnatal toxicity, 160
Postresection diarrhea, 217
Preclinical pharmacology, 65
Propoxyphene
  castor oil test, 80, 94
  tail-withdrawal test, 80, 94
Psychoactive properties, 236

R

Radioactive testmeal, 67
Radiotherapy-induced diarrhea, 219
Reduction of fecal output test, 67
Reinforcers, 247

Relative antidiarrheal specificity, 49, 101
Reproduction studies, 158
Ricinoleic acid, 68
Rotary motor excitement in mice, 113
Ruminal motility, 67

S

Safety evaluation, 155
Self-administration, 250
Straub-tail, 101
Structure-activity relationships, 49
Subacute toxicity, 156
Subjective effects, 239
Succus entiricus, 9, 12
Symptomatic treatment
 acute diarrhea, 207
 chronic diarrhea, 213

T

Tail-withdrawal test, 75
Teratogenesis, 159, 187
Tolerance, 241
Traveller's diarrhea, 207
Trendelenburg's method, 115

U

Ulcerative colitis, 217

V

Vagal section, 20

W

Withdrawal syndromes, 244, 245